HANS GERTH

C. WRIGHT MILLS

character and social structure

the psychology of social institutions

A Harbinger Book

HARCOURT, BRACE & WORLD, INC.
New York   Chicago   Burlingame

ISBN 0-15-616759-X

JKLMN

First Harbinger Books edition 1964

Library of Congress Catalog Card Number: 53–12721

Printed in the United States of America

CONTENTS

Part Three   Social Structure

Foreword

NEW findings and new ideas in a field of knowledge, especially when they come rapidly, generally produce numerous efforts to work out new theoretical formulations. Various perspectives develop, each differing in its view of the central problems of the field and the major conceptions that illuminate these problems. This is plainly the dynamic and hopeful condition of social psychology today.

Among this varied array of perspectives on social psychology, there is one which, while acknowledged to be important, has been greatly neglected in systematic expositions. This approach considers not only the psychological nature of social interaction but also, and primarily, the psychological nature of the major social institutions that constitute the historically significant forms of such interaction. It is the chief objective of this book to present a systematic statement of just this approach, one in which political, economic, military, religious, and kinship institutions, and their historical transformations, are connected with the character and personality, with the private as well as the public lives, of those living in the society. This book might therefore be described as an historically oriented psychology of social institutions.

Of late general works of social psychology have paid scant attention to the historical changes of social institutions. This has happened, it seems, not so much by design as by inadvertence: the emphasis—quite understandably—has been upon experiment, direct observation, and statistically controlled comparisons of behavior. This book should help restore the balance. Whether use of the book precedes, accompanies, or follows intensive study of the short-run present in the laboratory, field, and clinic, it should broaden the horizon of the student who generally comes into social psychology either through the gateway of psychology or of sociology. It should help him cultivate his powers of observation and analysis to understand the behavior of men, not merely in small groups literally before his eyes, but also in relation to the larger institutional structure, with all its complexity and historical meaning. And the wide range of comparative materials included in this book should do much to curb any tendency on the part of the student toward the provincialism of thinking in terms only of his own society or his own time.

For all their emphasis on the shaping of character by the social structure, the authors avoid dogmatism. They refuse to be drawn into the position, rapidly grown archaic, of maintaining that *everything* about human conduct must be explained by the organization of social institutions, or of assuming that even differences in the native endowment of men must be denied as a fact in order to lend seeming support to the sociological approach as an idea. On occasion, the authors do examine, compactly and fairly, some of the theoretical controversies which have raged in the field—for example, the long-lived debate over the use of instinct as an explanatory concept. In this way a new generation of students becomes acquainted with these early victories of the mind and is kept from unwittingly resurrecting some of these controversies in the mistaken belief that they have come upon a genuine intellectual problem. As the authors remind us, such spurious problems are usually solved by being outgrown.

Any book with a theoretical focus must select its materials and problems in terms of that focus, and selection of course involves omissions as well as inclusions. Omissions, therefore, do not necessarily constitute defects. The important thing is to inquire whether an omission is the result of careless and faulty thinking or of a considered judgment that the material is not directly germane to the logical structure of the book. The omissions in this book are of the second kind. On some matters, treated at length in other books of social psychology, the authors maintain deliberate silence; on some matters, found not at all in other books, they expound at length. Thus, if they make only passing reference to the experiments on social factors in perception, to learning theory, or to recent studies of voting behavior, they pay close and systematic attention to the comparative psychology of political and military life, of religious institutions, social stratification, and business enterprise. And they make use of every species of social psychological data.

The authors lay no claim to having achieved a fully rounded synthesis which incorporates all the major conceptions of psychology and sociology that bear upon the formation of character and personality in the context of social structure. Such a goal, they make it clear, is still a distant objective rather than a currently possible achievement. Nevertheless, they have systematized a substantial part of the field and have provided perspectives from which to examine much of the rest.

But perhaps above all else this book has the merit of giving the reader a sense of the intellectual excitement that comes from using the trained imagination to study the psychological meaning of social structures. In the world of social psychology as we know it, this is no small accomplishment.

ROBERT K. MERTON

Columbia University
July 30, 1953

Preface

THE shock of world events has hit the social sciences harder than many social scientists recognize. In most areas of the world, historic changes have been apparent to anyone who wished to look at them; if they have been attended to more by journalists than by social scientists, that has been to the loss of the social sciences. During the last half century there have been two world wars, and in Europe several political revolutions. The social structures of Russia and of eastern Europe have been thoroughly revolutionized; great changes continue to shake Asia, Africa, and South America. If the people of the United States have not known the tang and feel of revolution, it may be due to the fact that elections have continued to take place here within a political order that is over one hundred and fifty years old. In the meantime, the United States has become the creditor country for half the world and the naval and military protector of all her debtor states. It would, accordingly, be provincial of Americans not to think about the diverse possibilities latent in all modern social structures. For war has widened our view, and now the whole world lies before us, polarized between the U.S.S.R. and the U.S.A. Before such world events as we have known, it is not surprising that there is an uneasiness concerning the adequacy of the viewpoint and the equipment of the social scientist.

World War II and its aftermath compelled thinkers in the United States toward a larger view of the range and conditions of mankind. For better or for worse, the mind has followed the army and navy. Members of academic institutions who, till now, had never considered Europe and Asia in connection with their respective social studies have found themselves teaching courses about the peoples and resources of these areas. Social scientists have been asked questions which they cannot answer, and some of them, even as all thoughtful men, have asked themselves such questions.

Along with the historical transformations of whole societies, what must be described as a vacuum of loyalties, as a deep-seated malaise, has come about in the public life of the Western democracies.[1] Whatever its social-historical foundations may be, this malaise is of course experienced on the psychological plane. Socialism's theoretical crises, for example, are held by many to rest upon psychological misjudgments rather than upon misjudgments of the course of economic affairs. The radical and the liberal in America today are often more interested in psychological than in material exploitation, more interested in problems of soap opera than of child labor.

Due in part to the rise of totalitarian societies, we have become acutely aware of patterns of external constraint which are in tension with the impulses of man as a willful animal. Various schools of sociology have viewed man as a mechanism adjusting, or trying to adjust, to all sorts of overpowering "environments" and "conditions"; whereas positivist[2] psychologists have increasingly tended to lose sight of the individual man as an actor in the larger social and historical scene. Those schools of psychology, especially Gestalt and Psychoanalysis, which do try to bring man as an understandable actor into focus are not primarily interested in sociological problems. They are, however, greatly suggestive to the social scientist who while looking at social constraints is thinking about human freedoms.

[1] For an elaboration of this theme, see C. Wright Mills, *White Collar: the American Middle Classes* (New York: Oxford, 1951); Leo Lowenthal and Norbert Guterman, *Prophets of Deceit: A Study of the Techniques of the American Agitator* (New York: Harper, 1949), esp. pp. 11-20; and Karl Mannheim, *Man and Society in an Age of Reconstruction*, Edward Shils, tr. (New York: Harcourt, Brace, 1940).

[2] For one meaning of "positivist," we refer the reader to the jingle allegedly written by the distinguished T. H. Huxley:

> "There was an ape in days which were earlier;
> Centuries passed and its hair it grew curlier;
> Centuries more and its thumb gave a twist,
> And he was a man, and a Positivist."

Problems of the nature of human nature are raised most urgently when the life-routines of a society are disturbed, when men are alienated from their social roles in such a way as to open themselves up for new insight. When social affairs proceed smoothly, "human nature" seems to fit so neatly into traditional routines that no general problem is presented; men know what to expect from one another; their vocabularies for various emotions and their stereotyped motives are taken for granted and seem common to all. But when society is in deep-going transformation and men are pivots of historic change, they challenge one another's explanations of conduct, and human nature itself becomes problematic.

Several twentieth-century schools of psychology originated in conflict-ridden Central Europe, centering on notions of Gestalt or the Unconscious, or in types of body builds or in the projective tests of specialists like Rorschach. And there is the philosophical legacy of Kierkegaard and Nietzsche which lives on in the psychiatric work of Karl Jaspers and Ludwig Binswanger. Nietzsche —in one sense a precursor of Freud—felt himself to be in intellectual kinship with the psychological essayism of such French thinkers as Montaigne and La Bruyère, La Rochefoucauld and Pascal, who had observed men and their ways in comparably profound periods of transition. And we should not forget that the social psychology of such a man as Le Bon concerned the revolutionary action of man in crowds and mobs.

II

In our historical situation the hybrid, "social psychology," has come increasingly to appeal to those who are eager to understand social structures in such a way as to see how they have shaped the character of individual men and women.

Back of the interest in social psychology is the desire to answer simple yet momentous questions: What do given societies mean for men? What sort of creature is man in this or that political and economic condition? Are there limits to his manipulatability? Many of the new strivings and demands of social science seem to us to come to fruition in a psychology that is relevant to the processes of history and to varying types of social structures.

The challenge of social psychology, and its great appeal to modern scholars, is that in a time of intellectual specialization and of social and political disintegration, it promises a view of man as an

actor in historic crises, and of man as a whole entity. These promises and challenges become all the more compelling as social life
becomes a set of abstracted specialities, which various authorities
would motivate for the disciplined mass conduct of war and peace.
In such a context, it is one of the special obligations of the social
psychologist again and again to bridge the departmentalized gap
which unfortunately separates the sociological and psychological
approaches.

Our general purpose is to study the personalities of men in connection with types of social-historical structure. We wish to analyze
conduct and character by understanding the motivations of men
who occupy different positions within various social structures.
And we wish to understand how creeds and symbols contribute to
the motivations required for the enactment of given roles by persons within institutional structures.

III

No matter how we approach the field of social psychology, we
cannot escape the idea that all current work that comes to much,
fits into one or the other of two basic traditions: *Freud*, on the
side of character structure, and *Marx*, including the early Marx
of the 1840's, on the side of social structure. Of course, we use
both "freud" and "marx" as uncapitalized adjectives: they refer to
great perspectives and great bodies of work rather than solely to
the books of Freud and Marx. We have no objection, if the reader
prefers, to use the names George H. Mead and Max Weber, although of course they differ from Freud and Marx in many important ways.[3]

The reason we are drawn, again and again, to Sigmund Freud
and George Mead, is that they try, more effectively than others,
to show us man as a whole actor—instead of man as a set of traits,
as a bundle of reflexes. It was Freud's contribution to raise the
question of the nature of human nature in its larger framework.
That is also the reason, from the sociological side, that we are
drawn, again and again, to such men as Marx and Weber, who
would do no less than articulate a society as a whole inside an historical epoch.

Both the structural sociologist and the depth psychologist prom-

[3] The relevant books of these four thinkers will be found in the Bibliographical Note, pp. 481-85.

ise to help us locate modern men—and ourselves—as historical
actors. This promise motivates modern social psychologists, whose
present theoretical task is set by the availability of two such perspectives—of character and of social structure—and by their own
desire to see man intimately, yet as an historical actor. If their
theoretical task is to round out and to bring these two perspectives
together, then the theoretical significance of recent work in this
field must be judged accordingly: detailed research must be viewed
as contributing to one or the other of these two conceptions, and
at the growing edge, contributing to the linking of them into a
working model of man and society.

I V

On the psychological side, the explanations that have been advanced in the brief history of our discipline fall into two main
types: on the one hand, there has been the attempt to reduce social
regularities to universal constants, rooted somehow in man as
man; and on the other, the attempt to connect man's conduct and
nature with the social roles which he enacts.

The idea of some constant, lying back of conduct and in man's
universal human nature,[4] has been the most frequent and persistent
error of psychology, including that of Freud. It is as if this quest
for some constant element has served as a compensation for the
enormous relativity of human nature which anthropology and
world history make so evident. It runs through the older eight-
eenth- and nineteenth-century rationalist psychologies, to reach its
climax in the instinct school. Half of the American life of our
young discipline has been spent debating the notion of instinct in
all its various guises.

Nowadays, however, the idea of immutable biological elements
recedes and is no longer a problem engaging all our energies. We
did not solve the problem; we outgrew it. At best, all we learn
when we study man as a mere animal are his limitations when
stripped of all technologies. If we are imaginative, we learn also
that his "dispositions" are open-ended and capable of development. We learn that his "human nature" is not given to him once
and for all, but as a continual series of tasks. The establishment

[4] See Chapter I: Perspectives, Section 1: The Biological Model.

of the reality of the social and plastic nature of man is a major accomplishment of U.S. social psychology.[5]

The function of American behaviorism in the history of our discipline is found precisely here: it opened up the problems of human nature, by allowing us to see the great modifiability of man; it opened up our minds for explanations that are not tautological blind alleys. But the behaviorist's image of man "adjusting" to all sorts of overpowering circumstances is also in line with the modern temper of those who would manipulate without understanding closely. Behaviorism, as advanced by John Watson, eliminated instincts, but in the process social psychology was often made shallow. For as an explanatory model, behaviorism lowered our chance to understand motivations. Behaviorism's most fruitful outcome was George Mead's work, especially his daring effort to anchor personal consciousness itself in the social process.

Mead's concept of the generalized other, and Freud's superego—their closest point of contact [6]—enable us to link the private and the public, the innermost acts of the individual with the widest kinds of social-historical phenomena. From a logical and unhistorical point of view, Freud's work at this point may be seen as a specification of the social and biographical locus of the generalized other. For he indicates how, in the early phase of development, the family is important for the social anchorage of conscience, and thus makes his central hookup of love and authority.

Various philosophical assumptions that had crept into Freud's work have been torn out with little or no damage to what remains as usable heritage. More importantly, the conceptions of Freud have been made socially relative by the work of such writers as Bronislaw Malinowski,[7] Abram Kardiner,[8] Karen Horney,[9] and Erich Fromm.[10] Instincts have been formalized into "energy," in

[5] See Fay B. Karpf, *American Social Psychology* (New York: McGraw-Hill, 1932), for a detailed account.

[6] See Chapter IV: The Person, Section 4: Generalized Others and Section 5: The Social Relativity of the Generalized Other.

[7] Cf. *The Father in Primitive Psychology* (New York: Norton, 1927) and *Sex and Repression in Savage Society* (New York: Harcourt, Brace, 1927).

[8] Cf. *The Individual and His Society* (New York: Columbia University Press, 1939).

[9] Cf. *The Neurotic Personality of Our Time* (New York: Norton, 1937) and *New Ways in Psychoanalysis* (New York: Norton, 1939).

[10] *Escape from Freedom* (New York: Farrar & Rinehart, 1941).

order that we can better understand how various goals of conduct are socially fixed and socially changed. Indeed, that is why we believe Kardiner's and Fromm's work, as well as Harry Stack Sullivan's [11] on the significant and the authoritative other, is so much in the central stream of what is most promising in recent social psychology. In fact, work on the superego or generalized other is now at the growing edge of our studies, for such conceptions enable us to link traits deep in the individual with facts that lie in a widespread sociological perspective.

George Mead had no adequate notion of emotions and motives, no dynamic theory of the affective life of man; Freud's notion of the personality certainly tends to be socially inflexible. And neither Freud nor Mead presents a conception of social structure that makes it inherently, directly, and intimately relevant to psychological problems.

But from the side of depth psychology and of the mechanisms of personality formation and change, enormous advances have been made. Freud and George Mead, when appropriately integrated and systematized, provide a well-articulated model of character structure, and one of the most fruitful sets of ideas available in modern social science. It is our aim, especially in Parts I and II of this book, to construct a model of character structure that enables us to systematize some of these ideas and make them available for more sociologically relevant use.

v

From the other side, that of structural, comparative, and historical sociology—although there are notable exceptions—less has been recently accomplished. The tradition of Marx and Sombart and Weber, as well as of the late Karl Mannheim, who met so many of these problems with such great insight, has not advanced as we might wish. Yet, the urge to compare large social entities in their historical epochs with one another is one of the bequests of the founders of modern sociology, of August Comte and Herbert Spencer,[12] no less than of Marx and Weber. Quite apart from the problem of how much and what portions of their work are of

[11] See *Conceptions of Modern Psychiatry* (Washington: W. A. White Psychiatric Foundation, 1947).

[12] See especially the great, much neglected work of Spencer, *Principles of Sociology* (New York: D. Appleton, 1896).

merely historical interest, the impetus and the breadth of focus of such men should not be lost in otherwise legitimate and necessary criticisms of their work. In our endeavor to share the reawakened interest in studying world societies comparatively, we look to the outstanding work of such contemporaries as Arnold Toynbee,[13] A. L. Kroeber,[14] and P. A. Sorokin.[15]

If it seems to be a shortcoming of many eminent Europeans to be absolutist in certain phases of their work, it is a distinct contribution of American pragmatists to purge sociological thinking of such rigidities and to open our minds to the exploration of reality. As Karl Mannheim has written, "There were hardly ever two different styles of study as fit to supplement each other's shortcomings as are the German and American types of sociology."[16]

We think a signal danger to further advance in much good work now going on in social psychology is the use of inadequate notions of "society." In place of social structure, many students would use the concept, "culture"—one of the spongiest words in social science, although, perhaps for that reason, in the hands of an expert, enormously useful. The concept, "culture," is often more a loose reference to social milieu than an adequate idea of social structure.[17] Nevertheless, unhindered, as they have been, by aware-

[13] Cf. *A Study of History*, 6 vols. (London: Oxford Univ. Press, 1946).

[14] See his *Configurations of Cultural Growth* (Berkeley: Univ. of California Press, 1944).

[15] See, for an introduction to the sociology of history, the good summary of doctrines in Sorokin's *Social Philosophies of an Age of Crisis* (Boston: Beacon Press, 1950).

[16] Cf. Karl Mannheim's review in the *American Journal of Sociology*, September 1932, p. 281.

[17] We do not wish to dispute the various conceptual distinctions involving "society," "culture," and "civilization," as severally paired with "personality." To us, the term "culture" and its derivations refer to "nature worked over by man," which of course includes man's own nature. A gymnastically developed body and an intellectually trained mind are "cultural" attainments; so are various forms of interpersonal relationships, social institutions and organizations of all sorts. Indeed, all the "works" that man builds in his exchange relations with nature as well as in his endeavor to expand the meaning of his world, are part of "culture." And in all this work, man is himself shaped. For man's nature is not given; it is a task and a challenge. During recent decades, scholars in all the social studies have by their work brought out the social-historical determination of man's ideas and works, as well as of man himself.

It is one thing to accept, as we do, this very general perspective; it is

ness of "complexity" and of "methodological" difficulties, cultural anthropologists *have* sought to grasp the interdependence of preliterate cultural wholes.

What is needed to make such work more usable is a conception of social structure as an articulation of various institutional orders and functions; we must study each segment of a social structure psychologically, as Freud studied the kinship institutions of the upper classes in certain Western societies. We need to study men enacting roles in political, economic, and religious institutions in various societies; we need to form theories of how, on the one hand, types of personalities are variously anchored in each of these institutional orders; and, on the other hand, how the institutional orders themselves are variously combined, to form historical types of social structures. In the course of this book we shall set forth a general model of social structure which will help us carry out these aims.

VI

Intellectually, social psychology has become the main area of contact between the decisive intellectual traditions of our time; politically, this field is crucial, because now, when profound crises shake mankind, our urgent interest in the larger problems of man and society requires that we understand man as an historical actor.

The structural and historical features of modern society must be connected with the most intimate features of man's self. That is what social psychology is all about. And that, we think, cannot be done by dealing only in microscopic observations. If ever there was a field needing above all else imaginative theory, that field is American social psychology today. Only by such work, rather than by delving into unrelated specialities, can we at once avail ourselves of our intellectual opportunities and avoid slivering our image of man.

Our book is intended to offer some ways into the central issues of social psychology. We deliberately omit any discussion of numerous sidelines, and we do not attempt to offer encyclopedic

quite another to try to use the term "culture," which we do not, for more technically precise constructions. For an unduly depreciative assessment of recent literature, see Alfred R. Lindesmith and Anselm L. Strauss, "A Critique of Culture-Personality Writings," *American Sociological Review*, October 1950, pp. 587-600.

information, which no single volume can embrace—not even a one-volume encyclopedia. We wish to teach, not to engage in commentaries, polemical or complimentary, on what others have written or left unwritten. And we do not offer a history of ideas and concepts; accordingly, we have not burdened our pages with historical references to theoretical literature, which professionals already know and laymen often do not need. With all diffidence, we hope not to swallow up, but to contribute to an on-going work.

In our work, we do not make any formal distinctions among the several social sciences or their varying national manifestations. Indeed, we have constantly felt the need to think through various problems with the aid of all viewpoints which seem available, regardless of their departmental or national source. This does not mean that our explicit aim is to show how the concepts of the various human disciplines may be theoretically related, or how their "fields" might be integrated. Social scientists, although perhaps not deans, have got beyond the need of such formal discussions, or at least have come to believe that such discussions are no longer adequate. What we are trying to do is actually think about concrete problems of social structure and personality, with a set of perspectives drawn from the work of the various social sciences. For such thinking is necessary if we are to face up to the type of questions which confront us.

The range of data with which we attempt to answer these questions is thus wider than Western society and the world fringe of preliterate groupings. In time, it includes examples from ancient China and modern Russia; in location, it extends to Japan and Latin America, the United States, and the several European countries. Our central aim is to build a working model in terms of which we can use the data of world history and the perspectives of the social sciences and psychologies in an effort to understand the types of human beings that have risen in varying kinds of social structure.

Our book is arranged in four parts, in the first of which we introduce our general manner of explanation and lay out in a preliminary way the major components of our working models of character and of social structure.

In Part Two we analyze the conception of character structure, breaking it down into its elements, discussing each of them, and indicating how they are variously related to one another. In this connection, we pay particular attention to problems of motivation as well as to the development of character structure as a whole.

In Part Three, we turn to social structure, taking up, first, the general mechanisms by which persons and institutions are related and then examining, in turn, the range of institutions in the political, the economic, the military, the religious, the kinship, and the educational areas of a society. After relating these institutions to systems of social stratification, we suggest and illustrate various ways in which institutions may be integrated to form going social structures.

In Part Four we deal with social-historical change, explaining how our idea of social structure leads us to construct a model of social change, and how within this model we are able to locate such dynamic forces as leadership and the various forms of collective behavior, including crowds, publics, movements, and parties. We end by a general consideration of the world trends that now seem most importantly to shape the types of character that prevail in modern social structures.

PART ONE

INTRODUCTORY

C H A P T E R
I
Perspectives

THE social psychologist attempts to describe and explain the conduct and the motivations of men and women in various types of societies. He asks how the external conduct and inner life of one individual interplay with those of others. He seeks to describe the types of persons usually found in different types of societies, and then to explain them by tracing their interrelations with their societies.

The explanations generally offered by social psychologists have proceeded either from the side of biology or from the side of sociology.

The biologist, as George Mead said of Watson, writes with the animal before him, viewing the individual primarily as an organism, a live creature of bones, muscles, and nerves, each of which fulfills certain animal functions. To the biologist, the organism is a more or less unitary system, and so in explaining its behavior, he pays attention to what goes on inside that organism—to its biological and physiological mechanisms. The guiding thread of his work is the physiological process, the biological conditions of behavior.

The sociologist, on the other hand, tries to "locate" the human being and his conduct in various institutions, never isolating the individual or the workings of his mind from his social and historical setting. He explains character and conduct in terms of these institutions, and of the total social structure which they form. He draws upon the experience of people as social persons rather than upon the physical and organic facts about people as animal organisms. Since he is interested in the social setting and motivations of conduct, rather than its physical conditions and organic mechanisms, he does not attempt to explain conduct as if it were the realization of some fundamental condition within the individual.

The sociologist tries to explain character and conduct as a fulfillment of social function within an already established, although usually open-ended, network of social relations.

These two viewpoints—within which the explanations of the social psychologist are developed—are not mutually exclusive; nor do we believe it wise or fruitful to understand them as competing schools of thought. In the end, we can—in fact we must—use both viewpoints; but in the beginning we must think in oversimplified ways, in order the better to see just how to complicate our viewpoint most profitably. We must, therefore, examine the biological and the sociological models of conduct, each in its turn.

1. The Biological Model

The biologist is interested in what goes on in man's animal organism when it acts in certain ways or reacts to certain experiences; he reconstructs certain elements and sequences of internal events which are then used to explain the external behavior observed.

One of the simplest explanations from this general point of view proceeds in terms of the "conditioning" of reflexes. Here is an organism equipped with certain reflexes; there are certain changes in the environment which stimulate these reflexes to action. If a bright light is flashed into a human eye, the pupil of the eye will mechanically contract; if a blow is struck just below the kneecap, the lower limb will spring out; if an edible object is presented to a dog with an empty stomach, the dog will salivate; or if a small object is shoved into or near an infant's mouth, the infant will start sucking. Such automatic reactions, or reflexes, occur because the organism is a mechanical structure of muscles, chemistry, and nerves. Different animal species have different sets of such reflexes. They are simply built that way.

Now, if a light is flashed into the human eye and at the same time a little puff of air is shot at it, eventually the puff of air by itself will evoke the pupillary reflex. The puff of air replaces, so to speak, the light as the stimulus that makes the pupil contract. Such replacement of a biologically adequate stimulus by an artificial one is known as conditioning.

One may generalize this idea of conditioning—these mechanical changes in the reactions of the organism—and attempt to explain all of man's behavior in terms of various series of conditioned responses. Even such complex actions as getting married or planting corn are then broken down into intricate sets of conditioned responses. According to such explanations, man is a complex mechanism: when a given button is pressed a given action follows.

Since man is an animal organism, we may well believe that all changes in conduct and experience are accompanied by neurological changes. From the biological viewpoint, at any rate, it is assumed that mental processes are based on physiological processes —though much of the physiology is actually unknown. This does not, however, mean that the conditioning of reflexes is necessarily *the* most important, much less the only, mechanism by which changes in behavior take place. Many experiences of the human being are not readily explained or understood in such terms.

As a matter of fact, actual work on conditioning has, in the main, been limited to attempts to explain small "involuntary actions," like the eye blink, or of certain animal behaviors and the activities of small children who have not yet acquired speech. A generalization of "conditioning" into an over-all explanation of human behavior—which overreaches the delimited conditions and actions on which it is observationally based—confuses the biologically necessary conditions of animal behavior with the sufficient conditions of specifically human conduct. By "explaining" the differing activities and experiences of Panamanian politicians and Chinese children, Spanish generals and French peasants as due to the "different conditioning" of their originally similar reflexes, we are really explaining away the specific problems which each of these types of persons present to us. Conditioning as a master explanation of human conduct is so general that it accomplishes little more than to inform us that all animals, the human as well as the ape and the rat, have neural biographies, that all men are neuromuscular structures, and that these change as men are confronted with different physical environments.

But the mechanical changes in neuromuscular behavior which conditioning explains are not all there is to man. The idea of man as a mechanism is useful in understanding the how of his physical activity, but for the why of his conduct, and for the why of the mechanism itself, we must look further. In this search we can learn one point from the view of man as "nothing but" an ani-

mal organism. If man is a neuromuscular structure, all his conduct is controlled, in the sense of being limited, by the mechanical
structure of his skeleton, muscles, and nerves. Without mechanical
aids, man cannot fly; he cannot sit down upon his own stomach.
The range of his possible actions and the co-ordinations of his
body are limited by the kind of animal structure that he happens
to be. Different species of animals are variously limited. The
grasshopper, unlike most men, is not equipped to distinguish red
from yellow objects; his world is probably all gray. But the grasshopper can hear sounds that men (without mechanical aids) cannot, for his ears are differently made. Later we shall see that all
men do not realize the structurally possible range of perception
to the same degree or in the same way—that the possibility, for
example, of color discrimination is variously realized according to
such social conditions as the vocabularies we learn. But to explain
such varying sensitivities, we must avail ourselves of sociological
as well as biological explanations.

In their common biological limitations, then, men differ from
members of other animal species; yet man's own structural range
is quite broad. Within the limits of man's animal form lie the rich
diversities of conduct that make up history and differentiate men
from one another in different societies all over the world. Insofar
as such constitutional differences, inherited by men in specific organic structures, may be used in general explanations of behavior
and personality,[1] we must rest content with the view rather widely
held among clinical psychiatrists: "It is with mixed feelings of distrust and uneasiness that psychiatrists introduce factors of constitution into a case study. If, after what is believed to be a 'dynamic
approach' has been exhausted and found wanting, 'constitution'
becomes an insecure refuge." [2] What is here referred to as a "dynamic approach" definitely involves a sociological model of explanation.

Within the strictly biological viewpoint, then, we see that man
as an animal species is structurally limited. The species limits the
motor behaviors which its members are capable of performing

[1] We shall discuss such organic or constitutional differences as they affect
differing character structures in Chapter III: Organism and Psychic Structure.
[2] Fritz Kant, M.D., "Integration of Constitution and Environment in
Psychiatry and Psychotherapy," Diseases of the Nervous System, Vol. IV,
No. 9 (September 1943).

and the range of sensory perception to which they are open. Furthermore, these structural limitations vary from one individual organism to another within the species, according to individual constitutional differences.

When we say that man is an *organism,* we imply that he is something more than a mechanical structure with differing limitations. Seeing the infant wiggle and twitch about, we impute impulses or will to it; and as its wigglings and twitchings become more definite and co-ordinated, we tend to ascribe various urges, instincts, or drives as lying within the organism and impelling it to action. The fact that the organism sets itself in motion is then explained by one or the other of these driving forces which we have imputed to be naturally within the organism. Such an explanation, as Gordon Allport has put it, is intended to answer the question: "What is it that sets the stream of activity into motion?" [3] It is the problem of motivation taken *in general,* usually put on the level of biological factors. It is, as John Dewey has said, "absurd to ask what induces a man to activity generally speaking. He is an active being and that is all there is to say on that score." [4] The very asking of the question in such a general way assumes that the organism is naturally in a state of rest, and hence, like a machine, requires an "external" force to move it, to push "it" into action.

But man is not an inert machine: *organism* implies movement; our characterization of it as possessing impulse or will is an essential inference.

This spontaneous movement characterizes not only the organism but also each of the various organs that make it up. Even in sleep man seldom rests like a log, and when he is awake his perceiving eye is naturally in motion. By altering the direction in which he looks, and by changing his focus to cover near or distant objects, he scans his world. He must learn to fix and manage his gaze, like the lens of a camera. The school child does not naturally hold his eyes on the teacher nor keep his hands at rest. To sit still is an accomplished effort for which he must be disciplined.

The explanation of conduct by "instinct" carries us beyond the general inference that the organism is impulsive. If we observe

[3] *Personality: A Psychological Interpretation* (New York: Holt, 1937), p. 110.
[4] *Human Nature and Conduct* (New York: Holt, 1922), p. 119.

the organism engaging in sexual behavior or the ingestion of food, we may say that these specific activities are caused by instincts: biologically fixed ways of behaving which are innate within the organism. The term instinct thus includes more meanings than any one term properly should: it is used to refer to (1) the cause of an activity; (2) the goal of the activity; and (3) the rigid activity itself.[5]

The theory of *instincts,* when logically assessed, does not possess any explanatory value. First, one observes men engaging in a certain activity. From this observation one infers the existence of an instinct. Then, this inferred element is separated from the observed activity and posited in the organism as a force or cause of its activity. By this procedure one treats an alternative name for some activity as an explanation of it. Thus, if we say that men eat because of the "instinct to eat," or build houses because of the "instinct to build houses," we are merely giving another name to the observed activities of eating and building. Such "explanations" are tautological. Instincts, once supposed to be biological entities, are actually hypothetical inferences from observed activities. As such, they cannot be taken as logical explanations, nor held to be "causes" of behavior.[6]

The notion of instinct encompasses awareness of the goal of activity. Thus, since instincts are held to be biologically innate, goals must be biologically innate.[7] And this cannot be the case. For while normal men are everywhere quite similar physiologically, the conduct patterns which make up the behavior of men are everywhere quite different. The biological structure and capacities of man seem not to have changed conspicuously for some thousands of years, yet man's behavior and feelings have varied widely. One

[5] Abram Kardiner, *The Individual and His Society* (New York: Columbia Univ. Press, 1939).

[6] This statement draws upon A. F. Bentley, who in 1908 saw clearly the logical deficiencies of explanation by instinct. See his *The Process of Government* (Chicago: Univ. of Chicago Press, 1908), Section 1. A brief but acute résumé of the argument against the conception was written in 1921 by Ellsworth Faris, "Are Instincts Data or Hypotheses?", reprinted in his book, *The Nature of Human Nature* (New York: McGraw-Hill, 1937).

[7] Thus, William James defined the term as follows: "Instinct is usually defined as the faculty of acting in such a way as to produce certain ends, without foresight of the ends, and without previous education in the performance."

returns from a survey of ethnography and history with a fuller realization of the relativity of men's acts and experiences. "*Homo sapiens* of the modern type," Morris Opler puts it, "has changed physically hardly at all in the 30,000 years or more of his existence," yet, especially in the last 6,000 years of this period, men's behavior and character, his technical accomplishments and social techniques have changed in deep-going and rapid ways. The cultural may not be reduced to, and hence explained by, the organic.[8]

The enormous variety of specific activities which make up the histories of biologically similar men forces us to acknowledge that the objects and goals of behavior are not biologically given, but are derived from the environment in which men act. Both ends and means of conduct are diverse and changeable. Neither man's values and purposes, nor his ways and means of achieving them are common to all men, nor stable in the sequence of generations. Indeed, such regularities of behavior as we may observe in men are best described in terms of their goals or end-situations rather than in terms of any constant set of "urges" somehow "lying in" the organism and "back of" their conduct regularities. What we are aware of through our bodily senses is limited by the specific societies in which the human animal is born and how and what this society trains him to see and hear and act toward. To act one must have the proper apparatus; but this apparatus only limits and facilitates; it does not determine man's actions.

There is usually a direct correlation between an act and its object: we act towards something when it is a goal, away from it when it is not. As we have seen, the range of objects to which an organism is sensitive varies from species to species and varies further within given species. These objects involve, as George Mead has said, a "content toward which the individual is susceptible as a stimulus."[9] It is these objects, toward which man learns to be sensitive, that are important in explaining the diversities and regularities of the specific conduct of man. No inventory of conveniently catalogued biological elements in man's organism

[8] See Morris Opler, "Cultural and Organic Conceptions in Contemporary World History," *American Anthropologist,* Vol. 46, No. 4, October-December, 1944, which contains an excellent discussion of A. L. Kroeber's classic 1917 essay, "The Super-Organic."

[9] "Social Psychology as Counterpart to Physiological Science," *Psychological Bulletin,* Vol. VI, pp. 401-08.

will enable us to predict or account for the varied and changing activities in which men in different societies engage. The diversity of conduct cannot be adequately explained by a study of men merely as individual organisms. At an early age, infants lose the ability to discriminate between poison and edible food. Possibly man—like domesticated animals—has lost the complex instincts of his "natural" orientation. At any rate, domestic animals differ from their "wild" counterparts essentially in that domestication has disintegrated the instincts which linked them to their natural habitats.

From the biological point of view, then, man as a species and men as individuals are seen as organisms (1) whose action is *structurally limited,* who are equipped with certain mechanical responses, and (2) who possess *undefined impulses,* which may be defined and specified by a wide range of social objects. What these objects may be is not determined by man as an organism.

2. The Sociological Model

If we shift our view from the external behavior of individual organisms and from explanations of such behavior in terms of physiological elements and mechanisms, and view man as a person who acts with and against other persons, we may then (1) examine the patterns of conduct which men enact together, and (2) avail ourselves of the direct experiences which persons have of one another and of themselves. At its minimum, social conduct consists of the actions of one person oriented to another, and most of the actions of men are of this sort. Man's action is interpersonal. It is often informed by awareness of other actors and directly oriented to their expectations and to anticipations of their behavior.

Out of the metaphors of poets and philosophers, who have likened man's conduct to that of the stage actor, sociologists have fashioned analytical tools. Long-used phrases readily come to mind: "playing a role" in the "great theater of public life," to move "in the limelight," the "theater of War," the "stage is all set." More technically, the concept "role" refers to (1) units of conduct which by their recurrence stand out as regularities and (2) which are oriented to the conduct of other actors. These recurrent interactions form patterns of mutually oriented conduct.

By definition, roles are interpersonal, that is, oriented to the conduct and expectations of others. These others, who expect things of us, are also playing roles: we expect them to act in certain ways and to refrain from acting and feeling in other ways. Interpersonal situations are thus built up and sets of roles held in line by mutual expectation, approbation, and disfavor.

Much of our social conduct, as we know from direct experience, is enacted in order to meet the expectations of others. In this sense, our enemies often control us as much as our friends. The father of a patriarchal family is expected by his wife and children to act in certain ways when confronted with given situations, and he in turn expects them to act in certain regular ways. Being acquainted with these simple facts about patriarchal families we expect regularities of conduct from each of their members, and having experienced family situations, we expect, with some degree of probability, that each of these members will experience his place and his self in a certain way.

Man as a person is an historical creation, and can most readily be understood in terms of the roles which he enacts and incorporates. These roles are limited by the kind of social institutions in which he happens to be born and in which he matures into an adult. His memory, his sense of time and space, his perception, his motives, his conception of his self . . . his psychological functions are shaped and steered by the specific configuration of roles which he incorporates from his society.

Perhaps the most important of these features of man is his image of his self, his idea of what kind of person he is. This experience of self is a crucially interpersonal one. Its basic organization is reflected from surrounding persons to whose approbation and criticism one pays attention.

What we think of ourselves is decisively influenced by what others think of us. Their attitudes of approval and of disapproval guide us in learning to play the roles we are assigned or which we assume. By internalizing these attitudes of others toward us and our conduct we not only gain new roles, but in time an image of our selves. Of course, man's "looking-glass self" may be a true or a distorted reflection of his actual self. Yet those from whom a man continually seeks approval are important determinants of what kind of man he is becoming. If a young lawyer begins to feel satisfaction from the approval of the boss of the local political machine, if the labels which this boss uses to describe his behavior

matter a lot to the lawyer, he is being steered into new roles and
into a new image of his self by the party machine and its boss.
Their values may in time become his own and he will apply them
not only to other men but to his own actions as well.[10] The self,
Harry Stack Sullivan once said, is made up of the reflected appraisals of others.[11]

The concept of role does not of course imply a one person-one
role equation. One person may play many different roles, and each
of these roles may be a segment of the different institutions and
interpersonal situations in which the person moves. A corporation
executive acts differently in his office than in his child's nursery.
An adolescent girl enacts a different role when she is at a party
composed of members of her own clique than when she is at her
family's breakfast table. Moreover, the luxury of a certain image
of self implied in the party role is not often possible in her family
circle. In the family circle the party role might be amusing, as a
charming attempt at sophistication "beyond her age and experience," but at the party it might bring prestige and even the adulation of young males. She cannot, usually, act out the self-conception
of a long-suffering lover before her grandfather, but she can when
she is alone with her young man.

The chance to display emotional gestures, and even to feel them,
varies with one's status and class position. For emotional gestures,
expected by others and by one's self, form important features of
many social roles. The Victorian lady could dramatize certain emotions in a way that today would be considered silly, if not hysterical.
Yet the working girl who was her contemporary was not as likely

[10] The mechanism by which persons thus internalize roles and the attitudes
of others is language. Language is composed of gestures, normally verbal,
which call forth similar responses in two individuals. Without such gestures
man could not incorporate the attitudes of others, and could not so easily
make these attitudes a condition of his own learning and enactment of roles
of his own image of self.

These conceptions will be discussed in greater detail in Chapters III:
Organism and Psychic Structure and IV: The Person. Here we are only
concerned with setting forth in the most general way the sociological model
of explanation.

[11] "Conceptions of Modern Psychiatry," *Psychiatry*, Vol. III, No. 1 (February 1949), pp. 10-11. Compare also C. H. Cooley's *Human Nature and the
Social Order* (rev. ed.; New York: Scribner's, 1922). The tradition is well
documented by Fay B. Karpf, *American Social Psychology* (New York:
McGraw-Hill, 1932).

to faint as was the lady; there would probably not have been anyone to catch the working girl. During the nineties in America it
was expected that women who were also ladies, that is, members
of an upper status group, would faint upon very exciting occasions.
The role of the delicate and fainting lady was involved in the
very being of a lady.[12] But the "same" occasions would not elicit
fainting on the part of the ladies' maid, who did not conceive of
her "place," and of her self, as a fainting lady; fainting requires a
certain amount of leisure and gentlemanly attention, and accordingly offers opportunities to the gentleman to demonstrate that
chivalry is not dead.

The roles allowed and expected, the self-images which they
entail, and the consequences of these roles and images on the
persons we are with are firmly embedded in a social context. Inner
psychological changes and the institutional controls of a society are
thus interlinked.

An institution is an organization of roles, which means that the
roles carry different degrees of authority, so that one of the roles—
we may call it the "head" role—is understood and accepted by the
members of the other roles as guaranteeing the relative permanence
of the total conduct pattern. An *institution* is thus (1) an organization of roles, (2) one or more of which is understood to serve the
maintenance of the total set of roles.

The "head role" of an institution is very important in the psychic
life of the other members of the institution. What "the head" thinks
of them in their respective roles, or what they conceive him to
think, is internalized, that is, taken over, by them. In a strictly
patriarchal family, the head, the father, is looked up to; his is that
most important attitude toward the child that may determine the
child's attitude toward his, the child's, own conduct and perhaps
toward his self: in taking over this attitude the child builds up an
"other" within his self, and the attitude he conceives this other to
have toward him is a condition for his attitude toward his own self.
Other persons in other roles also have attitudes toward him and
each of these may be internalized, and eventually form segments of
his self-conception. But the attitude of the head of the major institution in which we play a role is a decisive one in our own maturation. If "he says it is all right," we feel secure in what we are doing

[12] Cf. Ralph Linton, *The Study of Man* (New York: Appleton-Century,
1936).

and how we are conceiving our self. When his attitudes are taken over into the self, this head constitutes in a concrete form, a "particular other." But he is not seen merely as a particular person; he is the symbol and the "mouth piece" of the entire institution. In him is focused the "final" attitudes toward our major roles and our self within this institution; he sums them up, and when we take over these attitudes and expectations we control our institutional conduct in terms of them. It is by means of such internalized others that our conduct, our playing of roles within institutions, is "self-controlled."

By choosing the social role as a major concept we are able to reconstruct the inner experience of the person as well as the institutions which make up an historical social structure. For man as a *person* (from the Latin *persona,* meaning "mask") is composed of the specific roles which he enacts and of the effects of enacting these roles upon his self. And society as a *social structure* is composed of roles as segments variously combined in its total circle of institutions. The organization of roles is important in building up a particular social structure; it also has psychological implications for the persons who act out the social structure.

Most of the various interpersonal situations in which we are involved exist within institutions, which make up a social structure; and changes of social structure make up the main course of human history. In order to understand men's conduct and experience we must reconstruct the historical social structures in which they play roles and acquire selves. For such regularity of conduct, and of the motives for this conduct, as we may find will rest upon the historical regularities of these social structures, rather than upon any suprahistorical, biological elements assumed to be innate and constant within the organism. From the sociological point of view, man as a person is a social-historical creation. If his view of his self and of his motives is intimately connected with the roles which are available to him and which he incorporates, then we may not expect to learn much that is very concrete about individual men unless we investigate a number of his specific roles in a number of varied social-historical settings.

Rather than constant elements within a physiological organism, the sociologist rests his primary model of explanation upon the interpersonal situations, and in the last analysis, the social structures within which persons live out their lives.

If, due to changes in the organization of institutions in a society, the patriarchal family should decline in importance, the weight of the father as a social control in the inner life of family members would decline. Thus, the institutional center of social control within ourselves may shift. This is what happens as a child matures, grows up. For, sociologically, "growing up" means the relinquishing of some roles and the incorporating of others. With this objective shift in the institutional roles we play, there is an accompanying shift in the institutional center of social control within the person. The child may no longer look only to his parents, but also to the leader of a gang or to a star of sports or movies to sanction his new roles and the conception of his self which goes with them.

The inner feelings, the entire psychology and outlook, of members of a stratum of small entrepreneurs may vary enormously according to the historical positions and changes of such strata. In the growing cities of the American Middle West, in the middle of the nineteenth century, the hopeful outlook and expansive view which small enterprisers possessed were functions of what was occurring in the social, and especially the economic, structure of which they were a segment. The twentieth-century members of such strata may experience anxiety and depressive fear of being engulfed and pushed down in the social scale by the increasing power and scope of large corporations and big government. To grasp these different inner feelings—self-confidence or deep anxiety—requires a reconstruction of the historical shift from one phase of capitalist economy to another. For it is this shift that carries with it changes in the psychological processes of members of various strata. Just as economists often trace the shiftings of tax loads among various income groups in the processes of economic change, so, in a similar way, the social psychologist may trace the shiftings of psychic strains and stresses ·which are deposited in various groups within a society by the structural changes which it undergoes.

The difference between the primary interests of the social psychologist and the physiologist becomes obvious if we consider, as an example, their respective approaches to the matter of hunger. To the physiologist, hunger is always hunger; his task is to trace the possible connections between the cravings of hunger as stated by the subject and the physiological processes apparently going on in the organism. And he does this quite irrespective of the institutional context and social evaluation of "hunger" by the person. "Hunger" involves a relation between the tremblings of the stomach wall and the feelings of its pangs, but such hunger processes are relevant to the social psychologist primarily in specific varieties of social contexts. For whatever the physiological processes of hunger may be, the social psychologist is interested in the meaning of hunger to the persons involved. The use of hunger strikes by suffragettes in prison or by political criminals as a weapon against instituted authority, the famine imposed on inmates of concentration camps, the organized and periodic fasting of monks and nuns in occidental religious orders, the old-fashioned hunger of the poor and destitute, the commercial records of forty days and forty nights of hunger piled up by competing hunger artists, the feasts of a northwest Indian potlatch or of a Southern political barbecue, or a medieval European coronation meal—all of these types of feasting and fasting involve a wide range of meanings and hence of motivations, irrespective of the similarity of the gastric juices involved.

In similar manner, the anatomy and physiology involved in sex become of interest to the social psychologist only as the prerequisite for behavior. They must be mediated through love, eroticism, types of passion, or other institutionally elaborated patterns of conduct or feeling. In the perspective of physiological psychology, legitimate and illicit love involve identical processes, whereas to the social psychologist these two kinds of situations involve conventional and legal definitions which make for significantly distinct motivation and conduct.

Aging is a physiological process, as is hunger. But age is important to the social psychologist not as a chemical and biological process, but as the object of insurance tables or as relevant to the chances of being employed in given occupations. Old age, in short, is sociologically interesting for what people make of it, whether they honor the grand old man, or despise the mean old fogey.

Certain biological capacities and traits, of course, often become particularly relevant to the demands set up by new roles. Thus, if a society needs aviators in order to fight an air war, those individuals who have good biological capacities for "balance" have increased chances to assume these roles. The sense of balance is located in the biology of the ear. Swiftly changing atmospheric pressures also affect in rather different ways different types of human organisms. In societies with such technologically determined social roles, such organic differences become relevant prerequisites, whereas in preindustrial societies the same individual differences would be irrelevant. What specific aspects of man's biological nature become prerequisites for role-taking are socially and technologically determined, and accordingly, those aspects which become relevant to our explanations of conduct, are thus determined.

In a somewhat similar way the biological differences between men and women are taken into account by the social psychologist only insofar as they become relevant to conduct by virtue of their evaluations in different societies. A woman is not only a woman: she is a wife, a nun, a railway conductor, or a parachutist with a bright new deadly weapon. She may drive a four-ton truck or nag an unsuccessful husband. There are greatly differing roles for men, too, ranging from those which gain a living, and which the Japanese honor with a two-handed sword, to the eighteenth-century fop with his effete gestures and niceties of taste. No doubt there are roles which women cannot fulfill and others which men are incapable of enacting. Although a man may be the sociological mother of a child, catering to its needs, he cannot actually give birth to one—although he may, in practicing the couvade, hysterically experience birth pangs. Most women cannot stand physical exertions of bodily work as long or as intensively as can most men. Yet many statements about psychological traits believed to be due to sexual differences appear on second thought to be ideologies which identify or at least confuse social traits with biological differences.[13] For apart from the reproductive functions and extremely heavy work, the range of conduct patterns which are interchangeable between the sexes is very broad, and it may become broader as social history unrolls.

The differences between biological and sociological types of explanation may be further revealed in the matter of authority and leadership. In an external, behaviorist manner, the term authority describes a situation in which one or several organisms will obey

[13] See Viola Klein, *The Feminine Character* (New York: International Univs. Press, 1949).

another one. Thus, groups may jump to rigidity when one man shouts "atten-tion." This is a purely objective definition. It grasps what is observed in the behavior of two or more individuals. This might be further explored biologically: We might try to correlate the size of the organism who is obeyed with the probability that he will be obeyed; the larger he is, the higher the probability is that he will be obeyed; or we might try to compare some measure of the vitality of the leader's constitution with the hypothetically lesser vitality of the bodies of the followers. Such external observations and physiological hypotheses are about all that we can do with animals and with prelingual children.

We have, however, another source of information when we deal with persons who possess language, and we would be foolish not to avail ourselves of it. It is simply the direct experience such persons have of the authority situation by those who enact it. Why do they obey? What feelings do they experience when they do so? Do they feel compelled to obey, do they experience fear? And, if they do not obey, are they full of enthusiasm or anxiety, remorse or elation? Such questions as these cannot be answered merely by observing the external behavior of the organisms, nor by probing their physiology. We must study the inner experiences and feelings of the persons who play various roles in the interpersonal situations of authority. And to do this adequately we must reconstruct the roles of followers and leaders in different societies, and the symbols they use and believe in.

The view that the biological or constitutional aspects of man are irrelevant and that everything depends upon social acquisitions and training may be just as dogmatic—however fashionable—as the view that such biological features are the major determinants of man's character. The conflict of these two viewpoints is not resolved merely by the slogan that personality is, "after all," an integration of biological constitution and sociological environment. "Though proportion is the final secret," E. M. Forster has remarked, "to espouse it at the outset is to insure sterility." What we want to know is precisely how one or the other of these two general forces influences the total individual.

CHAPTER

II

Character and Social Structure

BIOLOGICAL explanations of human nature and conduct center upon the notion of the organism; sociological explanation upon that of the person. In connection with the organism, we have discussed conditioning and instinct as explanatory mechanisms; in defining and elaborating the notion of the person we have discussed roles and institutions. Now, both organism and person—or other terms standing for similar viewpoints—must be understood and used in any adequate conception of the human individual. But each of them must be broken down and linked with other terms, and each must be more precisely linked with the other. If we did not so elaborate and refine them, we would find that our vocabulary was too gross for the sort of work we want to undertake. In this chapter, which completes our introduction, we shall lay out, in an over-all and hence a rather general way, other features of character and of social structure, which will enable us to complete our first view of these conceptions.

1. Components of Character Structure

To try to understand the individual only as organism and as person is to leave out an area of experience and observation that is very much a part of any adequate portrayal: the direct world of emotion and will and perception, of rage and determination and anger, of sight, sound, and fury. Physiologists,[1] of course, do study such phenomena, but psychiatrists and psychoanalysts have been most directly concerned with man as an emotional and willful creature, in short, as a "psychic structure."

[1] See Chapter III: Organism and Psychic Structure, Section 3: Feeling and Emotion.

We shall use this term, *psychic structure,* to refer to man conceived as an integration of perception, emotion, and impulse. Of course there are other psychic functions, memory and imagination, for example; but we shall limit our term at this point. For our purpose, "psychic structure" will refer to when, how, and why man feels, perceives, and wills.

If the human organism did not possess a chromatic eye, it could not distinguish colors; if it were not equipped with a certain glandular and nervous apparatus, it probably could not experience rage and hate; without undefined impulses, what is experienced as purpose or willfulness could not occur. Clearly, sensation, impulse, and feeling are in some way rooted in the animal organism and in its specialized organs; it may not be so apparent that they are also linked to man as a person, where they are revealed to us as perception, purpose, and emotion.

I. In order for inner feelings to become emotions, these feelings must be linked with socially recognizable gestures, and the person must become aware of them as related to his self. The same physical environment and the same physiology, for all we know, may be present, but in one case these conditions may lead to fear and flight, and in another, to rage and attack. The difference between the two experiences and behaviors cannot be adequately explained physically or organically. The social definition of the occasion, the meaning it comes to have for certain types of persons, provides the clue to which emotion and which conduct will arise.

II. For sensation (the physical and organic event, for example, of light waves impinging in a certain way upon a certain kind of eye) to become perception (the seeing of the object as a red light) certain meanings must be added. The sensation must come "to stand for" or to represent something: stop the car—a rather complex sequence of near-automatic behavior which as an aspect of a social role must be learned by the person as a driver. Sensations are organized into perceptions, and this organization goes on in close unity with the social organization of the person as an actor of roles.

III. For impulse (the undefined and generalized urge to movement) to become purpose (the more or less controlled striving toward a specific object) the objects so specified and defined must be learned. Impulses are specified and directed in terms of the expectations of others; they are socially defined, linked with socially available goals and thus sustain the person in enactment of his roles, and in turn, the institutions of which these roles are a going part.

The way in which each of these three elements of the psychic structure is joined to the other elements in some sort of unity; the way each is linked to activity; and the way each element, and thus the psychic structure as a whole, is socialized in man as a social actor—these linkages must be examined if we are to understand the integration of the organically based psychic structure with the person and his social experiences.

With the acquisition of language, we learn to experience our conduct and ourselves in relation to the expectations of others. We learn to distinguish ourselves from objects and from other persons by referring to ourselves by the personal pronoun, "I." With these distinctions, we acquire a self-awareness which henceforth accompanies many of our psychic acts; in fact, if our perceptions and impulses are experienced as alien, automatic, or compulsive—as not emerging from our self—we speak of the pathological phenomenon of "depersonalization." A sense of our own unity, of our identity, in time, and of our contrast to the world outside us, is characteristic of our very awareness of self. The person, accordingly, should be understood to involve two things: toward the outside world and in relation to others, we act out roles which, by virtue of our own feelings and consciousness, we ascribe to ourself. At the same time, we "enrich" our self by accepting the challenges of external tasks and by taking over into our selves the expectations of others.

In our attempt to understand the human individual, we shall find four key conceptions useful. Each of these conceptions stands for one aspect of man; no one of them exhausts our interest; together they may be adequate to form understandable models. In discussing the ways in which they may be integrated, we will also be assessing more precisely the relative weights of biological and sociological elements making up different types of human beings. The four key terms are organism, psychic structure, person, and, finally, character structure itself.

I. The human *organism* refers to man as a biological entity. The term invites attention to structural mechanisms and undefined impulses.

II. *Psychic structures* refers to the integration of *feeling, sensation,* and *impulse.* These elements are anchored in the organism, but their specific integrations into emotions, perceptions, and purposes must be understood with reference to man as a person.

III. *Person* refers to man as a player of roles. Under it we view man as a social actor and try to grasp the results of this social acting and experience upon him. By his experience in enacting various roles, the person incorporates certain objectives and values which steer and direct his conduct, as well as the elements of his psychic structure. Viewing man as a person we try *to understand his conduct* in terms of motives rather than *to explain his behavior,* in terms of stimuli and responses, or as an expression of physiological constants in the organism.

IV. *Character structure,* in our vocabulary, is the most inclusive term for the individual as a whole entity. It refers to the relatively stabilized integration of the organism's psychic structure linked with the social roles of the person. On the one hand, a character structure is anchored in the organism and its specialized organs through the psychic structure: on the other hand, it is formed by the particular combination of social roles which the person has incorporated from out of the total roles available to him in his society. The uniqueness of a certain individual, or of a type of individual, can only be grasped by proper attention to the organization of these component elements of the character structure.

Each of these four terms represents an abstracted dimension of man, a manner of looking at him, a suggestion of what to look for. Such differences as are found among men may be attributable to the constitution of their organisms, to the specific role-configurations incorporated in their persons, or to the peculiar integration of their perception, feelings, and will within a psychic structure. An adequate portrayal will direct our attention to all three as they come together to form a character structure within the limits of a given organism and the institutional confines of a specific social structure.

2. *Components of Social Structure*

The concept of role, the key term in our definition of the person, is also the key term in our definition of institution. It is, therefore, in our definitional model, the major link of character and social structure. We have already examined the formal components of character structure; we must now elaborate and classify the organization of roles into institutions.

We speak of roles as organized or instituted when they are guaranteed by authority.[2] Thus, the cluster of roles enacted by the members of a household is guaranteed by "parental authority": the "head" of the household may use sanctions against infractions of the role pattern. Thus, employees are subject to the control of owners and managers; soldiers are subject to the authority of the commanding officer; parishioners stand under the jurisdiction of church authorities. Whatever ends the organized and interacting partners may pursue and whatever means they may employ, "authority" exists: and whenever a role configuration is so guaranteed or stabilized by a "head" who wields authority over the "members" who enact the roles, the configuration may be called an institution.

The head of the institution, the king of a political order, or the father of a patriarchal kinship system is the most significant "other," of the persons following the institutional patterns. The kind of external sanction this head may take against those who do not meet their expected roles in expected manners may range from disapproval to expulsion or death. His expectations are treated as most important by persons so long as they are really involved in the institution as a going concern. In this way, then, as well as in others which in due course we shall take up, institutions are deeply relevant to our understanding of the person, and in turn to the entire character structure.

Just as role is the unit with which we build our conception of institutions, so institution is the unit with which we build the conception of social structure. There is more to a social structure than the interrelations of its institutions, but these institutions, in our view, do make up its basic framework. Our immediate aim, then, is to classify institutions in such a way as to enable us to construct types of social structure.

There are many possible classifications of institutions; in fact, the main concern of sociologists has often seemed to be the making

[2] The conception of authority will be explained more fully in Chapter VII: Institutions and Persons; it will be elaborated in Chapters VIII and IX.

of such classifications. Many of these classifications are descriptively
useful; they help us sort out many items of social conduct and
experience and thus to handle them more neatly. But we need
more than this; we need a classification that will be relevant and,
we should hope, fundamental to our general concern in understanding character structure on the one hand and social structure on
the other.

First we shall briefly examine two very simple classifications of
institutions: a classification by size and a classification by recruitment of members.

I. If we classify institutions according to size we end, for example,
with large families (households comprising three generations under
one roof—as among the Chinese), small families (comprising two
generations—parents and children), and incomplete families (of one
generation only—the childless couple). Even such a simple classification as this may be relevant to the types of social structures as a
whole, as well as to the milieu in which persons grow up and live.

Classifications of institutions by size, in fact, are sometimes used
as a basis for far-going descriptions, for example, the shift from
business institutions of very small size to those of great proportions.
The difference between the classic laissez-faire capitalist and the
monopoly capitalist eras rests upon this simple numerical fact. It
is also clear that the types of entrepreneurial roles typical of small
business institutions differ from those of the giant firm; and hence
the personalities of men, selected and trained for their roles, vary.

Classifications by size, then, can be very important: a sense of
numerical proportion is always indispensable for the understanding of social structure and character. But size by itself does not
seem to us useful enough to be a fundamental classifying device.
The size of institutions is more often a subsidiary than a fundamental distinction.

II. Institutions may be classified according to the way in which
their members are recruited. Compulsory institutions—those which
enroll members without the members' choice—include churches
which recruit their members essentially through infant baptism and
modern states, in whose territory we are "born" as citizens subject
to state authority. Where "compulsory education" exists we become

members of a "public school," from which we can steer clear only under special regulations.

Voluntary institutions—those which one may join or not, according to one's will—include the modern childless family, as well as most American civic societies and clubs. Indeed, most of the institutional drift of postmedieval society has been in the direction of an enlarged area of voluntary associations in social life as a whole. The United States is distinguished by the wide range and number of such voluntary institutions; it is with reference to them that Americans are known as joiners.

It is obvious that personality development in a society based primarily on voluntary associations differs from that in a society based primarily on compulsory institutions. In the former, one has to make many decisions on his own, for better or for worse; in the latter, one has no opportunity to make such decisions and hence is not burdened with the personal responsibilities which they may entail.

There are other ways of classifying institutions that are descriptively useful. For instance, the roles composing institutions may be permanently or only temporarily played by given individuals; they may be provisional or at once secure. But there is no need to parade additional classifications. Although we shall introduce and use them for various purposes as we need them, we do not believe they are adequate for our general purpose.

III. The classification of institutions that we shall take as fundamental to our model of social structure is a simple classification according to objective function, that is, to the ends which institutions serve.

An *institutional order,* as we shall use the phrase, consists of all those institutions within a social structure which have similar consequences and ends or which serve similar objective functions. However institutions may vary in size, recruitment, and composition of membership, in forms of control or proportions of permanent and transitory roles, as we examine the advanced societies of the modern Western world we can distinguish some five major institutional orders.

At least at first glance, we may classify most of the institutions as having to do with such ends as power, goods and services, violence, deities, and procreation. All those institutions which deal with the recurrent and collective worship of God or deities, for instance, we may call religious institutions; together they make up the religious order. Similarly, we may call those institutions that have to do with power, the political; with violence, the military; with procreation, the kinship; and with goods and services, the economic order. By delineating these institutional orders, which form the skeleton structure of the total society, we may conveniently analyze and compare different social structures. Any social *structure*, according to our conception, is made up of a certain combination or pattern of such institutional orders.

In the course of Part Three of this book, we shall concern ourselves with the social psychology of each of these orders in topical detail. In the present introductory statement we shall only present some of the mechanisms that hold generally for institutional conduct and some of the linkages of institutions with character structure.

(1) The *political* order consists of those institutions within which men acquire, wield, or influence the distribution of power and authority within social structures.[3]

(2) The *economic* order is made up of those establishments by which men organize labor, resources, and technical implements in order to produce and distribute goods and services.[4]

(3) The *military* order is composed of institutions in which men organize legitimate violence and supervise its use.[5]

(4) The *kinship* order is made up of institutions which regulate and facilitate legitimate sexual intercourse, procreation, and the early rearing of children.[6]

(5) The *religious* order is composed of those institutions in which men organize and supervise the collective worship of God or deities, usually at regular occasions and at fixed places.[7]

[3] See Chapter VIII: Institutional Orders and Social Controls, I, Section 1: The Political Order; Section 2: Nation and State; and Section 3: Democracies and Dictatorships.

[4] See Chapter VIII, Section 4: Economic Institutions; and Section 5: Types of Capitalism.

[5] See Chapter VIII, Section 6: The Military Order; and Section 7: Characteristics of Six Types of Armies.

[6] See Chapter IX: Institutional Orders and Social Controls, II, Section 3: The Kinship Order.

[7] See Chapter IX, Section 1: Religious Institutions; and Section 2: Characteristics of the World Religions.

Some four qualifications or cautions about this way of classifying institutions must be kept in mind at all times, and although they will become clearer as we proceed with our work, we must state them at once:

I. The conception of social structures in terms of such functional institutional orders is, of course, suggested by modern society in which various institutional orders have reached a high degree of autonomy and in which the relative differentiation of ends has gone very far; so far in fact, that business men often engage in the pursuit of profits without consideration for the effects of business institutions upon other institutional orders; that is, they posture as purely economic man. Yet few, if any, modern claims for the *pure* autonomy of an institutional order have been realized. If they were, it would mean that one order was wholly segregated from all others; no social structure is so mechanically composed. Moreover, during the last half century, modern social structures have definitely tended to become more tightly integrated, and their various orders interlinked under more total control.

There are social structures in which the specialization of ends and institutions has not been pushed as far as in modern society. Business and private life, or the economic and kinship orders, are not segregated in peasant society. Farms provide members of peasant families with a household way of life in which economic production and family living are not only interrelated but in many respects identical. We may isolate one aspect of a society from another for the sake of analysis, but we have to realize that often, as in the peasant village and the garrison state, this analytical isolation is not experienced; life is an inseparable fusion. For example, the fact that ancient Israel had no distinct term for "religion" did not mean that there were no religious functions; on the contrary, there was little in this society that was not at least indirectly related to Yahweh and his commandments.

Therefore, our first caution is: In "less developed" societies than the mid-nineteenth-century West, as well as in more developed societies, any one of the functions we have isolated may *not* have autonomous institutions serving it. Just what institutional orders exist in a more or less autonomous way is a matter to be investigated in any given society. In some societies the institutions of the kinship order may perform functions which, in more segmented societies, are performed by specifically political institutions. Any classification of institutional orders in terms of function should be seen as an abstraction which sensitizes us to the possibilities and enables us to construct and to understand the concrete segments and specific functions of any given social structure.

II. The classification of institutional orders according to the *dominant* ends of the institutions composing them should not blind us to the fact that the activities and and functions of an institution are not exhaustively characterized by its primary end. A religious institution, such as the Catholic Church, employs numerous specialized functionaries who devote themselves to the financial and property affairs of the institution; a monastery may specialize in the production and sale of "Chartreuse," an exquisite French liqueur; or it may engage in the brewing of beer, the printing of books, and so on. Yet, we shall not call such institutions "economic institutions"; for it is hardly satisfactory to account for the existence and shape of a "monk order" in terms of its economic pursuits, no matter how relevant economic activities may be for the religious organization. Monks who brew beer do not thereby constitute a brewery which just happens to recruit tonsured and celibate men as employees. The financial transactions of the Vatican do not make it a bank. That an army or a factory may employ religious leaders for morale-building purposes does not mean that the army or the factory becomes a religious institution, but rather that the military order is able to use religious personnel for its own ends. That the dispute concerning the dogma of the Trinity was settled at Nicaea in A.D. 325 by monks armed with clubs does not make "military institutions" out of monasteries. Neither is the employment of practitioners of violence by business corporations or trade unions sufficient to turn such institutions into elements of the "military" order. An institution may enroll numerous agents and may comprise many specialized roles for the implementation of its dominant goal.

Many and varied activities are required to operate large institutions, and these activities often overlap with those of other orders; accordingly, the ends of one order often serve as the means of another. Nevertheless, we must first set up a scheme in which we attempt to define and classify institutions by their *dominant* functions before we can consider such problems of "overlap" and integration in a fruitful and systematic way.

III. Our classification of institutions into orders is in terms of their objective, social functions, not subjective, personal meanings of their members or leaders. Concretely, this means that whether or not the persons who enact roles making up the institutions within an order are aware of the order's ends, nevertheless, their conduct is so oriented. A Catholic cardinal, for example Richelieu, may have been personally motivated to win political power, and may even have spent most of his life in political rather than religious activities; but this does not make the churches under his authority part of the political order. Nor does it necessarily mean that the more political bishops are less effective in their religious roles than "more religious" bishops. The motives that are typical of persons playing roles in a given order are matters to be investigated in every case; they are not in any way settled by any objective definition of the dominant functions of institutional orders.

IV. Not all social experience and conduct are included in this scheme of institutional orders. The "dating" of young lovers and the behavior of "the man in the street" are not institutional conduct—although, of course, they are affected by several institutional orders. Yet, if we aim to grasp total societies, it is convenient to focus first on institutions and their settings rather than on the more amorphous and ephemeral modes of social interaction, however crucial these may at times be.[8]

There are several aspects of social conduct which characterize all institutional orders, the most important being: technology, symbols, status, and education. All orders may be characterized by technological implements, by the modes of speech and symbols peculiar to them, by the distribution of prestige enjoyed by their members, and by the transmission of skills and values. We shall arbitrarily call these "spheres," in contradistinction to "orders," because they are, in our view, rarely or never autonomous as to the ends they serve and because any of them may be used within any one of our five orders.

(1) "Symbols" may be visual or acoustic; they may be signs, signals, emblems, ceremonial, language, music, or other arts. Without such symbols we could not understand the conduct of human actors, and normally, their belief in and use of these symbols operate to uphold or justify the institutional order. The religious order

[8] See Chapter XV: Collective Behavior.

has its sphere of theology, the elaboration, attenuation, and justification of God or deities; the military order has its startle commands; and the political order has its political formulae and rhetoric, in the name of which its agents exercise authority.[9]

(2) "Technology" refers to the implementation of conduct with tools, apparatus, machines, instruments, and physical devices of all sorts. In addition to such instrumentalities, the technological sphere refers to the skill, dexterity, or expertness with which persons meet their role demands. In this sense, "technique" is used by the violinist as well as by the skilled soldier; it is revealed by the surgeon's use of his tools, as well as by priest handling such paraphernalia of worship as the chalice or the prayer wheel. Whenever we concentrate on the degree, or the absence, of skill with which roles are enacted, we may speak of the technological sphere, regardless of what the institutional context may be. Technology is never autonomous: it is always instituted in some specific order or orders. In modern industrial society, it is centered primarily in the economic and military orders, which not only stimulate it and "supervise" its production and distribution to other institutions, but are the orders in which it is most often used.[10]

(3) The "Status" sphere consists of agencies and means of distributing prestige, deference, or honor among the members of the social structure. Any role in any institutional order may be the basis for status claims, and the status sphere as a whole may be anchored primarily in any one order or in many specific combinations of institutional orders.[11]

(4) The "Educational" sphere consists of those institutions and activities concerned with the transmission of skills and values to those persons who have not yet acquired them.[12]

A *social structure* is composed of institutional orders and spheres. The precise weight which each institutional order and sphere has with reference to every other order and sphere, and the ways in

[9] For the public role of symbol spheres, see Chapter X: Symbol Spheres; for the private role of symbols, see Chapter V: The Sociology of Motivation.

[10] See Chapter XIII: Social-historical Change, Section 3: The Technological Sphere.

[11] See Chapter XI: Stratification and Institutional Orders, Section 3: The Status Sphere; and Section 4: Class and Status.

[12] See Chapter IX: Institutional Orders and Social Controls, II.

which they are related with one another—these determine the unity and the composition of a social structure.[13]

The analysis of social structure into orders, as we have said, does not decide what "orders" exist; only concrete investigation of different societies can do that. We shall not be surprised, of course, when we have to elaborate or simplify the classification of institutional orders sketched here. Social structures are not frozen, they may be static or dynamic, they have beginnings, duration, varying degrees of unity, and they may disintegrate.

These problems of the interrelations of institutional orders and of social change will be dealt with in due course. Here it is perhaps enough to remark that the warp of one institutional order may be the woof of another. Military men, for instance, becoming conscious of a scarcity of manpower, may be concerned about the declining health of the working classes because they anticipate an increasing percentage of men unfit for military service—a thought that may not enter the mind of the businessman, still thinking of the abundance of labor force. Similarly, businessmen, interested in educated labor for clerical jobs, may become much concerned with tax-supported high schools.

In their ramifications, then, institutional orders have definite bearings upon each other; tensions and conflicts arise, and practices lead to results which the practitioners neither intend nor foresee.

It is often convenient to examine these interrelations of institutional orders in terms of ends and means; often the activities which fulfill one institutional order's ends serve as means to the dominant ends of another order. When we focus upon such subsidiary aspects of institutions, we may see the ramifications of another order. What dominates in one order may, in a different order, merely implement. The political activities of businessmen and corporations may thus be understood as "political ramifications of the economic order." The religious order or the educational order may also have political ramifications: the political activities of religious and educational institutions and personnel. Similarly, we may speak of the educational and religious ramifications of the political order when focusing upon educational activities of politicians in party schools or the role of prayer and other religious

[13] See Chapter XII: The Unity of Social Structures.

activities in politics. Any given order may thus become the ramification of any other order. "Ramifications" may thus be defined as those activities which are ends in one order but which are used as the means of another institutional order. In total war, for example, all orders become ramifications of the military state, for the military impinges upon all other orders which thus become prerequisites for realizing or for limiting military ends.

3. The Tasks of Social Psychology

Throughout this book we shall be engaged in elaborating and refining the various elements noted in our general model of character and social structure, and in tracing the possible linkages connecting one element with another. The various components of character and social structure are diagrammed in the following chart:

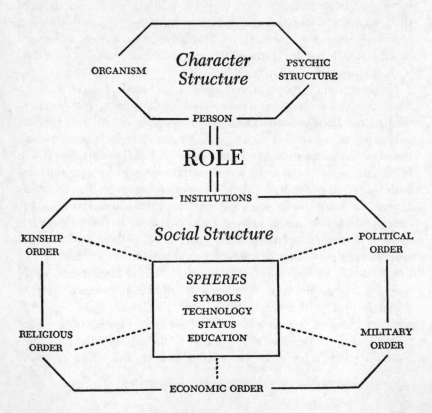

With this model in mind we wish to construct features of various institutional orders and their interrelations, in connection with the psychology of the individual. Now that we have presented the general features of our model, we are in a position to set forth, in a preliminary way, the tasks which it allows and invites.

I. The numerous roles organized into various institutional orders must be analyzed. Obviously, our goal cannot be the examination of all the roles, past and contemporary, which men have enacted. This would involve a complete rewriting of the universal history of mankind! Nor would a formal dictionary of possible roles be tied closely enough to institutional orders and social structures to be revealing and realistic. We shall have to use two general criteria for our selection of roles, and of persons formed and selected by them, which we shall analyze:

First, we shall select those roles which are of pivotal significance in the maintenance and transformation of given types of institutional orders. Of course, what order or orders we think most important in historical transformations will influence our selection of roles.

Second, the roles we select for analysis will represent the polar or extreme types within given institutional orders, thus affording us a chance to see the widest range of possible conduct.

II. We wish to focus upon the type of person selected and formed by the enactment and internalization of the roles which we analyze. Since a person participates in the roles of various institutional orders, and the dominant roles of given types of persons may be role-segments of one type of institution within a given institutional order, we shall pay attention to the various effects on the persons so formed and selected by institutions.

Our expectation of finding regularities in human conduct, experience, and motives is keyed to the role configurations forming institutions. We seek (a) to analyze roles as segments of institutions; (b) to discern the typical motivations which are required by individuals as necessary and sufficient for the enactment of these roles; and (c) to show how the central ideas and beliefs of a society, its communications and symbols, contribute to the formation, maintenance, and effectiveness of these motivations.

III. With reference to each institutional order, we need more adequately to characterize the primary and secondary functions which it may fulfill in the full range of social structures. In order to do this in an historically adequate way, we must lay out the range of institutional types which are available in each order. We shall then find it convenient to select polar extremes and analyze them in some detail. In this way we hope to grasp the possible *scope* of the character and functions of political and military, kinship and economic, educational and religious institutions.[14]

IV. We need also to gain a view of the major ways in which various institutional orders are related to one another in different types of social structures,[15] and changes in these relations.[16] For types of social structure may be constructed and compared by examining the specific combinations of institutional orders which make them up, the varying importance each of these orders has, and the definite ways they are interrelated. In a parallel way, working models of various kinds of historical change can be developed by viewing types of social structure in terms of their dynamic movements and shifts rather than in static cross section. For history is of course only the changes of social structures and their component parts.

Our general aim, then, is to display, analyze, and understand types of persons in terms of their roles within institutions in given orders and social structures within various historical eras; and we want to do this for each institutional order. We cannot, for example, rest content with the assumption that the kinship order, with its tensions of early love and authority, is necessarily the basic and lasting factor in the formation of personality; and that other orders of society are projective systems from this until we have studied the selection and continued formation of personality in the economic and religious and political institutions of various social structures. The father may not be the *primary* authority, but rather the replica of the power relations of society, and of course, the unwitting transmitter of larger authorities to his spouse and children. We must set forth institutional orders in a systematic way, relate them to one another within a social structure, and trace their impact upon persons and psychic structures.

[14] See especially Chapter VIII: Institutional Orders and Social Controls, I; and Chapter IX: Institutional Orders and Social Controls, II.

[15] See Chapter XII: The Unity of Social Structures.

[16] See Chapter XIII: Social-historical Change.

PART TWO

CHARACTER STRUCTURE

Organism and Psychic Structure

TO understand the psychic structure we must understand how it is both rooted in the organism and linked with the person. For there is nothing within the psychic structure itself which enables us to understand how impulses are transformed into purposes, impressions into perceptions, feelings into emotions. These psychic elements are linked with one another, and each of them, as well as the unity they form, is socialized in such a way as to sustain or to restrict the social roles that the person enacts.

1. The Social Relevance of the Organism

Human organisms are different in size, shape, and color. People who are lean and tall, with flat, narrow chests, who seem to be thinly made with bonelike arms and legs, have been called leptosomes. Others, whose organic constitutions appear to center around their abdomen, who have plump bodies, rather short limbs, deep-vaulted chests and magnificent paunches, have been called pyknic. And then there are the athletic men, tall and broad of shoulder, thick-skinned and coarse-boned, with big hands and feet. In sum, different individuals may be classified according to such body types. But can we go further? Can we state that these constitutional types are correlated with types of character, temperament, or with specific traits of personality? Is the appearance of the individual "expressive" of different psychic traits and qualities?

The physical signs of aging appear to us as signs of physical change, just as the trembling, sweating, swollen features of an alcoholic indicate somatic processes, and no more. But other bodily features and processes are often "read" as indicative of spiteful resentment, happy disposition, or other character traits. We experience our body externally by touch and sight, and internally by feeling tone; our psychic and our somatic life are thus intimately fused. But since, once we have grown up, our physical structure changes very little, this structure serves as a reference point in physiognomic observations of psychic life, in a twofold manner:

I. In observing the general appearance, the gestures, deportment, and conduct of the individual, one can assume that they are documentary evidence for an essential unit: The "nature" of this or that man, comprising his organic, psychic, social, moral, and other qualities. This current of romantic thinking has been elaborated in a broad literature. Yet however plausible and attractive the morphological types constructed may seem, one has to allow for so many exceptions and so many contradictions that the endeavor always seems to break down.

II. In the morphological approach one tries to intuit the essential nature of a type of individual as a unit. In a second approach, one measures certain traits, which one then correlates with one another. These elements and their correlations do not always possess the plausibility of the unitary whole or Gestalt. For in the process of such detailed research the idea of providing materials for physiognomic documentation loses its symbolic overtones.

Now, physiognomic propositions usually follow one or more of three principles: (1) Individual traits, being read as "signs," are understood as "symptoms" of character. Karl Jaspers,[1] whom we follow in this matter, points out the absurdity of this approach, which is perhaps best revealed in Lombroso's work, to be discussed presently. (2) By intuitive understanding, the observer tries to grasp the totality of the body, which at the same time is held to indicate a certain psychic type. The bodily form, the head and the hands, are artistically composed into a configuration that is "seen" as a whole of psychological quality. (3) The body build provides the observer, not with any psychological meanings, but with a form which the artist may take up and use in shaping his image of man. The human form—the thick and the thin, the angular and the round, the tall and the short, the straight and the lopsided—is thus put to essentially artistic rather than psychological use.

Much physiognomic literature—going back to ancient India and

[1] *Allgemeine Psychopathologie* (Berlin and Heidelberg, 1946).

Mediterranean antiquity—has since the eighteenth century been subject to intellectual fashions. In the recent past, two such works stand out: the "degeneration" literature connected with Lombroso's name, and the psychological elaborations of "bodily types" of Kretschmer.

In Lombroso's conception,[2] bodily deviations—such as inordinately long legs in comparison with the length of the entire body, strange skull shapes, absence of a proper chin, excessive hairiness or the absence of bodily hair, ingrown earflaps or big, protruding ears—are considered as signs of the "degeneration" of the psychic structure, and are alleged to stand for the degenerate nature of the respective individuals, of their dispositions to neurosis and mental disease and especially to criminal behavior. This sort of approach brings physiognomic intuition into spuriously scientific form, the "symbolism" of old assumes the form of "symptomatology," and medically nothing can be proven.

Kretschmer's attempt is comparable.[3] Its content differs, of course, but the method of relating body build and psychic traits allows us to place him near Lombroso, although he happened to be more concerned with geniuses than criminals. He distinguished three types—the leptosomic, the athletic, and the pyknic—and assigned the few unclassifiable individuals to the residual category of dysplastic men.

One of the most recent large-scale and careful studies designed to answer physiognomic type problems—the study of Sheldon and Stevens [4]—concludes with this comment: "If anything is demonstrated conclusively by the study as a whole, it is this: that neither the somatotype [type of organic constitution] alone, nor any other single factor, will suffice to 'explain' a personality. Persons of the same somatotype frequently develop into singularly different kinds of people. . . Furthermore, although the correlation between somatotype and temperament [of two hundred young American men], taken at large, is [moderately high] . . . so many [apparently secondary] variables are at work that the specific manifesta-

[2] Cesare Lombroso, *Crime, Its Causes and Remedies*, H. P. Horton, tr. (Boston: Little, Brown, 1911).

[3] E. Kretschmer, *Physique and Character: An Investigation of the Theory of Temperament* (New York: Harcourt, Brace, 1926).

[4] W. W. Sheldon and S. S. Stevens, *The Varieties of Temperament: A Psychology of Constitutional Differences* (New York: Harper, 1942).

tions of temperament can be predicted from the somatotype [only] within very wide limits . . ."

Such studies, we believe, do not result in more definitive findings because (1) they do not succeed in isolating, or in making fine enough distinctions among, the various elements of the total character structure. Usually working with such "constitutional traits," as size and proportions of abdomen and legs, on the one hand, and with "temperamental" items such as "love of comfort" or "desire for action" on the other, it is not odd that the results are gross and generally unrevealing.

(2) The total character structure, in which such "temperamental" factors are included, involves more than the organism. If attention were paid to the specific social constellation in which "love of comfort" was attributable to given individuals, it would be realized that the person as well as the organism must be studied if we are to grasp the integration of types of character structure, or even of "temperament."

(3) We might say that the tall constitution is organically correlated with "traits" or "abilities" of leadership (Abraham Lincoln) and that the short physique is accompanied by a lack of these social or psychic traits (Corporal Napoleon!). We would then search for something about the organism that makes for aggressive leadership or for its absence. So far, those who believe in such *organic* correlations of constitution with psychic traits have not isolated its mechanisms. And no statistical correlations have been found to be adequate as long as the organic mechanisms of the imputed influence were not set forth, for there are other ways to explain any correlations which might exist between types of constitutions and temperamental or personal traits.

Insofar as "leadership" is an accompaniment of big or of little physiques, for example, the connection may be in terms of others' reactions to such men, rather than *through* the organisms of the individual leaders. Biological capacities and deficiencies, as mediated through the reactions of others to them, influence the child's reactions to others and, in turn, his attitude toward himself. In given societies, the "social burden" of some organic deficiency may lead to the development of certain character traits. The person with a deficiency of some organ may be more preoccupied with himself than are organically normal persons. In compensation, he may increase his striving for superiority and supreme recognition.[5] On the other hand, defects, such as those of vision may be the basis, not of compensatory striving for superiority, but of alibis and justifications for feelings of inferiority.[6] How organic conditions are related to the development of personality traits and conduct patterns depends on how the whole structure of the character is *socially* estimated.

For the social psychologist, those features of the organism which are to be studied must be relevant to the social situation of the actor and to the actor himself. For that seems to be the way in which the type of body and other "constitutionally determined characteristics need to be taken into account in any successful effort to interpret a personality." The same principle of interpretation holds for *races*.

Race refers to a statistical type of constitution which a group of organisms approximate. The members of a race vary as individuals, but they vary around a norm or type: they are characterized, in E. A. Hooton's words,[7] by a "certain combination of morphological and metrical features, principally nonadaptive, which have been derived from their common descent." The anatomical features chosen as the bases of classification are biologically useless ("nonadaptive"); they usually include the shape of the head as measured in various ways, the type of hair, the proportions of the nose. Skin color is no longer generally used by biologists and anthropologists as a primary classification trait.

Given the type of organic traits seized upon for racial classification, it would indeed be fortuitous if organic correlations between these types of anatomies and any character or psychic traits were discovered. So far, they have not been: there is no conclusive evidence of difference in "native" intelligence or in types of personality between biologically defined racial types.[8]

The social and psychological irrelevance of the biological traits used by anthropologists in classifying races does *not*, however, abolish the "reality of race" or the "psychology" of races. It *does*

[5] Cf. Alfred Adler, *Understanding Human Nature* (London: Faber, 1927), pp. 69 ff.

[6] See I. E. Bender, *et al.*, *Motivation and Visual Factors* (Hanover, New Hampshire: Dartmouth College Publications, 1942).

[7] *Up From the Ape* (rev. ed.; New York: Macmillan, 1946).

[8] Cf. for example, Otto Klineberg, *Race Differences* (New York: Harper, 1935).

change the bases on which these matters are open to fruitful study. For if we use as racial criteria those anatomical traits characterizing a people, or even a portion of them, to which others pay social attention, we do find types of "racial personality." The personality traits which may become typical of members of races are then sociological in origin and operation. They will be traits which are socially visible and socially used as "badges" by other persons and by members of the race itself in social relations. In the United States, for example, color is obviously a primary criterion.

"Racial psychology" is most fruitfully understood as a social psychology of racial relations.[9]

Our emphasis on the causal irrelevance of the organism, individual or racial, to character traits and conduct patterns should not blind us to the direct intrabody effects of constitutional differences which do exist. We have said that the emotions, purposes, and perceptions which make up the psychic structure are "rooted in the organism"; this means that constitutional differences and changes in the organism may directly affect the elements of the psychic structure:

I. Feelings and gestures, the alertness and clarity of perception or the strength of impulse, may be changed by modification of physiological processes. Thus, physical exhaustion and fatigue may limit the control of one's speech in a court hearing or a police-directed interview. The organism may be so exhausted, due to prolonged worry and sleeplessness, as to be incapable of resisting suggestion. The speed with which one throws up his guard and collects his wits may thus be reduced. In this way one's physiological condition may be modified in order to open one up for ease of psychic manipulation.

II. Toxics may be used so to modify the physiological process and guarantee certain predictable psychic states. A candidate for an examination may use unusually strong coffee in an effort to heighten his alertness and forestall the slackening effects of fatigue and overlong concentration. Resources are thus mobilized for a supreme effort. The lowering of conventional inhibitions against aggressive impulses by the use of alcohol is another case in point.

[9] These matters will be examined in Chapter XI: Stratification and Institutional Orders, Section 3: The Status Sphere; and Section 5: The Status Sphere and Personality Types.

It should be noted that the economic position of persons may affect their type of diet, and deficiency in diet may lower the alertness of their perception, the intensity of their emotions, or the persistence of their will.

III. In certain role contexts, the physiological foundations of the psychic structure become especially relevant. The opera singer thus abstains from smoking, which is detrimental to the voice, and athletes who are in training are exhorted not to spend their "energy" with women. The history of religion is rich in examples of ascetic practices which lead to psychic states which are appraised as holy. There is the cultic chastity of the priest, and the abstentions from food, sleep, and sex of a variety of monks and holy men. And there are the practices of Buddhists which are productive of extraordinary psychosomatic states, which, in turn, are subject to elaborate interpretations.

IV. The general organic changes involved in maturation, puberty, and aging determine changes in performance in emotional state or perceptual clarity. But what is "childish" in the life-cycle and what is "mature" and "senile" vary widely in different societies.[10] Yet this variation is limited, and in part may be constituted, by biologically fixed and directed processes of maturation and aging. The link of physiological changes and psychic sequences is not set by external or chemical manipulations of the physiological state of the organism, but is rather a result and an aspect of the natural conditions and changes of man's body in the cycle of its life-span.

CHARACTER STRUCTURE

Organism			Person
PSYCHIC STRUCTURE			
structural limitations	impulse ..... impression... feeling	...purpose ...perception ...emotion	roles, meanings, gestures

[10] See Chapter VI: Biography and Types of Childhood, Section 7: The Relevance of Childhood; and Section 8: The Social Relativity of Childhood Influences.

The physiological foundations of the psychic structure, then, have intrabody effects; and within certain social-historical conditions they also have social effects. The way people feel, perceive, and will is rooted in the animal organism, and is influenced directly by its changing physiological conditions. The psychic structure is also linked to the person, most crucially by the way in which social expectations play upon the person to steer and control his impulses, emotions, and perceptions. The psychic structure (how, what, and when we feel, perceive, and will) is determined by the total character structure, but the "executive" of the character structure, the person, is a result of social experience and training.

2. Impulse and Purpose

Man is not merely a machine reacting to physical stimuli; he does not rest inert until he is jerked and pushed by outside forces. The use of such terms as "will," "volition," or "impulse" signifies the self-movement of the organism: the infant organism moves and wriggles and, in due course, gains a purposive control over the directions and objectives of its conduct.

From the rather abstract "standpoint of society," the question of impulse is: How can a person be produced who wants, or "wills," what is socially approved, demanded, or premiumed? How can impulse be trained to fit in with role-demands? The problem of social control is not merely one of coercing persons to act against their own wills, but rather to offer socially approved goals which will be incorporated as objectives of the will.

When the impulses of a psychic structure are directed toward socially approved objectives, they support and sustain the person in his roles. Then he wants to do what is expected of him. These roles of the person, many of which are segments of institutions, are then supported by the trained impulses of the person.

There is a cycle involving undefined impulses and socially available goals; and, by repetition and suggestion, punishment and reward, impulses are integrated with goals. Persons incorporate the goals and link them with impulses, which then sustain the continued operation of the conduct patterns that form various institutions. It is of course also true that persons may invent goals in order to deal with challenges which frustrate their impulses, and these may become social objectives.

The internal stimulation of hunger, thirst, or pain may excite the infant organism to general action and sensitize its perceptions toward certain classes of objects. This activity is impulsive and blind; when it is defined by external objects, when animal restlessness fuses with social objects, it is socialized. And in due course, if it becomes deliberate, it may be purposive.

At feeding time the baby raises its head, waves its arms, opens its toothless mouth. Its mother says that it is hungry, inferring "hunger" from the activity she observes. The correctness of her imputation is shown by the eagerness with which the baby grasps the nipple, firmly holds it, frantically sucks. By the choice and control of the food that is offered, the baby's food preferences are patterned. It *learns* what is "good" to eat and what is "bad," that food is good and feces are disgusting; and in due course, it will want the one and reject the other. Impulses for food are thus disciplined by sensations of sight and touch, of taste and odor, and more importantly, by the norms of others expressed in the child's presence: the social definitions of appetites and thresholds of disgust. Through her expressions of disgust and her gestures of approval, the mother patterns the baby's "taste." Organic disposition —the baby's "need" for food—its dependence upon whatever is provided, and the experience of gestured approval and disgust by those who care for it merge into the formation of the appetite and tastes of the social novice.

If several activities are possible and the individual chooses one and refuses the others, we ascribe will, purpose, or volition to him. Such a mastery of one's movement, a use of it as a means of acquiring what is wanted, involves the awareness and the anticipation of goals. Purpose, desire, or intention, as one stage in the development of impulse, exists when impulses have found objects.

Such anticipation of goals, as distinct from the "pushes" of bare impulses and needs, plays a decisive role in man's conduct. The anticipation of goals which will realize our impulses is often in terms of symbols. So purpose or intention may be termed "symbolized impulse." Wishes or desires are *for* something. Impulses which are not so attached to an object which would satisfy them may be said to be irrational and/or undefined. We cannot fruitfully treat "desires" as standing in contrast with what is desired. In desire, content and impulse form an intrinsic unity. When the impulsive features of a psychic structure are not so linked and

integrated with objects, they may burst asunder in wild and random action or become attached to objects which are not socially
approved.

The definition of impulses accompanies the definition of social
situations. Organic impulse and social situations become linked so
that impulse seeks the situation as an outlet, and the situation furnishes the cue and sets the type of conduct that will satisfy the
impulse. Such social transformations of impulses into conduct patterns are important aspects of the *social* integration of a psychic
structure. The internalization of social values and objectives gives
direction to impulses and, to some extent, even sets the intensity
of these impulses. When impulses are not disciplined into com-
municable purposes, conduct is irrational: it cannot readily be understood in terms of a rational calculation to attain some end,
although it may of course be predictable to the psychiatrist in accordance with his scheme of diseases. In fact, only certain areas of
social life, for example, the rational calculation of men bargaining
in a market, typically lend themselves to strict interpretation in
terms of the rational choice of expedient means for explicit ends.

Because undefined impulses become desires only by the importation of social values, we cannot take "desires" at large, nor lists
of specific desires, as explanations for specific conduct. The conditions of concrete desires and impulses must themselves be explained, and this explanation requires us to pay attention to interpersonal situations which train and which steer impulses.

When the adult observes the baby's overt activity and then says
that it "manifests" desires, he is treating this activity as a symptom
or a sign of desire. For the baby, no connection between the activity and the goal may at first exist, and unless it does we cannot say
that the baby is acting "out of desire." Eventually, activity and
goal will be linked: the child will learn to elicit an activity on *our*
part which completes *his* impulsive activity. He will then be acting
"in order to" experience the satisfaction accruing as a consequence
of his action. He will be acting purposively. When his stomach is
empty the baby squalls impulsively. Later, he will link this squall
to the touch of the mother's breast and later to the visual perception of the mother. When the tactual and visual consequences of
the squalling are linked with the impulsive spasm of squalling,
the baby will have learned to cry purposively. He will experience

his cry as a sign, just as the mother had previously interpreted it.

We learn to desire by having our impulses frustrated; purposes arise out of deprivations; they involve a duality; we strive against something; to have will, as C. S. Pierce put it, we must encounter resistance.[11] But before the physiological deprivation of an impulse can become a desire, experience must enter to connect the deprivation to a meaningful object that will satisfy it. The object of our desires and purposes will obviously be selected from among the objects that are socially available or offered to us, however oddly they may be combined in fantasies which arise from lengthy deprivations. Our desires for particular things are often placed in us by the fact that others desire them. "Emulation," wrote Spinoza, "is the desire of anything which is engendered in us from the fact that we imagine others to desire it also." [12]

Objects which are offered to, or withdrawn from, the infant, become the objectives of his impulses. Not having an adequate notion of space and the limits and burdens which it places upon man, the child will literally reach for the moon. A glaring disproportion between the child's impulsive movements toward objects that would hurt him and his insufficient fear of these objects Ferenczi has called "the magical hallucination of omnipotence." For the sake of the physical security of the child, his guardians train him to avoid dangers and to acquire adequate fears. In his interaction with others and with things, the child thus acquires purposes which determine the direction of his conduct and perception. Impulses are thus socially linked to perceptions of anticipated goals and are turned away from harmful traps.

The ascription of purposes to others on the basis of our own purposes may be quite complicated, but in terms of our awareness of our own purposes and our ascription of these purposes to ourselves or to others, there are four types of situation. (I) We may, in rational self-clarification, know our own purposes and ascribe them to ourselves as ours. (II) Our purposes may be unknown to us, although we ascribe them to ourselves, as in undefined states of "longing" or "cravings" or "free-floating anxieties." (III) We may

---

[11] *Collected Papers* (Cambridge, Mass.: Harvard Univ. Press, 1934), Vol. I, Book 3.

[12] Benedictus de Spinoza, *Origin and Nature of the Emotions*, Boyle's translation (Everyman's Library, New York, 1934).

know our purposes and yet deliberately ascribe them to others, as imperialist statesmen in modern propaganda have been known to do just before they launch their attacks. (IV) We may not know our purposes and at the same time unconsciously ascribe them to others. In this case, we speak of "projection," as when the anti-Semite believes himself to be persecuted by a world conspiracy of Jews, against which he then "defends" himself: he projects his aggressiveness to Jewry, in order to be "free" or to be justified in releasing his own aggressiveness.

The straightforward understanding of the purposes of others on the basis of our own purposes is more likely to be accurate in socially standardized situations. For if two persons are similarly trained, the purposes which the one finds in himself are likely to be similar to those in the other. But in a society composed of widely variegated situations, ascriptions of purpose are more often mistaken.

Men may treat anything which proves beneficent as motivated by benevolent purposes, and anything which hurts them as maliciously motivated. This may also occur with reference to physical objects, as when we curse a chair over which we have stumbled in the dark, or with reference to impersonally caused social upheavals, as when men curse the revolution or the reaction coming after a war.

3. Feeling and Emotion

All understanding of laughter and gaiety, of fear and trembling, and other expressive phenomena is often said to be based upon logical inferences from one's own psychic life to that of another. Actually, however, we seem to understand such expressive acts directly, we seem to understand even as we observe the activity.

In fact, before they have acquired language, infants—as well as some domesticated animals—seem to "understand" the facial expressions of adults. René Spitz, in exemplary experiments,[13]

[13] René A. Spitz with the assistance of K. M. Wolf, "The Smiling Response: A Contribution to the Ontogenesis of Social Relations," *Genetic Psychology Monographs*, Vol. 34, 1946, pp. 57-125. Cf. also, Weston LaBarre, "The Cultural Basis of Emotions and Gestures," *Journal of Personality*, Vol. 16, pp. 49-68, reprinted in *Personal Character and Cultural Milieu*, Douglas G. Haring, ed. (rev. ed.; Syracuse: Syracuse Univ. Press, 1949), pp. 487-506.

has shown that the smiling response can be elicited between the second and sixth month by the direct presentation of "another human being," or what the baby takes to be another, regardless of the facial "expressions" that are presented. After the second month, the smile is "integrated into the nascent pattern of the child's emotional needs on the social level. In the course of this integration the purely motor pattern of the smile is endowed with the psychological meaning inherent in the child's emotional relations with its human partners." In view of this, Dr. Spitz feels justified in calling the smile a semantic pattern, a genuine communication.

Dr. Spitz, dealing with the exceptions to the normal smiling response, holds them to be indicative of emotionally disturbed child-mother relation, which seems to indicate that this gestural pattern—the smile—is an acquired aptitude rather than the unfolding of an "innate disposition." At any rate, after the sixth month, the indiscriminate smiling response becomes more discriminate. The baby distinguishes friendly and unfriendly faces.

Not all bodily movements accompanying emotions are expressive phenomena. And we have no clear knowledge of which movements are and which are not understandable expressions. We do not necessarily and directly "understand" the dilated pupil as a phenomenon of fear, but if we know this meaning and have frequently observed it, then we seem to understand the enlarged pupil directly as fear.

Let us carefully sort out the various elements involved in the whole phenomena of feelings and emotions:

I. In observing the conduct and appearance of other persons, we notice on certain occasions that the postures of their bodies change, their voices are modulated or hysterical, offensive or inviting. Sometimes we see sweat break out on their faces. At others, the face before us suddenly goes white, or the play of its features is distorted. People look at us with aggressive eyes as if they wanted to destroy us. These types of behavior are called *gestures*.

II. Such conduct obviously involves *physiological changes* in the organism. When someone "blushes with shame," the distribution of blood within his body has concentrated in his face. When he feels strong in rage, his adrenalin glands have brought about an increased sugar content in his blood, thus strengthening his muscle power. In times of stress and danger the organism secretes adrenalin which, in co-operation with the sympathetic nervous system, elicits sugar from the liver and floods the blood with it; this sugar, in turn, eliminates fatigue in the muscles and strengthens the action systems of the organism. Within ten seconds the heart beats faster; within three minutes after an "emotional experience" there is 20 to 30 per cent more sugar in the blood. These processes increase muscular efficiency; physiologically, the body prepares for exertion in anticipation of action.[14]

III. From certain gestures and expressive movements we seem to know that those who make them are experiencing certain *feelings,* and looking within ourselves we experience the fact that our own gestures often involve feeling states. These feelings of pleasure, pain, or satisfaction seem to belong to the feeler alone. Our feelings can only be ascribed to us by others on the basis of our gestures and appearance. We do not read these signs unerringly and thus *know* the feelings of others; sometimes, even often, we do not know directly, nor can we name, what we ourselves feel.

Simple feeling states, or moods, or "affects," may be diffused: we feel tiredness or buoyancy all over; or, these feelings may be localized in the organism: we have an acute toothache. When feelings are localized, we can sometimes deflect attention away from them, and thus diminish the intensity of our awareness. Normally, feelings of hunger and thirst are localized signals of general bodily needs, but as hunger becomes starvation our whole psychic life is affected, and all our declining energies are marshaled to serve our craving for food. And as we sink into a state of general drowsiness, food becomes the all-absorbing concern of our phantasy life and thought, of our feelings and consciousness. Feelings of sexual attraction are usually diffused, but in severe tension they may be heavily localized in specific erotic zones.

Both localized and diffused feeling states may be classified in terms of their respective intensities of pain or pleasure. Thus: There is the intense, localized feeling of a broken bone; the intense, general feeling of starvation; the mild yet localized pain of a small

[14] A good account of the physiological changes involved in emotions is available in Walter B. Cannon, *Bodily Changes in Pain, Hunger, Fear, and Rage* (2d ed.; New York: Appleton, 1929), pp. 194, 196, 220, 225, 343. For a comprehensive examination of the literature, see H. F. Dunbar, *Emotions and Bodily Changes* (New York: Columbia Univ. Press, 1935).

cut; the mild, general feeling of tiredness; the intense, localized pleasure of the loving kiss; the intense, general feeling of bliss or euphoria; the mild, localized feeling of a pleasant taste in our mouth; and there is the mild, general awareness that we just feel good. Of course there are thresholds of intensity: climactic pain may become so unbearable that we faint to save ourselves from further awareness. And with palliatives, drugs, and ethers, modern medicine has made the intensities of pains and our awareness of them more manageable.[15]

It is possible to approach "emotions" in terms of the *gestures* of the person, in terms of *physiological conditions* in the organism, or in terms of our awareness of *feelings* in the psychic structure. To understand emotions, we must avail ourselves of each of these levels of description. We must see how they are each experienced, how social factors are involved in the experience of their operations, and precisely how the various levels may be linked.

One statement of the occasion and nature of emotions runs as follows: If an organism acts immediately and adequately in the presence of some stimulating occasion, no emotion is engendered. The action proceeds smoothly and no gestures, no feelings, and no physiological changes need occur. If, however, the response is in some way blocked or the impulse behind it is frustrated, emotion occurs; then gestures and feelings will make their appearance. The urgency of the feelings may be reduced by the expression of emotional gestures. Emotions occur, the statement runs, when the organism is disorganized; when it has no ready response. When behavior is running smoothly no emotional outbursts occur.

Such a formal physiological scheme does not tell us how we are to distinguish between different emotions, nor does it inform us

---

[15] There is another type of feeling which involves an awareness of our self as well as of our body. We feel ashamed or guilty or generally insecure. These experiences may be called *self-related feelings:* we shall call them *emotions*. They involve the psychic structure, just as simple feelings of pleasure do, but they also involve the person. Our image of our self, which is reflected from the social experiences which form the person, is involved in them. (See Chapter IV: The Person.) The emotions which are related to this self-image are linked with situations and social occasions in which emotional states are experienced. They are related to the position of the self within the social circle of others. Such self-related feelings, or emotions, may react upon and elicit more simple awareness of general feelings.

of the social occasions which for different types of persons engender the feelings, gestures, and physiology of emotions. Emotions, especially if they are intense, cannot be classified in terms of differing physiological conditions, nor in terms of different gestures. Both fear and rage may involve similar glandular secretions, similar facial contortions, and even awareness of similar feelings. Different emotions are identified in terms of the situations in which gestures are expressed. The vocabularies which are used as a response of others to our gestures define and give meaning to our emotion.

As "different emotions" become more intense, their gestural and feeling aspects become more similar. Psychic elements seem to take over the whole character structure. The control of emotions by the person is minimized, or even shattered. We cannot time and shape the gestural expressions nor the feelings according to defined occasions; we are overwhelmed. If the occasions which so upset us recur, we may develop ways of meeting them. If we can organize appropriate roles or rituals, and thus integrate and socially steer our emotions, our psychic structures will be less likely to take over the character structure as a whole and thus dominate our conduct.

To understand what "emotional experiences" involve, and what specific direction increased bodily power may take during such experiences, we must consider not only the physiological organism and the psychic structure, but also the person. In the face of "danger," flight is possible, but so is struggle and attack; fear, as well as rage or hate, may be felt. Adrenalin does not decide which of these emotions will be experienced and enacted. There do not, for example, seem to be noteworthy differences in the visceral accompaniments of fear and anger. In anger and in rage, in fear and in fury; there is adrenalin. The organism allows us, indeed helps us, to become truly fearful or full of powerful rage. But there does not seem to be any one stimulating condition in the physical environment of the organism that automatically produces awareness of any given emotional feeling or the expression of certain emotional gestures. We must go beyond the organism and the physical environment to account for human emotions. Physiological psychology has not reached a point at which it can claim to have established the identity or parallelism of physiological processes and specific emotional sequences and feelings.

"Emotional experiences" give the cue for physiological preparation; and after these experiences are under way the physical exertion produces further bodily changes. Socially induced worry, excitement, or anxiety, for example, may disturb the digestive processes, or cause peptic ulcers in the walls of the stomach. The mechanisms seem to include increased acidity as well as movements of contraction in the stomach.

The brain does not have any direct control over the viscera.[16] The autonomic nervous system and the system of our glands, according to modern medicine, are the links of physiology and the study of conduct and experience: they make up the sphere of the psychosomatic.[17]

The chief access we have to the autonomic nervous system is the experience of moods. These feeling-states, as Ives Hendrick has said, are thought to be an awareness of "changes in the muscle tone and blood supply of our internal organs produced by autonomic nervous stimulation . . ."[18] At times we cannot control such feelings. Physiologically this means that the central nervous system is "immobilized" so that we cannot control the "panicky feeling," or sometimes the excretory functions of the organism.

Whatever our theoretical assumptions concerning the complex relations between physiological organism and psychic structure, we know that externally produced physiological changes, for instance the consumption of stimulants or drugs like coffee, alcohol, marijuana, or aspirin, often becomes relevant. A society may avail itself, at conventionally and legally defined occasions, of these toxics; it may manage to suppress, or indeed, to impose them. In colonial societies, alcohol has been distributed to natives as a technique of "domestication." And as we have already remarked, suitable measures of alcohol have also, on occasion, been used to reduce conventional inhibitions, as between the sexes. Legal as well as conventional norms may define the range and direction of permitted consumption. In Western societies the habitual and medically unauthorized use of cocaine is prosecuted, and accordingly, trade in

[16] Cannon, *op. cit.*, p. 264.

[17] Ives Hendrick, *Facts and Theories of Psychoanalysis* (2d ed.; New York: Knopf, 1944), pp. 290-91.

[18] *Ibid.*, p. 289.

such stimulants is specifically licensed. Such norms have, of course, been violated, as when the British under the slogan of free trade imposed opium upon defenseless populations in China, as did the Japanese at a later date. When coffee was introduced into seventeenth-century England, there were attempts to suppress its use. The authorities feared the politically suspect sociability of literati and businessmen in the coffee houses; the women wanted their men to stay at home and away from the morally suspect female employees of such establishments.

The meaning of a situation to a person sets the experience and the nature of emotion. These meanings vary according to the person's past experiences; these experiences, in turn, must be explained in terms of the person's position and career within given kinds of social structure. Now, recurring situations become stereotyped in their meaning for emotion.[19] In some, it is "proper" to become fearful and run; in others it is cowardly so to feel and act. The American father is conventionally expected to gush joyfully at sight of a newborn baby; the Roman father could inspect it critically, deciding to accept or reject it. Persons internalize these social expectations of emotional display, which thus, at the proper occasion, are exemplified by the psychic structure. Even if we feel joy on some occasions, we may suppress the gestures of joy, should the occasion and our associates conventionally expect a display of sorrow.

[19] Gestures and mimic movements are of course socially and historically determined; they have, as it were, a grammar of their own, although the expressively gesturing person may know of this grammar as little as M. Jourdain knew of the fact that he had been speaking prose all his life. D. Efron has compared the gestural habits of East European Jews with that of first-generation Italian immigrants. He found that in Jewish arm gestures, the upper arm and elbow are held close to the body, that the lower arm and the hand are used at a close distance to the conversational partner; there is a sort of turtle movement of the head, a poking with the finger, or across the table with the fork; there are down strokes with the hand or chin and beard. By contrast, Italian gestures seek the greatest possible amplitude for horizontal movements of the outstretched arms and hands, to the right and left of the bodily axis. Efron attributes these differences to the ghetto, with its physical narrowness, in contrast to the Italian plaza, as delimiting and facilitating scenes of expressive behavior. Subsequent generations of immigrant Italians and Jews of course lose these gestural peculiarities as they take on the general Amrican pattern of expressive behavior. See D. Efron, *Gesture and Environment* (New York: Columbia Univ. Press, 1941).

Gestures of sorrow—stylized according to expectation—may become the basis for feelings of sorrow. Thus the person regulates the psychic structure, although of course psychic elements may burst out in uncontrollable ways. By our facial, bodily, and verbal gestures we make evident to others our psychic reactions. But when our feelings are vague and inchoate, the reactions of others to our gestures may help define what we really come to feel. For example, if a girl has been jilted at the altar and is generally upset about it, the responses of her mother may define the girl's feelings of sadness and great grief, or of indignation and anger. In such cases, our gestures do not necessarily "express" our prior feelings. They make available to others a sign. But what it is a sign of may be influenced by *their* reactions to it. We, in turn, may internalize their imputation and thus define our inchoate feeling. The social interaction of gestures may thus not only express our feelings but define them as well.

Moreover, our gestures may elicit or impose feelings which at first were not present. For example, a child may playfully heave a brickbat at another innocent youngster. The second youngster may not take the act as a playful gesture but treat it as an indication of meanness and aggression. This definition of the affective intent by another on the basis of the gesture or act may lead to a fight in which the first child acquires a feeling more socially appropriate to his own gestures.[20] The child thus links certain gestures and acts with their conventionally ascribed feelings. Children, or adults for that matter, may begin to feel angry *while* they are scuffling or fighting. "Hostility," as Bovet has made clear, cannot be abstracted and treated as a cause of fighting; it may just as well be an effect of fighting acts and fighting gestures.

We know our own emotions by observations of our gestures and actions, and more importantly perhaps, by what other people observe and report to us, directly or indirectly by their responses and gestures to the gestures we have made. Even if the external gestures from which persons normally infer the emotions felt by others are not available, as to the deaf or blind, the emotional agitations of others may be detected by feeling the tensions in the muscles of their arms and hands.[21]

[20] See Pierre Bovet, *The Fighting Instinct*, J. Y. T. Greig, tr. (New York: Dodd Mead, 1923), pp. 23-27.

[21] Helen Keller, *Story of My Life* (New York: Doubleday, 1903), p. 353 ff.

Normally, a certain skill of emotional expression is socially demanded. Because of traumatic shocks or slights, a person may at an early time seek spurious emotional security by what seems to him riskless withdrawal behavior. Accordingly, he may not learn how to "deal" with people. But this does not necessarily mean that he is insensitive, or has no feelings. On the contrary, he may be hypersensitive, and out of overwhelming fear of contact, prefer withdrawal and isolation.

Out of the social interplay of gestures a vocabulary of emotions emerges: the terms for the emotions and feelings which are supposed to accompany certain gestures bring out the meaning of those gestures for other persons. The vocabulary of emotions the person acquires is usually limited to the more common emotions experienced by all members of a language group in a similar enough manner to have been given common names. It is no accident that such phrases as "that leaves me speechless" exist in several different languages. At times, under severe emotional shocks, persons actually do lose their power of speech and may even become mute for life.

Skill groups, such as poets and novelists, specialize in fashioning and developing vocabularies for emotional states and gestures; they specialize in telling us how we feel, as well as how we should or might feel, in various situations. Many terms for our emotions become useless as they become banal or trivial through too frequent use. Stale words may not serve to designate fresh feelings. Thus, we find fashions in the vocabularies of emotion. We smile today at the direct way in which books given to young Anglo-Saxon ladies in the 1830's verbalized the sentiments of friendship and love, or at how Dickens described his heroines' feelings about their mates. We now shy at using words thus "loaded" with the gush of emotion of sentiment. Many twentieth-century European and American expressions were taboo in the Puritan past. Certain terms may be transferred from one sphere of emotion to another sphere in which they lose their appropriateness: by the incongruity of such shifts the terms are banalized and made "hollow." For example, political slogans meant to engage public sentiment and to implement national efforts have often been exploited for private commercial ends. Advertisements for eyeglasses have tried to exploit the emotions of a war, the eyeglass manufacturer implying that those who do not buy are saboteurs of the war effort.

Much contemporary literature and music deals with such "emotional masks," by means of caricatures; "Yankee Doodle," for instance, may be musically caricatured, distorting the harmonious features of the tune or chords or substituting words to deliberately produce incongruities. Prokofiev and e. e. cummings, Stravinsky and Bert Brecht are masters of such effects, as, for that matter, is Charlie Chaplin, in the incongruous opening of his *Modern Times*. Daumier's sketches may be said to have "dethroned" the Olympian figures before continental Europe. Karl Marx theorized about such matters when he stated that the end of an epoch repeats in comical form what at the beginning is enacted as heroic tragedy. He assigned a psychological function to this by stating that mankind could thus bid farewell to outlived forms, not with nostalgia, but with gaiety, and he viewed in this sense Napoleon III as the comical repetition of Napoleon the Great. If Beethoven's work belongs in the Napoleonic age, Offenbach's, for good reasons, belongs in the age of Napoleon III and the Empress Eugenie.

There are vocabularies for *gestures* and other vocabularies for *feelings,* but usually the two are combined. "Sadness" may thus refer to both the feeling-state and the drawn-down mouth and tearful eye. This double reference combined in a single term may be one cause of the social coincidence of gesture and feeling. For it symbolizes the expectation that the displayed feeling is genuine, an expectation based upon observation of the person's gesture.

But often emotional gestures may be "put on" without any "corresponding" affective feelings being present. Ranging from the expert professional actress to the insincere lover with the tender look, the stylization of emotional gestures may proceed without any development of corresponding feelings. We characterize as "spurious" those emotions which are not felt but which consist merely of gestural "expressions." Those gestures which do, in fact, reveal feelings appropriate to them we call "genuine." It should be remembered that the distinction is nice, and in many cases the inference from gesture to feeling is very difficult to make. Furthermore, in observing the gestures of others we often come to a point where *our* externally responsive gesturings invoke *their feelings* within us. Thus, we experience borrowed emotions, which, like our original gestures, may at first be spurious displays, put on for the purpose of dissimulation, but later be internalized and thus become quite genuine. The diffusion of the Nazi salute in Germany may be cited.

Emotional vocabularies of patriotism may be imposed upon populations who are thus denied the public "expression" of their own sentiments. Nationalist prospects may be sentimentalized as "Missions," and nationalist history becomes the hallowed memories of heroes and martyrs. In such cases, some persons may experience the imposed sentiments as spurious, although they may make the conventional gestures that express no emotion; others may withdraw even from the gestures, and some may even actively criticize and resist both the inner meaning and the outer expression.

For the degree to which persons can play roles involving emotional gestures without feeling the emotions conventionally appropriate to them varies widely, in terms of types of individuals and in terms of the frame of conventions. In the course of Western civilization, the rising lower classes have attributed greater truth and honesty in such matters to themselves than to the "sophisticated" upper classes. The rising plebeian almost always places a premium on "uprightness" and "candor" and "righteous indignation." Exclusive and high status groups, on the other hand, are apt to feel that if they owe truthfulness and candor to anyone, it is to their peers, but never to those "not on their level." Polite speech generally seems more important to them than honest speech. The language of righteous indignation is discounted as "rude" or "tactless," and in any case, "beneath them." And yet, the sense of responsibility of high decision-making circles in crisis situations makes them inclined to ascribe to themselves an extraordinary capacity to "face the facts," which they feel might unnerve the contemporary Little Man or the Common Man.

Autobiographical statements of actors and actresses [22]—experts in gesturing—indicate that the artistic enactment of prescribed roles may lead to an intense emotional identification of person and psychic structure with role and hence to deep feelings appropriate

---

[22] On the following autobiographical statements of actors, we quote from the following, in the order given: K. E. Behnke, *Speech and Movement on the Stage* (New York: Oxford, 1930), p. 166; John Barrymore, *Confessions of an Actor* (Indianapolis: Bobbs-Merrill, 1926), no pagination; Morton Eustis, *Players At Work* (New York: Theatre Arts, 1937), pp. 26 and 45.

to the role and the character played.[23] On the other hand, there are actors who interpret the gestures with which they act out a role in a detached and calculating manner; they do not feel that their own personality and psychic structure is fused with the enacted character, and they do not, therefore, experience the emotions which their gestures spuriously display.[24]

The fact that professional actors and actresses have different attitudes concerning the emotional feelings appropriate to the gestures of the roles they present has led to a variety of esthetic norms, held by professional critics and laymen. The social psychologist records the range and types of experiences and notes that no doctrine or rule *of the psychic structure* covers the matter. To understand the extent to which gestures correspond with feelings, one must know something of the persons involved and the conventions of the situation in which the gesture and emotion are presumably linked.

Emotional masks may be said to have a "tighter" or a "looser" fit for the social actor. Theatrical styles, as we have just seen, vary in this respect. Nowadays it would seem that critics and audiences prefer a "loose" fit and derive special enjoyment from realizing the self-conscious distance of the person of the actor from his presented mask. Bert Brecht has raised this attitude to a principle of modern staging, and has scored singular success with his performances in postwar Europe. A specific ethos informs this stand, basically holding that stage acting is after all "play," and that the art consists in being quite serious about the playfulness of the play, lest the presumption of sincerity become ridiculous. This whole

[23] Ristori, the great Italian tragedienne, claims: "I throw my whole passionate soul into my emotional scenes, because I know that my technique will never desert me." John Barrymore, playing Galsworthy's *Justice:* "On the opening night when I pounded with frenzy on my cell door, I broke right through the wood grating which was painted black as an understudy for iron."

[24] Helen Hayes believes that she follows this pattern: "At some time or other I must feel the role, but never in actual performance. There is usually one rehearsal in which I go through the part with real feeling. Thereafter, I *simulate* what I have felt." Such players as Alla Nazimova, Katharine Cornell, and Maurice Evans agree with Burgess Meredith who says: "You are conscious of the effect that emotion should produce, but you don't let it affect you." Ina Claire goes further: "The moment the actor lets himself feel the emotions, he begins to wallow in a role, he becomes a ham."

tendency has undoubtedly been influenced by the development of motion picture acting, which is best where the actor "acts" least, and which has trained the movie audience to new levels of critical appreciation, to the quick grasping of meaningful sights and sounds, of the weight and significance of gestures and words. So a slip of the tongue, which fifty years ago went unnoticed by all but psychiatrists, nowadays is understood by millions, when presented close-up and on a magnified sound-track.

Certain occasions conventionally require certain gestures. A person may cry and otherwise express grief, not because his relative has died, but because he is at a funeral. Crying may be a ritual of conduct, as is the wearing of black clothing. Gestures without feelings may also be simulated for the purposes of rational bargaining, as when sororities on college campuses send their very best "pleader" to a professor to inveigle better grades for a failing pledge who is not so adept at crying.

The gestures supposedly accompanying various emotions may be stylized without affecting any change of feelings. But this stylization of gesture may in time influence and stylize the effect. When you begin the ritual gestures of a funeral you may not feel grief, but in time the atmosphere of the funeral throng with its incantations of grief, its evocations of sorrow, may affect you quite genuinely.

When we ascribe feelings to others in terms of what we ourselves feel, the basis of our analogy is social. The correctness or falseness of such imputations does not have to depend upon any general biological similarity of human organisms. We can sometimes interpret correctly the behavior and gestures of others by ascribing to them sentiments, emotions, or purposes similar to our own because: (1) our interpretation of their external gestures, or of the situation they are in, influences and helps to define for them what they feel, and (2) because of the standardized expectation of certain gestures, and eventually of inner feeling-states, motives, and emotions, which are set up in recurring social situations within given societies. The measure to which we are correct in ascribing our feelings to others in any given case depends upon the extent to which these two conditions hold true.

Today, under conditions of mass movie-attendance, the stylizations of such emotions as tenderness, or various models of erotic allurement or approach, tend to be standardized and fashioned after the movie stars who specialize in such matters. And there are gestural fads which are related to fashions of clothing and make-up; the bent head with the eyes looking slyly out from under the brows goes with big brimmed hats or heavy bangs. Various gestures have differing prestige values attached to them, and insofar as inner feelings may develop from the repeated use of gestures in recurring roles, the emotions as well as the gestures of members of various status groups may be stereotyped.

On the other hand, gestures may be conventionalized precisely to hide inner feelings of one sort or another. In old Japan a code of deportment was elaborated in which it was a "mark of disrespect to betray, by look or gesture, any feeling of grief or pain in the presence of a superior." The code exacted very much more than impassiveness. It required not only that any sense of anger or pain should be denied all outward expression, but that the sufferer's face and manner should indicate the contrary feeling. Sullen submission was an offense; mere impassive obedience inadequate; the proper degree of submission should manifest itself by a pleasant smile, and by a soft and happy tone of voice. The smile, however, was also regulated. One had to be careful about the quality of the smile. It was a mortal offense, for example, in addressing a superior, to smile in such a way that the back teeth could be seen. In the military class especially this code was ruthlessly enforced. The women of the Samurai, like the women of Sparta, were required to show signs of joy on hearing that their husbands or sons had fallen in battle; to betray any other feeling was a grave breach of decorum.[25]

A person whose conception of his own welfare is deeply involved in the sacredness of religious objects will experience awe in their presence. He will become enraged at their desecration or destruction. A person who has not incorporated these objects as sacred, however, may be not at all awed, but, although externally respectful, amused at people who go mewling to the mosque. To the person whose security of self is deeply involved in the approval of a political party whose program includes atheism, the destruction of the sacred objects and the personnel who service them

[25] Cf. Lafcadio Hearn, *Japan: An Attempt at Interpretation* (New York: Macmillan, 1924), pp. 191 ff.

may produce the feelings, gestures, and the physiological changes which accompany great triumph and exalted joy.

A soldier genuinely imbued with a belief in the honor and correctness of his nation's cause and of the evil character of the enemy may experience hysteric joy or elation in "killing"; whereas two years before the "same man" as a clerk may have been revolted at even the thought of "killing." There are all types of killing. "You men are learning ranger fighting," said the lieutenant, according to a New York *Times* report.[26] "There are no rules of clean fighting that apply here. The dirtier you are the better we like it. A stab in the back is one of the finest principles we know of. Every time you think of a Jap, say to yourself, 'We must be more silent, cruel, and vicious than these little sons of b—'" A general ". . . watching with approval whispered: 'And that lieutenant used to be a clerk in Wall Street.'" The military training of the clerk for the situation of killing in war has given the thought and the act a different meaning to him. His immediate associates, and the patriots of his nation, have placed an honorable premium upon efficient killing.

Only rarely in history have *spontaneous* individual emotions and their expression been socially approved. When this does occur it is likely to be during great social transformations, such as the waning of the Middle Ages, the revolutionary turns of Italian city republics during the Renaissance, the upthrusts of the middle classes in Holland or in Cromwellian England, the peasant wars of central Europe during Luther's time, the American Revolution, and the French revolutionary and Napoleonic epochs. In such periods, the barriers of convention and status do not stand in the way of enthusiastic solidarity, but are broken down by the emancipated who spontaneously join with one another in the name of friendship or patriotism. There is much weeping, both spurious and genuine, and when such solidarity is religiously tinged, there is a renewed affirmation of the brotherhood of man. Thus during the 1820's mass revivals swept through the Western world, young lovers learned to trust their own hearts, and love became the prerequisite to marriage.

Such periods, however, soon give way to the re-establishment of convention, often to the point of rigid etiquette as we know it

[26] June 16, 1943.

from Victorianism or the court societies of the *anciens régimes* of prerevolutionary France and Tsarist Russia. Then elegant proprieties, rigidly prescribed forms of etiquette with "perfectionist" habituation of gesture and their ritual elaborations of spurious sentiments bespoke the underlying anxiety—in Western societies no less than in Confucian China.

The roles men play affect their physiology; the meanings of situations may be pointed up by ritual and ceremony. Football games in the United States are preceded by rituals which focus the players' and their followers' emotions on the game. Incentives of acclaim and censure are vividly presented to the players. An eminent Harvard physiologist has reported that such social keying-up of the players may result in their feeling such an "excess of strength" as to be able to crouch and then go breaking down a closed door. The physiologist is interested in discovering that such experiences increase the percentage of sugar in the player's urine; the social psychologist is attracted by the feelings, verbalizations, and consequences of such social interaction.

Many mass audience situations, with their "vicarious" enjoyments, serve psychologically the unintended function of channeling and releasing otherwise unplacable emotions. Thus, great volumes of aggression are "cathartically" released by crowds of spectators cheering their favorite stars of sport—and jeering the umpire. And in tear-jerking motion pictures, in the dark, the release of otherwise unwept tears is facilitated.

Eccentrist dances may have the same effects as football rallies and motion pictures. Religious manias and the jumpings and jerkings of the old Methodists may be more violent than "hysterical or epileptic fits." And dervishes can sometimes dance for days. In many displays of astonishing bodily strength, it has been noted that "crowds of witnesses" facilitate the exertion "beyond consideration of personal prudence." Music, especially martial band music and choral singing, may stimulate the physiology of emotion and bodily strength.[27] The meanings which the person incorporates from his expected roles are thus linked to his gestures, produce changes in his body, and influence the feelings of which he is aware.

[27] Cf. Cannon, *op. cit.*, p. 233.

4. Impression and Perception

The senses are those specialized parts or areas of the organism that are particularly sensitive to changes in the environment. The human organism, equipped with special kinds of sense organs, along with the intensity, duration, size, and movement of various stimuli, makes up the physical and organic conditions of perception.

We cannot see out of the back of our heads, although if we hear a very slight sound and whirl swiftly we may imagine we can. The body, insofar as it puts our senses in a position to record stimuli (the cocked ear, the peering eye) is involved in the act of attention. We bend down to smell a rose; we turn our heads in order to see to the side. These bodily postures put our sense organs into "contact" with the sights, sounds, and smells to which these organs are sensitive.

The pupil of the eye expands or contracts according to the amount of light reaching it; the eardrum vibrates with condensations and rarefactions of the air, and transmits these vibrations, tones, and noises, via three small bones, to the inner ear where different little hair cells are stimulated by high and low frequencies. The skin with which the organism is covered may be considered an organ of touch, but scattered through it are spots more sensitive than others to tactile pressure, pain, cold, or heat. When we move our arms, legs, or trunk, we are aware of these movements and of their extent, speed, and direction. The tastes of various substances in our mouths are received by virtue of our sensitive tongues. Smells come to us through our noses to stimulate olfactory areas. And by means of the nervous system these various perceptions are connected with the mechanisms of response and action, the muscles of which are hung and stretched over our skeleton.

What become stimuli to us are limited by the sensitivity of our sense organs. If sound waves are below or above a certain number of vibrations per minute, they do not stimulate our ears. We thus have physiological thresholds. The anatomy and physiology of the eye and ear and finger are part of the structure of the organism; how these organs are constructed limits and selects what we can see, hear, and touch. Thus, the eye is not merely a photographic lens which mirrors the world for the organism. Out of the total world of external objects, the nature of the eye cuts those which are visible to a particular organism. If the retina is not appropriately equipped for the job, colors cannot be distinguished. What is perceived is limited by the object itself and by the structure of the organism doing the perceiving.

The sudden and intense nature of some changes in the physical environment may completely dominate the organism so that the reaction is quite uncontrolled by the person. A noise of this sort, like a gunshot, will in most cases produce a definite pattern of startle.[28] Yet professional hunters or men very long in battle may have gained some control over such stimuli and over their organisms: they won't startle so easily. Within the limits of the organism, our sense organs may become habituated to paying attention to certain stimuli and to overlooking others. The crashing noises, fast-moving sights, and "queer" odors of a metropolitan area are different to men brought up there than to someone just arrived from the country. The soldier dozing off under ceaseless cannon fire, may be instantly alert to the faint signal of his field telephone; the young mother wakes from deep slumber at her baby's slightest whimper. What we are trained to pay attention to is related to our patterns of conduct and to the furthering of our purposes. Through repeated use of certain sense organs in connection with certain activities, the different organs and the different impressions derived from them become linked together or fused into a unit of social activity and perception.

The sense of smell, for example, must be understood in varying social contexts. There are, for instance, two ways of handling body scent. Conventions may encourage the covering up of body odor by artificially produced scents. This has been the historic way in Latin countries, notably France and Italy. Ladies may then choose a personalized perfume so as to have, as Georg Simmel has noted, a subjectively characteristic "scent" in ballrooms and in opera foyers. Or, in the second place, washing with soap may be the conventional way. Since the eighteenth century in Great Britain frequent use of the bathtub has been standard for certain classes in Anglo-Saxon and British-influenced societies.

Our sense organs are specialized, but they are also closely related to one another. Our taste and our smell of a peach, for ex-

[28] See C. Landis and W. Hunt, *The Startle Pattern* (New York: Farrar & Rinehart, 1939).

ample, form a close blend of perceptions; the odors we inhale stimulate the olfactory regions, but they also stimulate the gustatory areas in back of our mouths. Other evidence of the interrelations of our senses is shown when, one sense organ being defective, the others, being used more, seem more keen. If a person is blind and deaf, the sense of smell may become more discriminating and hence more useful in the orientation of the individual. Such a person may learn, as Laura Bridgram did, to select by smell her own clothing from the clothing of a hundred other persons, or to detect the differences between the recently washed socks of boys and of girls.[29]

In normal adults, "intersensory resemblances," as Charles Hartshorne has shown,[30] seem more typical than do isolated impressions from any one sense organ. We have already noted that the taste and the smell of a fresh peach may be closely blended. But that experience was organically based; the matter goes further. Our vocabularies themselves reveal two explanations of intersensory resemblances:

I. When we speak of "high" or "low" pitched sounds, or of the soaring, thin notes of the flute, we are translating perceptions of sound into vocabularies of anatomical and tactual experiences. When we speak of the "brightness" of high-pitched sounds, we refer to an intersensory analogy of the eye and the ear. When we speak of the "loudness" of certain colors or color combinations we are transferring the negative prestige value of talking in a loud voice in a "refined" atmosphere to visual perceptions that are "unrefined" or in "bad taste." By calling it "loud" one means that it is inappropriate. "Bad taste," used in this context, is itself an intersensory analogy of vision and taste. The eye and the tongue, vision and taste, are related when we speak of the darkness of bitter or of the brightness of salty. The tactual sense is related to the auditory in "the softness" or the "smoothness" of music. Poets and novelists are expert at describing colors and smells in terms of sounds, and sounds in terms of color, odor, or touch. But the matter

[29] See M. S. Lamson, *The Life and Education of Laura Dewey Bridgram* (New York: Houghton Mifflin, 1881).

[30] See his *The Philosophy and Psychology of Sensation* (Chicago: Univ. of Chicago Press, 1934), pp. 54 and 74. Our account is influenced by this excellent monograph, although it should be noted that the position taken does not at all points coincide with his.

is not reserved to them. Anyone can look at something, and without smelling it say, "It stinks."

II. But there is another view of such intersensory resemblances. Some psychologists hold that when we experience sweet music or sugary words, a sweet girl or a sour face, we are experiencing synesthetically the qualities of sweetness and sourness in manifold contexts. Thus, when we speak of a "cutting" remark, we do not, according to this view, transfer inferentially or by analogy the quality of cutting or sharpness from a knife to another context; nor do we transfer by analogy from taste to ear when speaking of a "bitter" tone or inflection of voice. Rather, the qualities of sharpness or of bitterness are directly available to us in diverse fields of experience. High life and "high-mindedness," "low thinking" and "base" feelings are in their contexts perceived qualities, just as is the "high" soprano voice or the "low" basso.

For the purposes of the social psychologist, it does not seem urgent that we commit ourselves to either of these views. Both, especially the second, have been elaborated on in a rich series of monographic work in technical psychology [31] and none of the inferences or constructions we wish to make rest upon explanations which go beyond these alternatives.

At any rate, the movement of the human organism differs from the physical movements of bodies in time and space. For, due to our body build, the forward position of our eyes and of our gait, as well as our upright posture, we experience our spatial world in terms of forward and backward, of high and low, of left and right. These dimensions have qualitative properties which differ from the purely quantitative dimensions of the physico-mathematical space. [32]

[31] We refer to the work of Wertheimer, Köhler, Koffka, and Lewin. See W. D. Ellis, *Source Book in Gestalt Psychology* (New York: Harcourt, Brace, 1938).

[32] Cf. Jerome S. Bruner and Cecile C. Goodman, "Value and Need as Organizing Factors in Perception," in *Readings in Social Psychology*, Newcomb, Hartley, *et al.*, eds. (New York: Holt, 1947), pp. 99-108; M. Sherif, "A Study of Some Social Factors in Perception," *Arch. Psychol.*, No. 187, 1935; J. Piaget, *Language and Thought of the Child* (London: Routledge, 1948); L. Postman and J. S. Bruner, "The Reliability of Constant Errors in Psychophysical Measurement," *Journal of Psychology*, 1946, XXI, pp. 293-299; A. I. Hallowell, "Cultural Factors in the Structuralization of Perception," in *Social Psychology at the Crossroads*, John H. Rohrer and Muzafer Sherif, eds. (New York: Harper, 1951), pp. 164-95; and Robert R. Blake and Glen V. Ramsey, *Perception: An Approach to Personality* (New York: Ronald Press, 1951).

Each of our sense organs contributes in its own way to our articulation of our own organism in space and time. As we know from studies of the blind and the deaf, the experience of space that is mediated through our eyes differs from that mediated exclusively through our ears. "The normal" way of locating our organisms in space and time is a complex integrative process of diverse sense experiences. Blind persons who learn to see have to reconstruct the experience of their own bodies, because the visual experience added to their previous tactile and acoustic orientations demands a new and more complex integration of perceptions. Similarly, unless we deliberately control our selves, we will not "naturally" walk in a straight but rather in a slightly curved line; our "rhythmic" experiences and activities (our gait, for example) will have more to do with the nonmetric regularities of the heartbeat and the blood pulsation, than with the chronometric exactitude of the pendulum stroke. The rhythm of language and of music is not identical with the metronomic "beat."

5. The Interrelations of the Psychic Structure

To understand how impressions are organized into perceptions we have to understand the interrelations of all elements of the psychic structure, for perception and feeling and impulse may be so closely linked that in the active experiences of each of them there is an element of the others.

By an act of attention, we connect our perceptions with our impulses. What we see is connected with what we want to see, and we tend to overlook what we dislike to see, or what is irrelevant for us. If we are beset by an impulsive need, we often dream the image of the object required for its fulfillment. We may see it in everything, as a man dying of thirst sees water everywhere in the desert. "All things look yellow to the jaundiced eye." Such mirages or hallucinations induced by our bodily deprivations are a subtle part of our waking lives. In a child the impulse of the moment will determine his action, his feeling, and even his perception of various objects. With a sudden change of impulse and feeling he will react quite differently to the same objects. His focus of perception will shift and race about as his impulse activities change. Feeling tone will lead us to see or hear the "brighter" or the "darker" side of things. The unpremeditated emotional effects that are socially trained into a person will determine his gestures and other conduct when he perceives a combination of colors in a flag or hears a national anthem.

Perceptions often have affective significance. The feeling tones of colors, sounds, and odors are imputed to them by virtue of the feelings which we typically have when we perceive them.[33] Thus we speak of the gaiety of yellow, the aggressiveness of red, the coolness of green, the distance of blue—or blue moods, hot scarlet, warm orange, and the melancholy of deep purple.

In live experiences not only visions but sounds seem to embody feeling tones: "There is the stillness of a city street at three a.m., the stillness of a Sunday, the startling quietness of the country after alighting from a train, or the muffling of sounds with a fall of snow. In each of these the stimulus is the same, a contrast, a lack of noise." [34] Yet each of these lack-of-sounds *feels* differently: we have linked different feelings and activities to each of them, and our psychic structure responds in a unity with the perceptions.

The interrelations of feelings, impulses, and impressions in the psychic structure form dynamic trends. The linkages of feelings with perceptions are parts of trends which involve expressive and purposive action within social relations. Impressions received from the various senses are fused with other features of the psychic structure—and they are linked with the social purposes of the person.

Just as our bodily postures are trained so that we can better see, hear, or smell different things, so are our senses trained by social directives and personal expectations. Since perception is linked to the values and norms incorporated by the person, the *commands* which literally direct a person's focus of attention tell him what to look for in a given field of perception. He will single this out and organize the field around it; the social *trainings* of his purposes and interests sensitize his view of the world. A carpenter perceives a different house than does its prospective owner; he looks

[33] On the affective significance of perceptions, see Charles Hartshorne, *op. cit.*, where he discusses these experiences under the term "affective continuum." The primary connection of sensing and feeling was suggested by C. S. Pierce who pointed out that both may involve relatively simple *unit* qualities; purpose, in contrast, is dual: we strive against something. See C. S. Pierce, *Collected Papers*, Vol. I, Book 3.

[34] J. T. MacCurdy, *The Psychology of Emotion* (New York: Harcourt, Brace, 1925), p. 52.

for those features of the house which will guide his construction work, while the owner sees an image of his finished house born of his desires and expectations.

What we see and hear and smell today, determined in small or larger part as it is by our social context and personal expectations, helps determine what we see and hear and smell in the future. The world we experience is in no small degree determined by our past experiences and future expectations, which form a "frame of reference" or "apperceptive mass," as it has been called.[35] Because of this, man cannot be said to receive passively the world of sensations; he is an active determiner of what he perceives and experiences. For not only his sense organs but his apperceptive mass, with its social organization of feelings and impulses, is part of his perception. In this sense, man as a person constructs the world that he perceives, and this construction is a social act.

Although they all have the same kind of sense organs biologically, people in different societies perceive things differently. Those who live on great plains develop visual capacities which inhabitants of Paris may not possess. Writes de Poncins: "I strained and strained and saw nothing until one of the Eskimos pointed with his whip and rather against my will I agreed that I saw what he saw. Soon what he saw became for me something as big as a pin-head; in a quarter hour the pin-heads were fly-specks; and in the end I could see that the fly-specks were in truth a camp."[36]

Expertness at fulfilling some role often involves psychic training; it involves learning what to look for as well as the meaning of what is seen. To one unaccustomed to an Eskimo trail, it seems that "nothing happens," yet for those who have long been on the trail, there is always work to be done. Every perception suggests something to do: "Watch the dog! She is getting ready to squat and stop, and if she does, give her the whip as the sled passes her (for her lead is long enough to allow the passage of the sled). Mind that stone! If the runner strikes it, the coating of ice may break . . ."[37]

Moral and social taboos, as well as interests and skills, pattern

[35] Grace De Laguna, *Speech: Its Function and Development* (New Haven: Yale Univ. Press, 1927).

[36] Gontran de Poncins and Lewis Galantière, *Kabloona* (New York: Reynal and Hitchcock, 1941), pp. 297-98.

[37] *Ibid.*, p. 55.

our perceptions. If the members of a group believe that children should not resemble certain relatives, it is unlikely that within the group any such resemblances will ever be remarked. The Trobriander, Malinowski has indicated, will not see resemblances between female parent and children, nor between two brothers. These resemblances are taboo and it is an insult to say that they exist.[38] These social norms may, in time, be internalized and actually block out the perception of resemblances. Proud mothers in American society will "see resemblances" between their offspring and themselves where the uninterested onlooker will merely see another infant. What we expect to see and what we should not see are selected and patterned by the various social norms that we have internalized.

Of all our social acquisitions, perhaps our vocabulary is most directly geared to our perceptions. Our perception is organized in terms of symbols, and our vocabularies influence the perceptions to which we are sensitive. The classifications we learn for colors, for example, enable us to distinguish between them, to pick out red from pink, lavender from gray. The Eskimo has so elaborated distinctions in his language that he is able to discriminate between types of "snow" which to the English or the Chinese seem to be the same.[39] Socially equipped with a color classification different from that of the West, natives of New Guinea, Margaret Mead asserts, "see yellow, olive-green, blue-green, grey, and lavender as variations of one color." [40] And a metropolitan woman, intensely interested in clothing fashions, can detect that slight difference in shade of blue which marks the difference between last season's and this season's style.

"In acquiring the vocabulary of his day," Grace De Laguna has written, "each adolescent youth is being fitted with a set of variously colored spectacles through which he is to look at the world about him, and with whose tints it must inevitably be colored . . . The lenses we acquire with language are not merely colored, but

[38] Bronislaw Malinowski, *The Father in Primitive Psychology* (New York: Norton, 1927), pp. 87 ff.; and *Sex and Repression in Savage Society* (New York: Harcourt, Brace, 1927).

[39] See Franz Boas, *The Mind of Primitive Man* (New York: Macmillan, 1927), p. 119 ff.

[40] "The Primitive Child," *Handbook of Child Psychology*, Carl Murchison, ed. (2d ed., rev.; Worcester: Clark Univ. Press, 1933), p. 638.

blocked out in more or less regular designs, so that the world we see through them is patternized to our earliest view." [41]

6. The Social Unity of the Psychic Structure

We have not been able to confine our analysis of emotion, purpose, and perception to the organism and the psychic structure. We have had also to examine the person and the roles and vocabularies he has acquired, and accordingly, we have had to discuss many relations between the different features of the character structure. [42]

At this point it is convenient to examine the psychic structure as a whole with a minimum of attention to the person. Points of view from which we may hope to observe the operations of the psychic structure in a relatively autonomous condition include: I. the child; II. severe organic deprivation; III. social crises, when

[41] Op. cit., pp. 287, 288-89.

[42] We are able now to make more precise a rather vague term—temperament—often used to refer to individuals. We speak of phlegmatic, melancholic, sanguine, or choleric temperaments. Such characterizations seem to involve two general facts about "the psychic structure": (a) the degree and manner in which it is socialized, and (b) the constitutional strength of the organism in so far as this affects the level, speed, and persistence of psychic reaction. The common denominator of all types of temperament and of temperamental actions seems to be the level of psychic reactivity. If it is generally high, emotional and impulsive reactions are quick and spontaneous. To slower paced individuals, the degree of emotionality experienced and expressed seems to be disproportionate to the occasion. In contrast to elation, when he is depressed, the individual loses this capacity for spontaneous feeling and impulse. The level, speed, and persistence of psychic reactivity, in relation to standardized situations, is the basis upon which we gauge and characterize types of temperament. Although these degrees of reactivity are limited in their speed, and certainly in their persistence, by the constitutional strength of the organism, they are also set by the degree to which and the manner in which the psychic structure is socialized. For it is only in terms of socially expected reactions to given situations that we can gauge temperament. Thus, if an emotional reaction to a given situation is disproportionate to the occasion's conventionally expected reaction, we speak of excitable or of flighty temperaments. If emotion or feeling is less intense than is expected, we speak of mild or of phlegmatic temperaments. Thus, although temperament involves the constitution of the organism, it is by no means an innate or wholly organic feature of the character structure. It is closely related to both organism and person.

instituted routines collapse; and IV. certain unsocialized aspects of particular individuals.

I. The psychic structure of the prelingual child has not yet been integrated with the person. And since its elements are not firmly integrated with one another, it is highly plastic. The unification of these elements is not a ready-made affair, but involves a long process; both the unification and the socialization of the psychic structure are major processes of human maturation.[43]

The psychic structure of the infant is more quickly translatable into activity than that of the normal adult. The infant has more immediate impulses which may be more immediately satisfied. If he is drowsy and you wake him up, he may begin to squall; but if you adjust his thumb back in his mouth he may quickly go to sleep again. His impulses have a limited range of objects and these objects easily satisfy. The pushes of impulse result in random movements and convulsive grasping at anything placed before him; if impulse and satisfaction are not tightly and quickly joined, he is upset. There is little or no poise in the gratification of his impulses, for they are not yet purposive.

His perceptions are not focused clearly upon definite objects, so he is easily distracted. The slightest sound may engage his attention in another direction. Since definite perceptions are not linked to impulses, his activities are not only random but they do not carry through. Stray impressions of sound or sight easily entice him, and his impressions of one thing are not linked to his impressions of another; impressions are not patterned into meaningful perceptions. He cannot see what is coming up. Perceptions of taste, for instance, may dominate the entire animal infant. A stick of candy will be slobbered over and bitten at with eager impulsive motions and gestures. When you take it from him, he will squall, with his mouth open and drooling, eager to engulf it again in an infant frenzy.

The reactivity of the infant's psychic structure is high, random, and very responsive. Since its various elements are not integrated into unities, its feelings, impressions, and impulses are not linked firmly with one another. It is, in short, not yet internally co-

[43] See Chapter VI: Biography and Types of Childhood, Section 2: The Psychic Structure.

ordinated, nor linked with activities, and much less with the person.

Bodily discomfort is not yet a sign for the motor apparatus to move into another position. All the baby can do is cry and maybe wriggle at random a little. That is what we mean when we say he is "so helpless."

The unification of impulse, feeling, and impression into a psychic structure occurs before the child has acquired language, by means of the interrelations of the various senses. An infant, or an adult for that matter, cannot visually perceive all the parts of his body. Usually he cannot hear his own heartbeat nor, without mirrors, see the middle of his back. Nor can he *hear* the beat of his own pulse. But what is not available through one sense organ may be experienced through another: not being able to *see* his rearward portions the individual can *touch* them with his hands and thus finding them to be round can *see* the image. Out of the feeling-awareness an image of the body develops.

Of many feelings and parts of his body the individual has access in two or more ways: he can *feel* his toe wiggle and he can *see* it wiggle. Just as he learns his motor capacity—what he can do with his arms and legs and trunk, through feeling them in action—so he can learn by vision, by seeing distances between what he grasps for and what he actually grasps. By the consequences of various bodily movements upon his feelings, he learns and his movements are integrated. The sight of his toes wriggling may become a sign to him for the bodily feeling which usually accompanies this sight. Thus a network of intersensory signs is set up.

The feeling-states which are consequences of various action also operate as signs. Through the systems of such signs the infant individual's psychic structure becomes unified. Impulses are linked with positive and negative feeling-states in the early history of the organism. The range of the infant's feeling-states, which follow from acting out various impulses, is probably set by and limited to the motor experiments which he has made.

Just as impulses are steered and limited by the circle of the baby's feeling-states, so is the horizon of his perceptions. Bright colors may feel gay to the baby, dark shades feel threatening. The positive and negative feeling-states accompanying acts of perception are circumscribed by the ranges of the stimuli, especially by the thresholds of sense perceptions and the "saturation points" of the organism; after a certain point what was "sweet" becomes "gaga." The increased sphere of a child's perception is steered by the limitations which the accompanying feelings set up.

Gradually, habituated feelings channel impulses and impressions into aversions and likings; the world is learned and divided into things for which to grasp and things from which to draw away. If impression, feeling, impulse, and motor behavior are linked and habituated into a positive unit, a channel of action is set up and we may expect a willful repetition of the unit. As it is repeated, sometimes over and over again, the psychic structure of the baby is being set into a "dynamic trend." Such repetitions, often rhythmic in the child, form patterns of impulse, impression, and feeling as a unit and as a part of a locomotion: they are often experienced as pleasure. And they are, in fact, the beginnings of play; for play begins when the baby beats his hands together regularly, or when he utters rhythmic noises.

Learning is anchored in the feelings and impressions which are both prerequisites and consequences of actions. We learn to ex-perience our self as an organized and mobile unit in opposition to inviting and challenging features of the environment. The realities of the world and the capacities of our own bodies are learned together; both come to us in terms of resistance and mastery, limi-tation and capacity. We get an image of what can be done with our organic equipment by learning what can't be done and some-times suffering from the consequences of trying.

II. In severe organic deprivation the impulse that is deprived of an object of gratification may temporarily dominate and shape the entire psychic structure. It may even operate autonomously, casting off the social inhibitions, patterning, and pose of the person. Thus, feelings of hunger, as we have seen, are intrabody signals that the stomach is contracted for ingestion. When we eat, gastric juices begin to flow and the feelings disappear. Eventually, if we fail to eat, this state of deprivation may dominate not only our bodily feelings but the entire field of our external perception. We will see and smell food everywhere as we walk about the city; all people may begin to look plump to us. We see objects that would satisfy the deprived impulse. Eventually, we may invent sights and sounds and smells; in sleeping, if we can, we may dream of suc-culent foods or even scraps of edible objects. Our experience, in all its phases, night and day, is dominated by the deprivation. In many ways, we are like the child, who does not have a unified psychic structure under the control of the person.

The norms which have been internalized and which have controlled the psychic impulses and regulated their operation may no longer be effective. Our pride, our sensitivities to what others will think, are drastically minimized or eliminated; we may simply go "all out" to satisfy our want. We will snatch food, eat garbage, go on the dole. The one deprived element of the psychic structure controls our conduct.

To what degree the person may lose control is shown by various accounts of cannibalism due to starvation. In California in the winter of 1846-47 a party of pioneers were trapped and isolated in the Sierra mountains. They were starving. Cannibalism occurred, even between members of the same family. When the survivors were rescued, one man, having lost the social prohibitions of the person, was so dominated by the bare psychic structure that he had apparently come to prefer the flesh of infants to that of mules, leaving the latter until he had consumed his supply of the former.[44]

On the other hand, there is ample evidence that concentration camp survivors facing extreme situations of mass starvation and death may regularly share what is to be had and "take it" together. They have been known to develop intense group solidarity and friendship, and to invent new codes of conduct to meet the challenge of traumatizing events, such as transportation to the camp and induction into its routine. Held together by religious faith or political conviction, the members of such groups jointly resist all attempts to strip them of man's nature as a "political animal," and reduce them by twentieth-century techniques to Hobbesian wolves. The available evidence of survivors strongly suggests that the chances for survival in the extreme situations of the concentration camp universe were greater for the socially attached person than the competitive lone wolf.

During prolonged sexual deprivation, a domination of the emotions, perceptions, and social incorporations of the person may

[44] For documentation on the Donner party, see C. F. McGlashan, *History of the Donner Party* (San Francisco: Bancroft, 1881) (Stanford: Stanford Univ. Press, 1940), especially pp. 88, 106, 129, 211; see also Quinn Thronton, *Oregon and California in 1848* (New York, 1848), Vol. II.

occur. The whole environment and most bodily feelings become sexualized. All the members of the opposite sex, regardless of their condition, look attractive, for their attractiveness is linked with deprivation. Conventional ways of winning the erotical partner may give way to bold aggression and physical coercion. In such deprived states, the sexual object to which the sexual aim is socially directed may be replaced by another, which may be a member of his own sex, or it may be himself. Every touch of his hand upon his own body may excite him sexually. In the prolonged absence of the socialized object the impulse of sex thus shifts its aim and tries to achieve another target. On the other hand, religiously motivated asceticism may condition celibate life to the point where sexual stimuli, objects, and impulses shrink and wither away.

III. In crises of institutional orders, as during a peasant revolution, when suppressed feelings of anger and aggressive impulses toward the landlord flame into cruel action, the social steering and traditional controls of the person may become ineffective, indeed, quite swept away. Peasants seem more likely to revolt when the lord is not present in person, that is, under conditions of absentee landlordism. The atmosphere of prestige and power which surrounds the lord is probably too strong an anchor of dutiful conduct for the repressed anger and aggression to be released directly upon him. His presence enforces the social roles which the peasant must enact; but in his absence, inhibitions collapse and repressions are removed.

During the enthusiastic phase of mass movements there may occur a mass transformation of character structures. Hitherto unsocialized and repressed psychic impulses may emerge on the field of social conduct. New norms are incorporated as new obligations, as features of a new duty and conscience, thus forming a stabilization and integration of character in terms of the new conduct patterns. Changes in the objective social structure are paralleled by changes in what psychic elements are accentuated in the character structures of man.[45]

IV. It should not be supposed that all the elements of the "normal" adult's psychic structure are socialized in terms of approved

[45] See Chapter XV: Collective Behavior, Section 2: Aggregates, Crowds and Publics; and Section 4: Revolution and Counterrevolution.

social roles. Various impulses and feelings which have been set into a psychic structure, perhaps before the emergence of the person, may not have become institutionalized, and cannot be socially placed in the roles available to the person. The steering process provided by role incorporations and social conditioning may not take care of all that there is in man; that is, the person's roles may not include all that is involved in his psychic structure. Through its specific systems of premiums and taboos, approbations and disapprovals, the social context may rule out the display of some features of the psychic structures of some persons.

Due weight must be given to that in man which institutions do not "place." To the conservative such impulses and darker emotions usually appear as destructive of organized social conduct. But they may also be viewed as the conditions of new beginnings in social organization and in man himself. These elements, upon which society places no premium, or places a negative premium, form the psychic stuff covered by the term "repression."

Now impulses, when they are socially disapproved, may not have become linked with social objects and roles. The emotion which wells up within us and for which we have no vocabulary nor outlet in conduct may form an extraconscious or an unconscious part of our character.[46] Nevertheless, such forces may influence our conduct. Blocked at one outlet, psychic elements may be directed through another; hatred and aggression toward economic and social superiors may enter into a man's cruel conduct toward his wife and children.

An easy socialization of impulses requires that their outlet be ordered in time and with reference to certain occasions. Thus, among their institutions most societies provide special occasions for the release of psychic elements not otherwise placed. Mass sports may thus be seen as a vicarious discharge of latent aggression, as well as a feeder of it. In other contexts, such aggression may come out in mass political rallies. But whether in sports or in politics, the expression of the latent aggression is socially channeled. By being released in these special ways, the psychic structure, experiencing catharsis, is relieved of otherwise unplaced impulses. The deflection of such mass emotions through the scape-

[46] For problems of the "unconscious," see Chapter V: The Sociology of Motivation, Section 4: Awareness of Motives.

goat mechanism or through warfare waged by tottering regimes has frequently been noted.

In discussing how the various elements of the psychic structure are rooted in the organism, we have found it necessary also to discuss the person and the society in which he lives. The organic features of men—individual or racial—do not in themselves enable us to explain man's psychic traits; in fact, we cannot adequately define psychic traits without reference to the social milieus and trainings of the person. This is not, of course, to say that the organism is not relevant to the development of psychic traits as well as of the person; it is to say that the organism is relevant only within the meanings assigned it in the roles men play.

Our undefined impulses are defined by goals that are socially acquired. Our perception is decisively conditioned by the social organization of our organic sensations in accordance with accepted symbols and vocabularies. And our feelings are socially transformed into the emotions of the developing child. We recognize such emotions by the gestures that are socially associated with them. Different societies and different social units have their verbal and gestural vocabularies of emotions which define approved feeling states: the emotions that individuals feel on given occasions are often socially stereotyped.

The development of the psychic structure—of impulse, perception, and emotion—thus involves the social roles that the person acquires and enacts. But in order to view the organization of the psychic structure with a minimum of social complication, we have examined it in the child, in severe organic deprivation, in social crisis, and in certain unsocialized areas of individual development. And, among other things, we have found out that nothing we can learn of the naked psychic structure necessarily enables us to understand the conduct of the person; that, in fact, we must interpret the psychic structure within the larger frame provided by the character structure as a whole.

CHAPTER

IV

The Person

IN discussing the psychic integration of emotion, impulse, and perception, we found it necessary to consider man as a person as well as man as an animal organism. The conception of the psychic structure is closely linked to that of the person, and the person as such, in turn, is predominantly a creature of interpersonal situations. Indeed, this integration of person with others—that is to say, the roles that persons play—is the key to the understanding of the concept: the person is composed of the combination of roles that he enacts.

Awareness, or consciousness, is a reference to the field of our experiences at any given waking moment; it is *what* we are aware of. Thus we may experience a crowd of people, or a forest of trees; or we may experience a certain body tone, a diffuse feeling of tiredness, the localized pangs of hunger, or a knife cutting our left hand. To be conscious of external events in just the way that we are, requires an organism with certain kinds of sense organs; the anatomy and physiology of these organs are as necessary for our consciousness of a brown dog as is the dog as a brown physical thing. Anyone who is equipped with the appropriate kind of eyes can be aware of the dog. But awareness of our toothache, hunger pangs, or body tone of buoyancy is restricted to each of us individually. Yet, our awareness of external and of internal events, is primarily rooted in the organism and the psychic structure.

In *self*-consciousness, or *self*-awareness, however, the person is also involved. Although our bodily feelings and our awareness of our toes, hands, and noses are involved in our image of self, or at least often color it with feelings and sensitivities, our total self-image involves our relations to other persons and their appraisals of us.

1. Language, Role, Person

The use of language is the most important mechanism of inter-personal conduct, and the major source of knowledge of our selves.

The speech apparatus of the organism is a necessary condition for the acquisition and use of language. As an organism, man can make a wider variety of articulate noises than any other animal. Moreover, he can control his noises, varying them according to tone, pitch, percussion, inflection, and intervening silences; he can gurgle, goo, squeak, and grunt in a wonderfully flexible manner. From this wide variety of sounds, certain patterns of articulate sounds are selected and socially fixed as units with definite meanings. Strictly speaking, there are no "organs of speech"; rather, as Edward Sapir put it, there are "organs that are incidentally useful in the production of speech sounds." [1] The controlled sounds of speech require delicate co-ordinations of an elaborate muscle and nervous structure; they involve the teeth, tongue and lips, the larynx and the lungs, as well as the auditory senses.

Yet these organic conditions are not sufficient for human speech. The human organism isolated from all other human beings probably would not develop intelligible speech, even though it had all the organically required equipment.

All men are biologically similar in their speech equipment, yet they learn variously to speak Chinese, Portuguese, Brooklynese, or English, according to which is spoken in the community in which they grow up. No doubt the larynx of a North Chinese peasant is not very different from the larynx of an East End Londoner, but the language they come to understand and use is quite different. When we say that the Londoners and the Chinese cannot "understand" the different articulate noises they have respectively learned to make, we refer to the fact that the sounds which one makes do not "mean" the same thing to the other. Now, what is meant by "mean the same thing"?

When a sound which one person utters calls out similar responses in those who hear it as in those who utter it, then the sound has a common meaning. It is then, as George Mead terms it, a significant symbol. When a given symbol means similar things to a group of persons, we may say that these persons make up a community of

[1] *Language* (New York: 1939), pp. 7-9.

discourse. In general, symbols will mean similar things to this community in so far as they are used by persons acting in co-ordination. If one person interprets a symbol differently than another, the common behavior in which they are involved may become uncoordinated. This mixup of conduct, arising from the symbol's failure to co-ordinate the actions of two or more persons, will check the wrong interpretation—that is, the one which is not usual and common to most of the participants. In this way, the meaning of a symbol, the response which it typically calls out in various persons, is kept common.

A community of discourse thus normally coincides with a community of co-ordinated activities. For the prime function of language is to co-ordinate social conduct. Very little truly human conduct could be successfully performed if for even a single day we could not speak or understand the speech of others.

Traditional theorists of language have held that the primary function of language is the "expression" of some "idea," or some feeling already within the individual. Although it is true that language enables the mature person to express ideas and feelings, modern theorists no longer agree that the prime function of language is expressive. It has been found more fruitful to approach linguistic behavior, not by referring it to prior states or elements in the psychic structure or even in the person, but by observing its objective function of co-ordinating social behavior.[2]

Language is primarily a system of signs which are responded to

---

[2] The shift in the general approach to language has been summarized by Edwin Esper in "Language," *Handbook of Social Psychology,* Carl Murchison, ed. (2d ed., rev.; Worcester: Clark Univ. Press, 1935). The shift is part of the larger drift to a sociological psychology, a connection traced by John F. Markey, *The Symbolic Process and Its Integration in Children* (New York: Harcourt, Brace, 1928). From a philosophical viewpoint, the neatest and most useful analytic scheme for the study of language is probably C. W. Morris, *Foundations of the Theory of Signs,* International Encyclopedia of Unified Science, Volume 1, No. 2 (Chicago: 1938). Among the many scholars responsible for the newer viewpoint toward language, see: Grace De Laguna, *Speech: Its Function and Development* (New Haven: Yale Univ. Press, 1927); Bronislaw Malinowski, Appendix in Ogden and Richards's, *The Meaning of Meaning* (New York: Harcourt, Brace, 1927) and *Coral Gardens and Their Magic* (New York: American Book Co., 1935), Vol. II; George H. Mead, *Mind, Self and Society* (Chicago: Univ. of Chicago Press, 1934); and John Dewey, *Experience and Nature* (Chicago: Open Court, 1925), Chapter 4.

by other persons as indicators of the future actions of the person speaking. A given symbol can thus mediate conduct only if it calls out a similar response in the one as in another, that is, if it has a common meaning. This point of view toward the function of language invites us to pay attention to the social context of language behavior, for the same sound may have different meanings when uttered in different contexts.

Words take on meanings from the other words with which they are associated. The United States Senate has been known to argue for several days over the insertion of the word "an" in a formal document.

But the context which lends meaning to words is social and behavioral, as well as linguistic. This is indicated by the meaninglessness of words which we hear without being aware of the context in which they are uttered or written. Most language situations carry unseen and unspoken references which must be known if the utterances are to be meaningful. In the case of the Senate debate, the full meaning of the inclusion or omission of "an" may require an understanding of the connections of various senators with their respective state organizations, and of pronouncements previously made by Republican and Democratic party officials.

A person is composed of an internalization of organized social roles; language is the mechanism by which these internalizations occur. It is the medium in which these roles are organized. Now, we have defined role as a conduct pattern of a person which is typically expected by other persons. It is an expected pattern of conduct. The roles a person plays thus integrate one segment of his total conduct with a segment of the conduct of others. And this integration of persons, and of the roles they expect of one another, occurs by means of language. For it is largely by a language of vocal gestures that we know what is expected of us. We meet the expectations of others by calling out in ourselves a response similar to the response which the other person has called out in himself . . . that is, both respond similarly to the same vocal gesture.

When we are learning a new role and do not know what is expected of us, our correct and incorrect moves are indicated to us by the approval and disapproval of others. By their vocal expectations they guide us into the conduct pattern. Various nonvocal gestures may also guide our performance: The frown and the smile deter or encourage us. But the vocal gesture is more explicit, for the gesturer himself is more readily affected by speech than by any other kind of gesture he can make. We can hear ourselves talk more easily than we can feel our eyes blink or our foreheads wrinkle. This means that we can manage the performance of our own roles by our own vocal gestures.

When we have internalized the vocal gestures of others, we have internalized, so to speak, certain key features of an interpersonal situation. We have taken over into our own person the gestures which indicate to us what others expect and require. And then, we can make certain expectations of ourselves. The expectations of others have thus become the self-expectations of a self-steering person. The social control and guidance which the gestures of others provide have thus become the basis for self-control—and for the self-image of the person.

2. Images of Self

The self-image develops and changes as the person, through his social experiences, becomes aware of the expectations and appraisals of others. He acts one way, and others reward him with food, warmth, and attention; he acts in another way and they punish him with inattention; when he fails to meet their durable expectations, they deny him satisfaction and give him their disapproval. "The approbation of the important person is very valuable," Harry Stack Sullivan has written, "since disapprobation denies satisfaction [psychic structure] and gives anxiety [person], the self becomes extremely important." [3]

If, as a child, the person does not meet the roles expected of him, he may be faced with two results: (1) Such impulses as impel him will not be satisfied, for other persons will not cater to his needs unless he meets the requirements they exact. He is dependent upon these others for nutrition and warmth and other bodily requirements. (2) He may also, in the course of his experience, know anxiety or insecurity, for he is dependent upon others for approval of himself as a person.

[3] *Conceptions of Modern Psychiatry* (Washington: W. A. White Psychiatric Foundation, 1947).

As he matures, the person's image of self is taken over from the images of him which others present to him, by their gestures of approval and of disapprobation. This general statement, however, must be qualified in two ways:

I. For the adult, it is more accurate to say that the attitudes and expectations of others facilitate or restrain the self-image. For by the time the person is adult, the image of self, although dependent in varying degrees upon the current appraisals of others, is normally strong enough to exist autonomously. This is possible because the person has already built his self-image on the basis of a long sequence of previous appraisals and expectations which others have presented to him.

The person learns to follow models of conduct which are suggested to him by others; in addition, as he comes to read, he chooses such models from the store of socially organized memory. These latter models, as well as those he imagines for himself, may be at variance with those whom others immediately around him appraise favorably. His own expectations and appraisals of self thus acquired may enable him to *accept, refract, ignore,* or *reject* the expectations and appraisals of the current others. Indeed, if this is not the case, if there is not some autonomy of self-image and the adult person is completely and immediately dependent for his own self-image upon what others may currently think of him, he is considered an inadequate person.[4] The self-image which we have at any given time is a reflection of the appraisals of others as modified by our previously developed self.

[4] Erich Fromm has aptly called such a person "the automaton": being completely dependent upon the appraisals of others the person conforms to their expectations in a compulsive manner; he does not have "a center in himself." Both Fromm and Karen Horney attempt to resolve the problem by invoking components of the psychic structure as "the real self." This does not seem to us an adequate solution: The psychic structure, if it is to operate in a manner harmonious to a social order, must itself be quite socialized in specific directions, even stereotyped in some. The answer to the "façade self" and the "real self" dichotomy is found not by trying to jump past the socialized portions of the personality and finding something more "genuine" in the psychic or organic "foundations," but by viewing the social process of the self in a longitudinal way, and "finding" a "genuine self" that is buried by later socializations. See Erich Fromm, *Escape from Freedom* (New York: Farrar & Rinehart, 1941).

II. The social idea of the self must be qualified in a second way: by consideration of who the "others" to whom we respond are. Only the appraisals of those others who are in some way significant to the person count for much in the building and maintenance of his self-image. In some societies and families "the mother" is the most significant other to the infant and child, since she caters most directly to the bodily needs and by her actions completes the impulsive beginnings of the child's activities. In such cases, the image which the child has of himself is perhaps at first the image which his mother has of him. But as the person grows up, a variety of significant others begins to operate. If we know who has been and who is thus significant to the person's image of self, we know a very great deal about that person.

Three general principles seem important in determining this *selection of significant others:*

(1) *Cumulative Confirmations.* The image of self which a person already possesses and which he prizes leads him to select and pay attention to those others who confirm this self-image, or who offer him a self-conception which is even more favorable and attractive than the one he possesses. This principle leads the person to ignore, if he can, others who do not appreciate his prized or aspired-to self-image, or who debunk his image or restrain the development of it. A circle of friends is typically made up of those who further, or who at least allow the other persons to retain, their respective self-images. As the ancients put it, "The friend is my other self." One avoids as best he can the enemies of the self-images one prizes. The cumulative selection of those persons who are significant for the self is thus in the direction of confirming persons, and the more he succeeds in limiting his significant others to those who thus confirm his prized self-image, the more strongly he will seek such persons as significant in the future. So there is a tendency in the biography of the person for a sequence of confirming persons to accumulate.

Now if this were the only principle involved in the selection of significant others, life might perhaps be a happy and spontaneous affair; but other considerations do interfere with its single action: a person cannot choose all his relationships. The child, for example, is less selective than the adult of the others to whom he pays attention—which is one reason that children are so easily "hurt."

Trusting children frequently experience disappointments, rebuffs, and slights, until they learn to stem their confident approach with some degree of "shyness." If the balance tips in the direction of withdrawal, a scale of orientations and traits are observable, from reserve through suspicion toward the friendliest guest; anyone and anything that is new may become fearsome, until the child is frequently misunderstood as "insensitive." In fact, he may not have learned how to deal with the new, and hence be relying upon total avoidance of all new challenges.

The image of self built up during childhood may thus contain negative elements so firmly integrated that they are never gotten rid of. During adolescence in Western societies, the child is "catching on" to the selection of confirming others as significant, and this involves the development of sensitivities to little cues which other persons present and which warn the person whether or not someone is likely to confirm or to threaten prized self-images. Between the polar opposites of the fear of always being "left out" and of "never being left alone," the maturing person seeks to win and move in his own "elbow room." The adult often sees a man and immediately "takes a dislike to him." Other persons he immediately likes; they are felt to be "considerate," which means that they defer to him in the direction of his desired self-image. They treat him as he would like to be treated: they are confirming others. But the child may not be so aware of those often unspoken cues which aid the strategic adult in his selection of significant others according to the principle of the confirmation of his desired self-image.

(2) *Selection by Position and Career.* In the construction and maintenance of a prized self-image, the selection of significant others is limited by the institutional position of the person and by the course of his career from one institutional position to another. This selection is not, of course, a simple mechanical process; in most positions there are various possibilities. The position of a nobleman within the status levels of a feudal society in revolt, and of a factory worker within the occupational hierarchy of modern capitalism may each be examined in this connection:

A nobleman may be (a) insulated against the harsh and negative appraisals of serfs or peasants by childhood segregation in which a strong and exalted self-image was built—an image which later enables him to deem the peasants' approval and disapproval as equally irrelevant. Only the judgments of his status peers count.

(b) The noble may interpret the peasants' negative appraisals in a wholly different way than they are intended. He may have become aware of the peasants' attitudes only from other nobles, and thus his self may refract and modify the appraisals before they are incorporated into his self-image. He may, indeed, force the obedience of the peasants to him, and then interpret their obedient gestures as confirming and facilitating his honorable image of self. (c) Under certain conditions, the noble may not be able to stand the real or imaginary disapprovals of the peasants. He may then change his own self-image, and the conduct which it involves, so as to permit kindness to the peasants, which his previous self-image permitted only to other nobles. He thus seeks to modify their negative appraisals and in the process of doing so, he gets from their appraisals another image of himself. In turn, he will now strive "to live up to it": the line of his confirming other has shifted, and the strategies employed by him to win such confirmation from persons who become significant have shifted. So did certain Russian noblemen in the nineteenth century "humble themselves," go among the peasants, and, on humanitarian grounds, seek to co-operate with them politically.

The class and status positions of a person may thus be restrictions upon his *selection* of significant others, as well as determinants of the *degree and kind of significance* and of the *angles of refraction* which other persons of differing status may possess for the person of a given status position.

If a factory worker rejects, on ideological or other grounds, the appraisals of members of the employing class, his image of self may not directly reflect their appraisals of him. If working-class parents proudly tell their children tales of how they, and their parents before them, were imprisoned for heroic violence "against the capitalists and their state apparatus," then upper-class appraisals are less likely to be positively significant to the construction and retention of a self-image of the child of the workers. Under such conditions we may speak of "class consciousness." Such class tradition and consciousness may be said to have considerable weight when it restricts to one's own economic class the community of others who are significant for the self-image.

On the other hand, if the upper classes monopolize the means of communication and fill the several mass media with the idea that all those at the bottom are there because they are lazy, unintelli-

gent, and in general inferior, then these appraisals may be taken
over by the poor and used in the building of an image of their
selves. The appraisal of the wealthy, privileged children may then
be internalized by underprivileged children and facilitate negative
self-images. Such images, if impressed early enough and continually
enough by all persons who are significant to these children may
cripple their chances to better their social position and thus obtain economic and social bases for more favorable self-images. An
outstanding example of such restriction in the selection of signifi-.
cant others as determined by class and ethnic position is found in
the self-images of many American Negroes.[5] If, on the other hand,
the Negro child is able to exclude the appraisals of various public
others, he may build up a more favorable self-image on the social
basis of the more intimate others of his ingroup of fellow Negroes.

It is worth noting that there are several ways in which self-
respect and social respect may be related:

Self-valuation and valuation by others may be in positive agreement. For example, a proud group of rulers may also be admired
by others—the feudal lords of the Middle Ages or the Roman
emperors come to mind.

The self and the other may be in agreement—but negatively;
an inferior group may accept the negative images imposed on it by
their status superiors. All ruling groups seek to impose such sentiments upon subject groups. Stereotyped images and unwarranted
generalizations from the worst case, which make him "representative" for all, are among the means used to breed inferiority feelings. Exacted deference is another. Thus, the despised serf comes
to think lowly of himself and of his fellows. The slave is despised
as chattel and, being powerless, seeks to hold his own by fraud,
which is despicable to those who esteem only violence.

Self-respect may be high, but the social esteem of others may
be low. Thus, the posturing of the "misunderstood" or "unknown"
genius and the dictum that the prophet is not known in his own
home town. In such cases, an invented or imaginary other may
be used to compensate for the denial of respect by a public and
thus high self-valuation be maintained. The misunderstood genius
assures himself that "posterity," if not his present colleagues, will

[5] See Chapter XI: Stratification and Institutional Orders, Section 5: The
Status Sphere and Personality Types.

surely come to honor and respect him and his work. Behind such a secularized theology of martyrdom there is often religious imagery of various sorts. Such sentiment may be entirely adequate to the situation—as it was for Schopenhauer, who published in 1819, but gained esteem only after 1848; or for Arnold Schönberg whose works for long years were not fully appreciated. On the other hand, a mere megalomanic, and hence groundless and spurious, attitude is also possible.

Finally there are situations in which, despite the great esteem of others, a man deprecates his own worth, and, in the eyes of his God he may—as did young Luther—go to extraordinary length in his sense of humility and his moods of penance.

(3) *The Confirming Use of the Intimate Other.* Thwarted in his public search for a confirming other, the person may restrict his search for confirming others to a few intimate others. Perhaps this is especially true of persons who occupy inferior institutional positions, who thus try to build durable, intimate relations with which to counteract public depreciation. The number of intimate others may even become drastically restricted and at times become a sole significant other. The person may then attempt to derive the image of his or her self entirely from the appraisals of this one particular other. These two withdraw socially: as far as other people are concerned, they are "in a daze." They integrate themselves in a situation of intimacy, and together face the broad and alien world which "does not understand." Fed by the warmth and security of such intimate closure, they have this larger world at their mercy and can discuss, debunk, and ignore it. This strategy may be temporarily successful—and in fact, expected—during certain phases of adolescence, when many others crowd in upon the person with new and less favorable appraisals than his family and school have offered.

Such a condition cannot usually last forever. Nevertheless, in the modern industrial metropolis in which private and public roles are rigorously segregated, a certain degree of such exclusion and refraction of public appraisals by intimate circles, and a more or less exclusive acceptance of the desired approval of intimate others, may be integrated into a rather enduring basis for personal images of self.

These three principles involved in the selection of significant others may be linked in this way: the social position and career of the person set limits, more or less broad, for the selection of significant others. Within these limits, the selection will proceed in the direction of those others who are believed to confirm the prized or aspired-to image of self. If the institutional position and career prohibits the selection of such others from public life, the quest for such confirmation of self-image by significant others may be narrowed down to a sequence of intimate others.

These principles do not, of course, exhaust the determinants of the process of selection. We shall encounter others, and further examples of these, in their proper institutional contexts.[6] For it is, in some major part, through the line-up of significant others that institutions form personalities in often intricate ways.

3. Unities of Self

"It has been said," writes Frank Jones in commenting on the contemporary painter, Marshall Glasier, "that everyone is three persons: what he thinks he is, what others think he is, and what he thinks others think he is. The fourth—what he really is—is unknown; perhaps it doesn't exist."[7]

If a man is what he thinks he is, his image of himself has a controlling function: he shapes himself in terms of his own self-image. But others may hold diverse images of a man, according to their own perspectives and roles. Both hatred and love may lead to exaggerated emphasis upon despicable or upon lovable features. The fighting caricaturist and the build-up specialist, like the disillusioned lover and the adoring lover, know this well. There are as many images of us in circulation as there are people who take note of our past, our present, or our potential relevance for their own actions and expectations. Some of these images may be of no concern to us—we may not even know of them; others we may "overlook" as irrelevant. Or a series of images may be known to us, and may matter to us in quite varying extents. Our awareness of the fact that others hold views about us, and our eagerness to be well thought of by those who matter to us most, naturally influences

[6] See Chapter VII: Institutions and Persons, Section 1: The Institutional Selection of Persons; Section 2: The Institutional Formation of Persons; and Section 3: The Theory of Premiums and Traits of Character.

[7] Reed College Brochure, 1952.

our behavior; and that is why to quite some extent we are what "others think of us."

But we are also to some extent what we think others think of us. For often there is a difference between what we think others think of us and what they actually do think. The entire machinery of "conventional lies" and "tactful proprieties"—along with the fact that most people do not feel any particular incentive to "tell the truth" to others—allows for a considerable, and often a typical, disparity between what people actually think of us and what they allow us to know of their true opinion. "Flattery," as we all know, is widespread in a society where people crave to be "popular."

Consider some of the ways by which other persons may have gotten the image of us which they hold: (1) Other people may get an image of us in terms of the role we play in a given stratum or group. Thus, no matter what other roles he may have played or may currently be playing, an American Negro is often viewed as a Negro. The image held of the person's self is based on experience with him only as a member of some social category, and no other aspect of the self which may exist outside this segmental role is considered. (2) Another person may "make allowances" or modify his image of us in terms of the manner in which we play some role. Variation in our enactment of even the most stereotyped role often results in another's calling us a "very intelligent Negro," or in our having *some* personal characteristics which lifts us out of the segmental role of the Negro. (3) Others may experience us in an intimate situation and build their image of us as we present it in this situation. We sometimes tend to believe that those with whom we are intimate accept our self-image, but this may be very far from the case! The concept of intimacy has to be handled with care. Mere intimacy does not guarantee that we know another's image of his or her self: There are many ways in which we can let our hair down, and we may appear differently in each. Two persons can integrate their selves in a most intimate—and quite false—manner; indeed, quick and mutual acceptance of presented or stylized selves, or of aspired-to selves, may be a requirement for certain kinds of intimacy.

We can have an adequate image of ourselves and it can be shared by our friends; but we can also share with them a false image of ourselves and thus be self-deceived hypocrites. Then again, we can have a true image of ourselves which is rejected by our friends—and thus be the misunderstood woman, the unknown genius or prophet. Finally, we can have a false image of ourselves which is rejected by our friends: we deceive ourselves but not others.

At any rate, the scale of impersonal, personal, and intimate does not seem to provide us with an adequate basis for predicting the chances of one person to know the self-image of another. The self-image we hold and the image we present to others are complicated by the appraisals of significant others with whom we are currently integrated, and by such appraisals as have carried over from our previous integration. A total view of even the presented images to current others would require us to tag along with a person and observe the selves he presents in all the situations in which he is integrated with other persons. But even if we had access to every image the person presented in every one of his relations, we would still have to choose which of these segmental roles in which the self is presented is the one most likely to coincide with "the genuine self-image," if any, held by the person himself.

The question of what really lies beyond all the imagery of self and of others, of what the individual really is—clearly that is one of the great puzzles of man. So the Buddhist pronounces his tat tvam asi, "Man become who you are"; so Socrates finds it a hard task for man "to know himself"; and so Nietzsche proclaims "Man is most remote from himself."

At any rate, we do know that in some situations the image a person holds of himself is more or less integrated with the images which significant others hold of him. The image of self which he presents to others and which he is trying to have them accept or confirm is identical with the image to which he aspires. In other situations, there may be great differences between self-image, presented image, and aspired-to image.

Such differences and similarities, though they often arise in the direct experience of the person, are determined by sociological conditions. We may attempt to systematize those varied conditions under which the different images *coincide;* and those under which they may *collide.*

To know another's self-image we have to study the others who are significant to him. It is convenient to refer to the circle of current significant others as "the *position*" of the person, and to refer to the sequence of previous significant others as "the *career*" of the person.[8] These terms enable us to simplify our terminology. With them—"position" and "career"—we knit interpersonal situations into social structures. For these concepts help us to locate types of persons within social structures.

Unity of self, occurring when all the images of self held by the person and by others coincide, will most likely occur when the position and the career of the person is composed of significant others who are harmonious in their appraisals and expectations.

In a society where roles are stereotyped and each man "knows his place," as do others, there is not much chance for differences to arise between self-images and the images others hold of him. The techniques of self-presentation, the problem of what others really think of us, and the possible differences between what they say to others about us and what they say to us, all compared with what they *really* think of us, do not arise. In such a society, the changing self-images which occur along the career are fairly well set, and hence calculable. The roles which different age groups are expected to play are well known by all significant others and are adhered to traditionally. So previous self-images do not conflict but blend with later self-images, just as the expectations and appraisals of others smoothly shift as the person passes through stereotyped stages of his career. Aspiration is also traditionally stereotyped, publicized, and accepted by everyone as appropriate; indeed, there is no alternative available. Both the self and all significant others know what the person would like to be at the next juncture, and what, under optimum conditions, he probably will be.

The type of society in which we may imagine various images of self to conflict is characterized by the fact that both the position and the career of the person involves conflicting expectations and appraisals by persons who are significant to him.

In such a society, according to the principle of the confirming other, persons will present themselves in one way to one set of persons and in another way to another set. The ways in which the person presents his self will vary according to what he believes these various others think of him. In general, his style of self-presentation will be a bridge from the image of self which he

[8] See Chapter VI: Biography and Types of Childhood.

believes others hold of him and the self-image he would like to have them confirm.

If he has the power, like the nobleman discussed above, the person may force others to defer to the image of his self which he desires, and then interpret their deference as a confirmation of this image. If he does not have the power and is not certain that someone accepts the image he wishes to publicize, he may run little tests, or have third persons spy for him in order to find out if his presented self has been accepted.

Hypocrisy and posing—the stylization of self-presentations—are the results of the status-ridden man's frantic attempt to get others to confirm his self-image in a society in which there is no common career pattern, no harmony in the shifting expectations and appraisals by others. Diversity of ascent and aspiration is thus possible; there is freedom to choose occupational roles and intimate others; there are many and often conflicting alternatives. People learn to feel that certain others would never accept the stylization of self to which they aspire, and so they refrain from presenting it, lest laughter hurt the image. In short, private persons go in for "public relations."

4. Generalized Others

The attitudes of significant others toward the person leave their mark upon his self-image; they form a residue from social experience which he may re-experience and use in evaluating his own self-image; when thus internalized, they form his "generalized other."

The experience of this generalized other—the experience of "conscience"—is not the experience of a self-image; it is the experience of the appraisals of others who are not immediately present, but who, nevertheless, restrain or facilitate our own appraisals and images of our self.

Significant others, as we have remarked, are those to whom the person pays attention and whose appraisals are reflected in his self-appraisals; authoritative others are significant others whose appraisals sanction actions and desires. The generalized other is composed of an integration of the appraisals and values of the significant, and especially the authoritative, others of the person.

The generalized other of any given person does not necessarily represent the "entire community" or "the society," but only those who have been or who are significant to him.[9] And some of those who have been significant others may not operate in the generalized other, but may have been excluded from awareness—a fact that is in line with the principle of selecting as significant those others who confirm the desired image of self.

The content of a person's generalized other generally depends upon the normative attitudes of "the society" only as these attitudes have been selected and refracted by those who have been and who are authoritatively significant to the person. Accordingly, persons who have moved along different career lines will accordingly feel quite different "pangs of conscience" in regard to given actions. And, on the other hand, persons who have occupied similar institutional positions will have similar generalized others.[10]

Both Sigmund Freud and Max Weber have attempted to explain the rise of conscience. Freud believed that the primordial parricide by the "brother horde" was the fateful event leading to religion and morality, to law and guilt feelings. Despite the in-

[9] This term, generalized other, is an invention of the late G. H. Mead. Our use of the term differs from Mead's in one crucial respect: we do not believe that the generalized other necessarily incorporates "the whole society." It may stand for selected societal segments. See George Herbert Mead, op. cit., pp. 154 ff. For a preliminary statement of our use of the term see Mills, "Language, Logic, and Culture," American Sociological Review, Vol. IV, No. 5 (October 1939), p. 672, footnote 12. Abram Kardiner, working with a modified version of Freud's concept of the superego, has made several very provocative remarks concerning the relativity of what we here call the generalized other to certain social relations bearing on the child; see his The Individual and His Society (New York: Columbia Univ. Press, 1939), pp. 74, 124, 130, 134.

[10] We may express the position of some Freudians by saying that they restrict the significant others who by their appraisals deposit a generalized other (or "superego") to one or two persons, and locate these influences in the childhood phase of the career of the person. The generalized other is thus believed to be composed of the forbidding or authoritarian parent. See Chapters IV and V on the temporal autonomy of motives, self-images, and generalized other. Freud's own position excluded such bases of the superego as we are considering. Only when social influences remain "properly within its assigned realm . . . [and] follows the path sketched for it by the organic determinant" are they to be considered. See Freud, "Three Contributions to the Theory of Sex," in The Basic Writings of Sigmund Freud, A. A. Brill, tr. and ed. (New York: Modern Library, 1938).

formed criticisms of anthropologists and historians, Freud did not modify this view.

Max Weber sought to trace the rise of conscience in the history of ancient Judaism and in the Judeo-Christian tradition. He examined the ethical and religious compromises of this tradition, its reformations and revivals, and its sequence of martyrs, saints, and priests. In his work, Weber highlighted the Torah teachers (the Levites) and the great scriptural prophets of Jewish antiquity, as well as the Puritans who, because of their "activist" concerns, influenced mass behavior in everyday life.[11] To this Western sequence, Weber juxtaposed that of the East. There religious elites, as aristocratic intellectuals in despotically ruled societies, withdrew to practice apathetic contemplation. These elites failed to shatter the massive growth of popular magic and to displace it by religious and ethical systems of action. In other words, for most people in such societies, the generalized other remained narrowly circumscribed by the particular groups—castes or ancestral families—to which the individual referred himself.

In the generalized other, the appraisals of many particular others are organized into a pattern. The contributions of any particular other are fused with the contributions of these various others, and thus form the generalized other. Accordingly, when the person performs an act that is out of line with expected norms he may experience a general disapproval of his self, which means that the generality of his significant and authoritative others expected an alternative act. He may not be able to locate and specify just which other forbids this act, for this particular other has become part of his generalized other.

If the others who have been most significant to a person have been very forbidding, the person may be burdened by feelings of unbearable guilt. In a restricting parental situation he may have incorporated a generalized other that is too narrow for the requirements of the larger institutional world of business and pleasure, and he may not have been able to integrate the appraisals and expectations of later others which are more appropriate to his adult roles. With psychiatric aid the person may be able critically to review his internal behavior and escape his generalized feelings of

[11] See Chapter IX: Institutional Orders and Social Controls, II, Section 1: Religious Institutions.

guilt by specifying and recomposing the significance of particular others within his generalized other. He may be able to add (or even to substitute) the authority of the psychiatrist to his generalized other in such a way as to gain genuine independence for rational determination of self.

As new appraisals are added to older ones, and older ones are dropped or excluded from awareness, the generalized other normally changes. Such changes in the composition of the generalized other may occur as an aspect of the person's growing up or maturing, which we shall discuss in a later chapter; [12] or the generalized other typical of an entire stratum or of an entire society of persons may change. If, for example, the norms of a society are smashed, new significant and authoritative others may emerge who define new values and loyalties, and there is a crisis in every person's conscience as his authoritarian others change. The person is reappraised, and he reappraises himself as well as the selves of others. Such "crises of conscience" [13] have occurred several times in the course of Western history, for example, in cases of political revolutions and religious revivals and conversions. In fact, crises of this sort are quite widespread in contemporary society, in connection with totalitarian parties. Such a recomposing of the content of generalized others may conceivably be initiated in any area of society. In political and economic revolutions, the authoritarian other of public figures and leaders may begin the process of reappraisals which gradually spread into other segments of the society so that parents and teachers will imbibe them and present them to the social novice. Or, changes of interpersonal conditions may force such reappraisals, which will then be transmitted to public figures and political leaders, so that a revolution in these institutions may be forced.[14]

5. *The Social Relativity of the Generalized Other*

Since the generalized other is relative to those others who have been and who are significant to a person, any area of the person's

[12] See Chapter VI: Biography and Types of Childhood.

[13] This phrase is used by H. D. Lasswell in a lecture reprinted in *Public Opinion and World Politics* (Chicago, 1933).

[14] We shall examine these processes in Chapter XV: Collective Behavior, Section 4: Revolution and Counterrevolution.

life may contribute to its content. This is so whether or not their appraisals have been presented in a sequence of interpersonal situations, or in various secondary symbols, in movie, play, or book. The content of the generalized other changes with shifts in the person's career and with changes in the norms of those institutions which the person enacts.

We may imagine certain sequences of roles in which no generalized other would be deposited, and, quite apart from such constructions, there are historical societies in which the generalized other is so minimized that its effects seem negligible. By inquiring into the types of condition which bear upon the chances for a strong and for a weak generalized other to develop, we are able to understand the concept in a more adequately sociological manner:

I. The most important of the conditions which favor the chances for an effective generalized other to emerge are found in the childhood and adolescent phases of the life history. To consider the mechanisms involved we must consider both the *career* of the person and the *maturation* of the psychic structure. For the infant and the child is typically helpless in both zones of his developing character structure.

The disciplining of the child's impulses by the appraisals of authoritative others may be internalized as expectations by which the child will come to control his own impulses. Although normally the psychic structure is socially integrated, its socialization may not direct all the impulses which are available, and accordingly some are excluded from the child's awareness. In this case, there might, in time, be no tension between the psychic structure and person. But if it is not the case, and authoritative others continue to forbid the realization of the impulse, the tension between the child's person and his psychic structure may in time lead to the experience of a repressive generalized other.

In terms of this view, we may say: look for a society in which the impulses of the child are typically allowed free sway, or even allowed to govern the conduct of others toward him—in such situations, the chances of a generalized other to develop are minimized, and the operations of the generalized other that may be deposited are, in turn, minimized. Or, to put it another way, which carries us beyond childhood: when the proportion of authoritative others to the total of significant others is high, the chances are increased for a maximum generalized other to develop.

II. A generalized other arises only with great difficulty when many contradictory expectations are exacted of the person, for under such conditions a given performance will be appraised by one significant or authoritative person quite differently than by another. When expectations and appraisals thus conflict, the person may choose between alternatives—or he may reject both. In the latter case, he may project a new generalized other in the name of new and wider groups, real or imaginary; or he may withdraw from the larger society into "criminal" behavior; or, in case of extreme tensions and value conflicts, into a privatized world of behavior disorders defined as pathological.

III. On the other hand, a conscience does involve a degree of individuation, which in turn requires a detachment from roles, a distance from the expectations others exact when we play these roles. Such detachment and individuation come about when there are conflicting expectations exacted, along the sequence of our careers and currently among our circles of significant others. Individuation of the self results from the variety and scope of voluntary actions which we undertake. It involves the reality of individual decision and being held responsible for personal choices.

Personal or joint "responsibility" exists socially when the individual, as an individual or as a member of a group, is held accountable for his activities, in short, when his acts are ascribed to his self or his group. In a society where roles are quite stereotyped, this reality of alternatives, and such conceptions as personal responsibility, may not exist. Only if they do may a person come to address himself in an attempt to secure "consistency" and unity of self-image on the basis of self-expectations. There must be an area of voluntary action, which normally involves the perception of open alternatives or of conflicting expectations. The chances for an *individual* to emerge and to control himself by a generalized other are decreased as the variety of voluntary choices and decisions which confront persons diminish.

In a society in which the roles certain persons may play are consistent, and in which few choices exist, the problem of the consistency of the self is socially solved. For then no one person may take it upon himself to achieve an individual integration of self. But in a society where there are inconsistent expectations exacted of the person, and hence alternatives offered, each person will have to achieve such consistency and unity of self as he can. In this process, man is individuated, and this individuation involves the building of a generalized other from the conflicting expectations of significant others.[15]

IV. One person may be integrated with another because they both feel themselves to belong together. This kind of relationship may be called "communal." But they may be integrated because both think that their special interests are facilitated by collaboration—the individual purposes of each are thought to be furthered by the other, and each thus uses the other. This kind of relationship may be called "societal." Nations and families, religious orders, and intimate playgroups are generally communal. Business corpo-

[15] The accountability of the individual refers to the ways in which societies ascribe responsibility to their members. They may do so (1) by ascribing the acts of the individual to a subcommunity, and holding all of its members responsible for what any single member does. In such cases, we speak of "joint responsibility." Thus, an army officer may punish a whole company for the misconduct of one GI, a school teacher may punish her school class for the misdeeds of one child, family clans in old Kentucky still engage in the blood feud, that is, punish the family for the behavior of one of its members. Ancient Jewry felt jointly responsible to angry and jealous Yahweh. It has taken Western civilization centuries to emancipate the individual from such joint responsibility. Among the forces involved have been Roman jurisprudence, canonical law, revolutionary movements of urban middle classes, the cumulative work of professional jurists, academicians and free intellectuals, as well as all the individualizing social, intellectual, and economic forces. All these stand behind (2) a situation in which no son should be punished for the trespasses of his father, no parent for those of their children, no wife for those of her husband. Indeed, not persons but specific acts of persons should be prosecuted under due process of law and punished with pedagogical or preventive intent rather than in vengeance or annihilative interest.

Much of the history of legal technology in the West is associated with this interest in ascribing responsibility strictly to the individual, only to acts proven to be his by due process of law. In many other ways the "crisis" of our times also means a recession from individual responsibility in favor of joint responsibility. Peace treaties and their punitive stipulations hold an entire nation responsible for war. Thus, the Nazis punish families for the political acts or thoughts of one of its members. During the late war, American-born citizens of Japanese descent were placed behind barbed wire. Thus citizens have to prove their loyalty to authorities, who may discriminate administratively against them as a group, without bothering to prove individual guilt, and without giving the individual information about, nor occasion for defending himself against, his civic disability.

rations and special interest organizations are generally societal. There may, of course, be elements of each type present in cases which are placed under the other.[16]

Now, if a society is predominantly composed of communal relationships, so that interpersonal integrations throughout the person's career are communal, there is less chance of experiencing a generalized other than if the careerline contains first communal and, at a later juncture, societal integrations. The mechanisms at work in this latter type of biographical sequence are as follows:

The career of the person will at first be composed of significant others with whom he is integrated communally. Their harmonious expectations will coincide with his roles, and each person will be his own end and his own means. The center of the self will thus coincide with the center of social expectations. But at a later stage of his career, the person will have to integrate the self so built with societal others, and in these societal integrations he will have to use these others—to be sure, under enforceable rules—for his own purposes; and he, in turn, will also be used by others for their purposes. Accordingly, there are more chances for conflicts between others' expectations and the purposes of the self. Out of the calculations involved in successfully meeting these conflicts, and out of the differences between the societal integrations and the previously integrated communal roles, a generalized other may emerge.

V. All the interpersonal conditions which lower or raise the chances for a generalized other to develop are themselves facilitated or restrained by broader conditions of social structure. When, for example, the rate of social change is so low that during their careers the members of one generation are not aware of significant changes, the career patterns of persons will not significantly change. Hence, no conflicting expectations arising from changing careers are experienced. In such stable societies communal relations are also more likely to prevail.

It is also true that where all persons are on very similar eco-

[16] Community (Gemeinschaft) and society (Gesellschaft) were invented as technical terms by F. Tönnies. See his *Fundamental Concepts of Sociology*, C. P. Loomis, tr. (New York: American Book Co., 1940). See also the twist given these concepts by Max Weber, *The Theory of Social and Economic Organization*, A. M. Henderson and Talcott Parsons, trs. (New York: Oxford, 1947), p. 136 ff.

nomic, political, and social levels, the individual cannot easily experience the drastic inflation and deflation of self-image involved in dramatic social ascent and descent. Since all positions involve similar deference, competition for status position does not exist. On the other hand, somewhat similar personal consequences, in terms of our problem, may occur where there is very rigid stratification. For if positions are fairly equal (no significant stratification) or hereditarily closed and endogamous (rigid stratification), the careers of all persons are likely to be settled and known. In neither case is there competition for positions, or status alternatives between different careerlines. As soon as the person is old enough to realize, he knows rather precisely what his future will be, and so does everyone else. Hence, the expectations exacted of him by various others are homogeneous and coincide with the person's image of self, realized and aspired to.

But where stratification is steep and open enough to permit ascent and descent, the chances for the development of a generalized other are increased. For then there are likely alternatives between the conflicting expectations of various significant others, along the different careers open to the person, and confronting him in the choice of positions for which he may strive. It becomes necessary to control the strivings for success and to train the failure to "be a good loser."

When the total society is stable, social change being so slow that the members of no one generation are aware of it; and when there are no strata in society or the strata are absolutely rigid and fixed by level of birth—then the norms of conduct are likely to be positive, and the approved virtues to be specialized. This occurs in Indian Hindu society, hereditary castes, or in some periods of feudal Europe with its legally privileged status groups—its Christian saints and kings, its lords and gentlemen, its Christian burghers and peasants down to its honorable prostitutes and Christian hangmen. There is, thus, little opportunity for any given person to face the strivings of ascent, the discomforts of descent, or the insecurities either may involve. The image of aspiration coincides with the image achieved, and in fact, there is little awareness of such a distinction. Auguste Comte of nineteenth-century France admired Indian caste society for its excellent integration, cohesion, and wondrous stability.

In summary: A strong conscience is likely to emerge when group controls are continuous, rather than sporadic, and when they extend over the entire way of life, rather than to only segments of it. This is most likely to be the case when the group's members are "up close" to one another in everyday life and hence, as in a small community, know one another well. It is also likely to be the case when to belong to the group is prestigeful or otherwise worthwhile for the member, as it is, for example, for the husband to be a good provider, or for the businessman to have a good credit rating. To be "a member in good standing" must be seen as a competitive task for the person. For example, he may be admitted only after investigation of his character and his record, threatened to be excluded for failure to abide by the code. Moreover, he must gain the respect of the group's members by following the code in all his roles; that is, the code must be total. In addition, all his merits and demerits, gained in various roles, should be ascribed by other group members to the role of the member in *this* group; it is his master role which, as it were, co-ordinates his motives for and his enactment of roles in other social areas. The collective aspirations of this co-ordinate group, which forms the frame of reference for the member's strong generalized other, should be to subject the rest of the world to its standards. Thus, although it is "exclusive," it must be actively exhortative or at least exemplary, seeking to extend its jurisdiction or to withdraw in exemplary perfectionism.

We may thus speculate about typological conditions for the generalized other, but we do not have available the kind of sensitive field and clinical observations necessary to discuss the matter in full detail for any given society. We can, of course, apply general conditions and mechanisms to various societies in an effort to see how they may approximate the typical conditions.

Certain of the conditions for the "particularization of conscience" seem to be present in the old Chinese peasant village. We do not hold that the Chinese peasant villager did not have a generalized other, but we do suspect that his chances to develop one beyond the enlarged kinship group were drastically minimized by the roles which his society laid down for him, and that if developed, his generalized other was not a leading feature of the person.

The peasant of classical China was so bound to his roles, so closely tied to rigidly conventionalized situations that the question of a center of self-expectations which would form the basis of an individuated self did not typically arise. So the Chinese never experienced a prophetic salvation religion which might lead him to self-repentance or train him for feelings of personal guilt. He never felt the need to "redeem the times because the days were evil." The growth of an individualized conscience in the Occident has been, to a very large degree, the result of Christian endeavor.

The Chinese peasant of course experienced occupational, social, and residential mobility, but he did not experience any prophecy of salvation—either salvation of the individual soul or of a suffering people. Therefore no ethical code shattered magic practices and ancestor worship. He was forever bound to his extended family, wherever and however high he managed to climb. His successes and failures, no matter how competitively won, were not "counted to his righteousness" but to the honor or blame of his family name. The multiplicity of functional deities and the ritualistic magical techniques which were professionally offered in the market for pay provided no central and unified anchorage for an ethical code.

It is also significant for our problem—the conditions under which the generalized other is minimized—that the significant others of the peasant's childhood phase, his extended kinship group, remained predominant among his significant others until he died. This continuity of homogeneous expectations throughout his life was extended by the cult of ancestor worship. Elaborate politeness and the "conventional lie" were socially secured and enforced patterns; they reinforced the stability and harmony of the expectations exacted of him. They enabled persons to avoid shaming one another, that is, from presenting an image of self to the person which would conflict with his self-image. The conduct of the person could thus be controlled by prudence and fear, but not by the internalized expectations of self which we know as the generalized other.

A man would accept another as significant only if this other was a member of his sib and local in-group. People from outside these circles, such as an imperial tax collector, had to perform their work without benefit of tax morality on the part of the peasant: tax collecting involved raids and flogging.

Were we to develop our point in detail we would have to consider the different sequences of roles played by men as compared with women, and of both men and women reared in households owning different quantities of land, and so on. The order of birth of the siblings and their sex would also claim our attention.

We should seek interpersonal conditions typical of Chinese society which would favor or disfavor the development and operations of a generalized other. For instance, when a woman was married she went to live in the husband's family abode and took the role of a daughter to his parents. The man stayed at home after his marriage and, although the wife became one of his others, her significance was precisely conventionalized, just as were the expectations she exacted of the husband. The woman, however, changed households and thus came into a new circle of significant others. If the expectations exacted of her were drastically shifted at this juncture, we might expect her to become aware of these conflicts and out of them to strengthen her generalized other. Operating against this was the fact that the pattern of her parental family was probably very similar to that of her husband's. Because of the conventional similarity of family integrations, the expectations along her careerline were harmonious, and thus permitted a ready transfer, or substitution, of one circle of significant others for a previous circle.

6. Types of Persons

When we speak of types of *persons* we do not mean types of character structure. Of course, any conduct regularly performed by the person doubtless involves the integration of his roles with components of his psychic structure; nevertheless, by types of person we mean only the variations of roles which compose the person, and the person's way of reacting to these roles. Here are three dimensions in terms of which types of persons may be constructed:

I. If in all his social relations, a person is subordinate—a subordinate bureaucrat, a henpecked husband, a docile newspaper reader, a willing soldier, a gullible consumer, or an avaricious absorber of advertisements—we may say that from a formal point of view this type of person is unified. This means that we can state a principle—submissiveness—which seems to underlie all of his reactions to the roles expected of him. Other persons, who react differently to their own roles, might consider such a man a dupe or a "sucker"; by still others this term of opprobrium might be sophisticated into the term "conformity neurotic," while for still others, and perhaps for the man himself, this type might be supposed to represent "Christian humility," as the man willingly shoulders all the crosses which others and he himself place upon his back.

If in all his social relations a person is domineering—self-assertive on his job, a tyrant of his family, a critical newspaper reader, a scoffer at advertisements—we may also say that he is unified. The principle of his unity is that of domination, which all his conduct and feeling seem to follow. He is a unified person, and if he is not a unified character structure he may become such should he continue to enact roles according to the unifying principle of his person.

There are, on the other hand, types of persons who have extremely diverse reactions to various roles. A man who is a self-assertive authority on the astronomical movements of the universe may, in the smaller orbit of his family circle, be a mere satellite of his wife. The subordinated and ingratiating peddler who has doors slammed in his smiling face all day may himself slam doors all the more viciously as his family trembles in fear. These types of persons seem to make up in one context what they give up in another. By exploiting their chances at self-assertion in one role, they "compensate" for the frustrations inflicted upon them in another. The organization which connects their reaction to one role with that to another is a network of compensations, and with this principle they achieve a sort of balance.

II. The reactions of a person to the requirements of a role may be classified in terms of the role's powers to make him feel restricted, or, on the other hand, anxious that he cannot meet the expectations upon him.

A man may feel restricted in playing certain roles; he may not be able "to place" all his energies, push, and drive within the conventionalized expectations his roles require. The image of self reflected from *other* roles (currently and previously enacted) may conflict with the image reflected from enactment of the restricting role. Hence, the person cannot "put his all" into their enactment, for by doing so he would be damaging his own image of self. Or some component of his psychic structure, which had been socially channeled, may now be blocked by this role. Hence, as the person strives to perform it, this role restricts his accustomed impulses and emotions. Or, his feeling of restriction may be due to ambition: the referral of his self to larger tasks ahead by anticipation.

On the other hand, the person may feel that in performing a certain role he must do his very utmost in order to satisfy its requirements. This reaction may arise from the fact that others involved in the role are very significant, yet their expectations are, from the person's standpoint, very hard to meet. Enactment of the role may, for instance, require energies and habits which his organism is not capable of developing, or it may require a type of temperament which his psychic integration does not enable him to develop, or again, it may be that he does not have the education or intelligence to meet the demands. Yet, since they are very significant to him, he continues to try, and hence he continually feels the strain. It is also possible that he is a "perfectionist" and thus holds an exaggerated view of the role demands exacted of him, even if others encourage him to "take it easy."

Either incongruity—the restricting or the straining role—may lead to personal dissatisfaction; in either case, frustration and anxiety may result. These mechanisms may, of course, operate in any role context—in the home no less than in the diplomatic conference.

III. However similar different men's external reactions to the requirements of their roles may seem, they may, in truth, have internalized different roles in quite varying degrees. The image of self reflected from one significant circle may be so satisfactory that men do not accept the significance conventionally assigned to appraisals by other circles.

A professional man, for example, may be so absorbed in his work, and be so satisfied with the self-image reflected by his colleagues that his love life may remain quite undeveloped, his reactions to it remaining quite stereotyped. Such men are among those who at the age of sixty speak to their wives in the same flowery vocabulary of romance that was current in their high school days. On the other hand, a man may dedicate his life to his intimate other, whom he has "chosen from all the world," and she may be the center of his life and of his person. His occupation may thus be a mere means of economic support for her, and for himself. It may be that when one has no such intimate other, he will be all the more sensitive to the appraisals of his professional role, since it is the deepest internalized; then those who are significant to him in this role will form the social basis for his central self-expectations. But if we were to take any one type of role, say the occupational, and attempt to classify persons solely in terms of that one type, we should fail to grasp what is essential to the kind of man whose job is merely a means of support and not significant to his self-image and personal integration.

Roles, we know, may be segments of various institutions and at the same time components of persons. The relationship between different roles may be construed as a scheme of means and ends. Certain political roles or family roles, for example, may be enacted in order to achieve or facilitate ends which lie in other institutional orders. Now, the integration of the roles which compose a given person may also be grasped in terms of such a means-end scheme. If, for example, political ends are all that matter to a man, he may act the role of the clerk only in order to make money in order to have pamphlets printed in behalf of a political movement. His personality is integrated around his political role, and the other roles he has incorporated facilitate this political role. The significances of family and of occupational others are instrumental, and his image of self and his conscience are primarily reflections of his political others.

Suppose, on the other hand, a professional career is the most significant basis for a man's self-image; then he may be willing to play the role of the husband in order to secure a typist. Or a woman may be willing to play the role of a wife because this role guarantees her membership in the household of a man who is a good provider and whose position enables her to borrow prestige.

Of course, the person—as built of roles and of his reactions to them—is not the complete character structure. The psychic structure, as we have seen, is linked with the person, and the two, along with the organism, form the dynamic whole of character. As we have just seen, one type of person may be more or less dominated by a key role, which is thus the hub of his character. But there is also the contrasting type of person in which no one role predominates. In all post-Renaissance societies, for example, the upper classes have produced certain models of representative men. The British gentleman, the Italian cortegiano, the French cavalier—these are images of men who are *not* dominated by any one role, but rather maintain a certain distance from all roles, even while playing them all with proficiency. Such excellent performances would seem possible only when the demand for special skills is not too rigorous. Whether they involve generalship or erotical conquest, statesmanship or economic bargaining, their contexts must be sufficiently personalized to permit what nowadays would seem amateurish. The images of such representative men, including as they do psychic elements as well as external demeanor, transcend any one role, and yet enable men to play all the roles required by their social position.

There is also what may be called the experimental man, who like Saint-Simon, takes up, one after the other, many roles, and puts the whole force of his character into each of them in turn. Such a man does not try to integrate himself in terms of all these roles, but rather to conquer all of them and to be above any one of them. Thus Bismarck asked: "Why should I be a harmonious personality?" [17]

In the analysis of institutional orders and social structures, one encounters many types of persons, integrated with roles in various degrees and in various ways. The discernment of such types, in fact, is a major part of the social psychology of institutions. For the person is related to society by the roles he acquires. These roles, in turn, are related to his psychic structure, primarily by the language of his group. The acquisition of language requires a certain kind of organic equipment, but the function of language is to co-ordinate the social activities and roles which the person enacts, for it is primarily by means of language that we learn what is expected of us in all the varied roles we play.

Our images of our self are facilitated and restrained by the expectations of others; we are sensitive to the expectations of those who are most significant to us. But our selection of significant others is limited by our positions in the varied institutions of which

[17] Alfred von Martin, *Sociology of the Renaissance* (New York: Oxford, 1944), p. 95.

we are members. Within these institutional limits, however, we will generally turn towards those whom we believe will confirm the desired image we would have of our self. And, if others' expectations and images of us are contrary to our desired image, we will try to reject them, and seek only confirmation among more congenial others.

Our unity of self—the secure feeling of what we really are—ideally occurs when the various images of our self—held by us and by others—are in some way reconcilable. In some societies, all the roles we play are stereotyped, so that it is easy for us to experience unity of self. In other societies, there is no set pattern, and we spend much of our life trying to get the images we hold of our self confirmed by others.

Our conscience—the generalized other or superego—is the product of all expectations of significant others in our life history. Many of these expectations are internalized during our childhood, and are below the level of our awareness; hence, in later life, as we become sensitive to new significant others, we often encounter conflicts of conscience. Social conflicts among the expectations and demands of various significant others thus become conflicts within the person. The consciences of men can only be similar in so far as they have experienced similar types of significant others. And, as we have shown, not all human beings have a strong conscience.

Types of persons can be deduced from the various roles that different persons play and the various ways they react to those roles. They may make up for restriction in one role by aggressive activity in another; they may expend more energy in some roles than in others; and, even though one person may seem to play a role in a similar way to another, he may have internalized this role in his psychic structure very differently. Accordingly, the similar objective social role may carry very different meaning in his character structure. In order to understand types of persons, we must know something of the motivations which prompt the acquisition and the enactment of various roles.

CHAPTER

V

The Sociology of Motivation

OUR threefold division of character structure enables us to set forth three theories of motivation. We can locate the center of motivation primarily in the organism, in the psychic structure, or in the person.

On the level of the *organism*, we might assume that "all organic processes are initiated by the need to restore a physio-chemical equilibrium which is experienced as health."

In terms of the *psychic structure* we might assume that "psychological processes are initiated by the need to restore an emotional equilibrium which is experienced as pleasure." [1]

In terms of the *person*, we might assume that conduct is motivated by the *expectations* of others, which are internalized from the roles which persons enact, and that important aspects of such motivation are the vocabularies of motive which are learned and used by persons in various roles. Motivation thus has to do with the balance of self-image with the appraisals of others.

1. The Sociological Approach

When motivation is viewed on the level of the organism, the processes and elements of the psychic structure are likely to be seen as mere epiphenomena, or at best, means to the attainment of some physiological condition. On the other hand, many who,

[1] These two quotations paraphrase the positions of the physiologist, W. B. Cannon, and of the psychologist, Sigmund Freud, respectively. They are from Ives Hendrick, *Facts and Theories of Psychoanalysis* (2d ed.; New York: Knopf, 1944), pp. 206 ff. See W. B. Cannon, *The Wisdom of the Human Body* (New York: Norton, 1932), pp. 306 ff. The formal similarity of the two writers is the more striking when we realize that they worked independently of each other and used very different methods.

like Freud, consider the psychic structure as a fairly autonomous and somewhat closed system, ascribe what they cannot otherwise explain to "the constitution" of the organism. "Organism" is thus used as a residual category to "explain" what cannot otherwise be explained. Operating on either of these two levels, the impact of the social roles of the person upon the psychic structure and organism is minimized or omitted.

For Freud, the psychic structure ("drives") may be socially canalized, but is not itself subject to basic social modifications. The concept of "sublimation," for instance, implies that role-conditioned forms of psychic drives are epiphenomena of "the basic drives." These "real drives" are assumed somehow to lie in the psychic structure or in the constitution of the organism. The split between man's primordial biological nature and man's cultured personality is thus retained and a metaphysical accent is placed upon the biological or the psychic level. Emotions, urges, or various physiological processes are "the real" motivating factors of conduct; the rest is sham, or at any rate distorted and ungenuine expressions of the real motives of the real individual.[2]

If we drop this metaphysical accent on the biological and the psychic and treat the person as just as "real" as, and in many ways more important than, the organism and the psychic structure, we are able to enlarge our conception of motivation. Although we shall give due weight to organic and psychic factors of motivation, we shall approach the topic primarily in terms of the person:

It should be clear from previous chapters that by "the problem of motivation" we mean the understanding and explaining of why and how human conduct takes a specific direction. It is a problem of *steered conduct* rather than a problem of *motive power*. And we stand a better chance of solving this problem in terms of the person than in terms of the unsocialized organism or psychic structure.

Moreover, only on the level of the person can we expect to deal with *understandable* motives. The restoral of the organic equilibrium of health or the impulsive squirmings of emotional balance experienced as pleasure are not understandable in terms of the

[2] The new psychoanalysis of Karen Horney and Erich Fromm, e.g., has not succeeded in entirely overcoming Freud's biological metaphysic. See below, this section.

organism or the psychic structure as such. Motives may be explained in part in terms of these levels, but they cannot be understood. It is clear that when we speak of understandable motives
or intentions, we must pay attention to the social function of
language in interpersonal conduct; we can speak of understanding
something only if it is meaningful, and language, a social acquisition and a personal performance, is the prime carrier of meaning.
Even dreams have to be deciphered or interpreted as a language
of "unconscious impulses."

We have also seen that the organism is relevant to our understanding of conduct and character only when its effects are mediated by the social evaluations of other persons; and that the
impulses, emotions, and perceptions of the psychic structure are
patterned and channeled by the social organization of the person.
Therefore, insofar as the organism and psychic structure enter into
understandable motivations, they may be most readily and significantly grasped in terms of the person, for it is in such terms that
emotional or organic equilibria are organized and attained.

The person acting out his roles in various situations is the
most immediately observable aspect of character structure. Although, like the psychic structure and the organism, the person is
an abstraction with which we conceive one aspect of the total
reality of man, it is that aspect which is typically what-is-to-be-
explained-and-understood. In ordinary life situations we do not
deal directly with the psychic structure or with the organism. We
deal with these indirectly, often without being aware of doing so;
we deal with them as they manifest themselves in man as he presents himself to us, and he presents himself as a social person.

Our "final" theory should be a model within which we can locate
the other theories, which is adequate to everyday experience and
to known data, and which allows and even suggests lines of reflection that are open to research test.

2. Vocabularies of Motive

Motives are generally thought of as subjective "springs" of action lying in the psychic structure or organism of the individual.
But there is another way to think of them. Since persons do
ascribe motives to themselves and to other persons, we may consider motives as the terms which persons typically use in their

interpersonal relations. To explain some line of conduct by referring it to an inferred and abstracted motive or to some psychic element is one thing; to observe the function of motive imputation and avowal in certain types of social situations is quite another.[3]

We have already seen that we cannot treat "desires" at large as motives, and yet, since persons do talk about their own and others' desires in this way, we cannot afford to ignore them. These avowals and ascriptions of motives—the differing reasons men give for their actions—are not themselves without bases. Rather than throw these reasons aside as "mere rationalizations," we may use them in understanding why men act as they do.

Avowals and imputations of motives seem to arise in interpersonal situations in which "purposes" are vocalized and carried out with close reference to the speech and actions of others; in situations in which one's conduct or intentions are questioned by other men or by one's self. We tend to ask questions in situations which involve *alternative* or *unexpected* purposes or conduct. Sometimes we refer to such situations as crises, however minor they may be. Men live in immediate acts of experience and their attention is directed outside themselves—until their conduct is in some way frustrated or fails to receive an expected response from others. Then there is awareness, questioning by others, self-questioning, and justifications to others and to self. And it is then that statements of motive perform their important function.

Conversations may be about the facts of a situation as they are seen by the participants, or they may be attempts on the part of various persons to co-ordinate social conduct.[4] By means of conversation, different roles are geared to patterns of expectations, but when a person does *not* respond to the expectations of significant others, he will typically begin to explain or justify his own conduct. Now it is in such conversations that statements of motive are often brought into operation. The function of such statements

---

[3] For a preliminary statement of the point of view expressed here, see C. Wright Mills, "Situated Actions and Vocabularies of Motive," *American Sociological Review* (October 1940). Cf. K. Burke, *Permanence and Change* (New York: The New Republic, 1935).

[4] On the "question" and on "conversation," see Grace De Laguna, *Speech: Its Function and Development* (New Haven: Yale Univ. Press, 1927), p. 37. For motives in "Crises," see J. M. Williams, *The Foundations of Social Science* (New York; Knopf, 1920), pp. 435 ff.

is to persuade others to accept our act, to urge them to respond to it as we expect them to, and to make them believe that our act sprang from "good intentions."

Sociologically, as Max Weber put it, a motive is a term in a vocabulary which appears to the actor himself and/or to the observer to be an adequate reason for his conduct.[5] This conception grasps the intrinsically social character of motivation: a satisfactory or adequate motive is one that satisfies those who question some act or program, whether the actor questions his own or another's conduct. The words which may fulfill this function are limited to the vocabulary of motives acceptable for given situations by given social circles.

Conceived in this way, motives are acceptable justifications for present, future, or past programs of conduct. But to call them "justification" is not to deny their efficacy; it is merely to indicate their function in conduct. Only by narrowing our view to the point where we see the isolated individual as a closed system, can we treat verbalized motives as "mere justifications." By examining the *social* function of motives, we are able to grasp just what role motives may perform in the social conduct of individuals. We know that even in purely rational calculations acceptable justifications may play a rather large role. Thus, we may reason, "If I did this, what could I say? And what would they then say or do?" Decisions to perform or not to perform a given act may be wholly or in part set by the socially available answers to such queries.

But the problem of the social function of motives goes deeper. A man may begin an act for one motive; in the course of this act he may adopt an auxiliary motive which he will use to explain his act to others who question it, or whom he feels may question it in the future. The use of this second motive as an apology does not make it inefficacious as a factor in his conduct. In such after-the-event explanations we often appeal to an acceptable vocabulary of motives, associated with expectations with which the members of the situation are in agreement. Accordingly, our statement of motive serves to integrate social conduct, in that the reasons we give for an act are among the conditions for its continued performance. By winning allies for our activities the motives we verbalize may

[5] *The Theory of Social and Economic Organization,* A. M. Henderson and Talcott Parsons, trs. (New York: Oxford, 1947), Chapter 1.

even be controlling conditions for the activity's successful performance. And by winning social acceptance, such motives often strengthen our own will to act. For the performance of many roles requires the agreement of others, and if no reason can be advanced which is acceptable to these others, such acts may be abandoned. Diplomacy in the choice of motives thus controls the conduct of the diplomatic actor. Strategic choice of motive is part of the attempt to motivate the act for the *other* persons involved in our conduct. Carefully chosen and publicized motives often resolve social conflicts, potential and real, and thus effectively integrate and release social patterns of conduct.

When a person confesses or imputes motives, he is not usually trying to describe his social conduct, he is not merely stating reasons for it. More usually he is trying to influence others, to find new reasons which will mediate the enactment of his role—and in so trying to influence others, he may often influence himself. The verbalization of motives for an act is itself a new act; it is a phase of role playing which lines up the role with or against the expectations of others. In such cases, accordingly, it is not necessarily wise to seize upon the differences between the conduct and the verbalization as a discrepancy between action and speech. There is simply a difference between two kinds of action, one verbal, one motor.

In terms of motives, conceived as acceptable grounds for social action, persons will alter, deter, or reinforce their individual conduct. To speak, for instance, of someone as having "scruples" is of course to indicate a complex type of internal behavior, but one index to it is that a moral vocabulary of motives is effective in controlling their conduct.

In the course of our biography, our motives are imputed to us by others before they are avowed by ourselves. Such vocabularies of motive then become components of our generalized other; they are internalized by the person and operate as mechanisms of social control. Thus the mother controls her child by imputing motives to him; by having certain actions called "greedy" and others "good," the child learns what conduct he may perform with approval; and he learns what he cannot get away with socially. He is also given standardized motives which sanction and promote some acts by placing a public premium on them, and which dis-

suade or prohibit him from other acts by publicly disapproving
them.

Along with the conduct patterns appropriate for various occasions, we learn their appropriate motives, and these are the motives we will use in dealing with others and with ourselves. The
motives we use to justify or to criticize an act thus link our conduct with that of significant others, and line up our conduct with
the standardized expectations, often backed up by sanctions, that
we call norms. Such words may function as directives and incentives: they are the judgments of others as anticipated by the actor.

Accordingly, when new roles are taken on, old motives may need
to be modified or new motives learned. For new motives may be
conditions for the enactment of new roles. We control another man
by manipulating the premiums which the other accepts; we influence a man by naming his act in terms of some motive which we
ascribe to him.

Vocabularies of motives have histories, as their various institutional contexts undergo historical change. The motives accompanying the institutional conduct of war are not "the causes of
war," but they do promote continued participation in warfare,
and they do vary from one war to the next. For vocabularies of
motive are modified, as the institutions in which they are anchored
undergo change.

Examine the shift from the laissez-faire to the monopolistic phase
of modern capitalism. The profit motive of individual gain may be
widely espoused and accepted by businessmen during a relatively
prosperous and free economic era, but such commercial vocabularies of motive may undergo severe modifications during monopolistic phases of the economy. For then, a vocabulary of public
service and efficiency may be added to the public motives of businessmen. Now, if a man finds himself unable to engage in business
conduct without joining a "liberal" business organization and
proclaiming its public-spirited vocabulary, it follows that this
particular vocabulary of motives is an important reinforcing feature of his social conduct.

The choice of a motive which is ascribed to some conduct pattern reflects the institutional position of the actor and of those
who ascribe motives to him. For example, the vocabulary of motives used by privileged groups for the conduct of persons in minority groups is different from the motives used for members of high

prestige groups. "Aggressiveness" on the part of a Jewish child may be "impertinence" or "pushing" to anti-Semites, who may entitle the same conduct, when it is displayed by a Gentile child, "independence" and "initiative." By thus ascribing different motives to similar acts, status lines are upheld.

The "success" or the power of an actor may drastically influence the vocabulary used in describing his character and motives. Lord Byron put the fact of these dual vocabularies of motive for identical conduct neatly in speaking of

> "Firmness in heroes, kings and seamen,
>   That is, when they succeed; but greatly blamed
>   As obstinacy, both in men and women,
>   Whenever their triumph pales or star is tamed . . ." [6]

"Events" may decide between which of two vocabularies of motive are used. Only great men can leave their reasons to the creative hands of their apologists, and some are famous because they have found apologists.[7] Yet, there may be a way to go behind the event and, by using the acceptable vocabularies of motive, understand successful-men-with-apologists as well as those who failing descend into the limbo of anonymity.

3. The "Real" Motives

Thus far we have been examining motivation on the level of the explanations people use and accept to account for their actions. But now we must ask whether such explanations are "the real motives" of the persons using them.

We have first to abandon the notion that merely because vocabularies of motives are acceptable they are necessarily deceptive shams. The very fact that many "sophisticated" persons doubt the validity of such motives is itself an historical phenomenon which must be explained. The Freudian theory of motives, for example, has been summarily stated by Ralph Barton Perry as the view "that the real motives of conduct are those which we are ashamed to admit either to ourselves or to others." [8] We can admit the truth

---

[6] *Don Juan*, Canto XIV, pp. 89 ff.

[7] See Chapter XIV: The Sociology of Leadership.

[8] *General Theory of Value* (New York: Longmans, Green, 1936), pp. 292-93. For another criticism of Freud on this point, see Karen Horney, *New Ways in*

in this statement in a more fruitful manner: the vocabularies which persons choose for their statements of motive tend to be those which are accepted by others. But whether this means (1) that these acceptable motives, stated to others and to self, are inefficacious in social conduct, or (2) that they are not to be considered "the real motives" of the person using them are further questions, the answers to which cannot be inferred from the principle governing the social choice of vocabularies of motive.

We have already indicated that acceptable vocabularies of motives may be controlling factors of social conduct, but under what conditions may they be considered "the real motives"? We may assume that the more deeply internalized in the person, and the more closely integrated with the psychic structure, a vocabulary of motives is, the greater is the chance that it contains "the real motives." In fact, that is what "real motives" may be assumed to mean. We must, in order to "test" motives, therefore, attempt to find out on what level of character structure a given vocabulary of motives is integrated.

But how can we find this out? What are the optimum conditions for the fuller integration of a vocabulary of motives with the psychic structure?

Those vocabularies of motive which are consistently used by the person when in public, when in private, and when alone have the highest chance—other things being equal—to become fully integrated with the psychic structure. If differing vocabularies are used by the person when with his wife than when with his coworkers, and still another vocabulary is used when he is by himself, we do not know what his motive may be.

Moreover, in terms of his life history, to the extent that the vocabularies of motive now used by the person are the same as those which were used in the socialization of his psychic structure, the chances are higher that they are integrated on deeper psychic levels of his character.

In other words: to probe for motives requires us to observe the function and the *context* of vocabularies of motive. It is from such observations that we may infer how deeply given motives are

Psychoanalysis (New York: Norton, 1939). The present discussion is not, of course, intended as a comprehensive statement or criticism of Freud's theory of motivation.

integrated with the character structure, and thus how "real" they may be.

Now, whether the same vocabulary of motives for given types of activity is used frequently in the life history and widely in contemporary contexts depends not only upon the internal condition of the individual but also upon the typical social-historical situation that prevails. Accordingly, we can imagine sociological conditions which favor or which work against the psychic integration of vocabularies of motive; we can in fact construct two contrasting types of society—(I) in one of which conditions maximize the chances, and in the other (II) minimize the chances that a vocabulary of motives coincides with "real" motives. We know that societies, as well as institutions within societies, differ in the extent to which the roles of their members may be classified into different sectors of the private and public. At one extreme, we may think in a simplified way, of a small preindustrial village; at the other, of a modern industrialized metropolis.

I. In the village the various situations in which men play roles are not so widely different from one another and are transparent to all. Even in his family group a person's talk and actions may not be very different from his talk and actions while working with other family heads. The variety of roles which any given person plays is not very wide, and each is translatable into the others. In such a society a single vocabulary of motives may be used by a person for all his roles, or at least he will use the same motives in speaking of some conduct pattern to his wife and to his neighbor, to his working mates and to the village head. His children will learn these same homogeneous vocabularies of motive. And these vocabularies of motive are not likely to be questioned, for they are used in public, in private, and when alone, and their chances of being integrated firmly and smoothly with the psychic structure of the character will be high.

In such a society, *if* a variety of motives is used, each set of motives is likely to remain associated in a stable way with its respective roles. The motives used to explain why one works will be the same before one's wife and friend as before one's working mate and village chief. So, different vocabularies for different situations are easily understood and relatively unquestioned by the different members of each situation.

The motives of a person are thus compartmentalized and ordered without conflict to their respective institutional compartment. So motives stabilize and guide conduct; the expectations of the several others with which the person is confronted are not in conflict when he uses the vocabulary of motives appropriate to a given occasion. Being typically unquestioned and being intertranslatable —and hence usable before everyone—the chance is great that stable and acceptable vocabularies of motive will be used when alone and that they will be linked with impulse and emotion during the socialization of the psychic structure. Appearance and reality are one; or if such be the case, the cant is completely shared and socially effective.

II. In an industrialized metropolis, the person is confronted with a variety of roles and situations. Not only is there a typical split between his more intimate roles and his more public appearances, but the differences between any two intimate roles or between any two public roles may be very wide. Different motives may be employed for roles involving one's wife and for those involving one's acquaintance on the commuter train.

This segmentalization of conduct means that the person will internalize many vocabularies of motive which may very well be in conflict. Then the individual must keep one set of motives secret from the others, for they may appear "silly" to some, even though "beautiful" to others. He compartmentalizes not only his conduct but also his reasons for it, and insofar as he cannot do so, his motives may be in conflict. He may have difficulties deciding whether he does this or that for love or for duty, for "selfish" economic gain or for civic betterment; perhaps he will not be sure whether he is marrying this woman because he loves her and she has such a pleasant voice, or because she is so wealthy.

No one vocabulary of motives is accepted by everyone, so the alert individual must use one or the other tentatively, until he finds the way to integrate his conduct with others, to win them as allies of his act. Different motives may integrate roles and release conduct in the same situation, and similar motives may integrate roles and justify conduct in very different situations. Then others and the person himself may be confused and not know just what motive does prevail.

Vocabularies of motive which are historically associated with one type of institutional conduct may spread to other institutions. The motives which are acceptable for economic enterprise may gain partial or entire acceptance in other institutions. And such spreading motives may become universally accepted as the comprehensive motives of man. The intricate motives of business conduct in America have spread in this way to other types of conduct. They have encroached upon the Victorian vocabulary of the virtuous relations of men and women: love, duty, kindness. Among certain strata, the romantic and virtuous vocabularies of motive have been "confused" with the pecuniary. To ask whether a woman or man is marrying "for love or for money" is to point to this overlap. The decline of the family relative to other institutions involves a questioning of the vocabularies of motive which accompanied the more stable family patterns. And Max Weber has remarked that what formerly was thought of morally is in our time thought of esthetically or psychiatrically. Whereas formerly maidens and ladies spoke of "wicked" men and of "good" and "bad" conduct, today they speak of "decent" and "indecent" conduct, or of "neurotic" and "stable" persons.

Due to the great weight which the economic order has in the American social structure, pecuniary motives tend to form a sort of common denominator of many other roles and motives. Other vocabularies are treated as shams, façades, and "rationalization," and "the wise guy" knows that *the real* motive is the desire for money which, as is commonly said, may not be everything but is almost everything.

Back of the motive-mongering and the self-doubts of persons as to their own motives is the fact that in modern life there is often no stable or unquestioned vocabulary of motives available. And back of this is the fact that the institutional arrangements of roles demand that we rapidly give up and take on roles and along with them, their socially appropriate motives. Back of these "mixed motives" and "motivational conflicts" there is going on a competition of varying institutional patterns and of their respective vocabularies of motives. Shifting and borderline situations, having no stable vocabularies of motive, may contain several alternative sets of motives originally belonging to different systems of roles.

Such institutional conflicts are internalized and, accordingly, are revealed in the confusion and self-doubt of institutionally marginal persons. Institutional conflict, in short, threatens the sense of unity and even the identity of the modern self. The rival demands of conflicting roles, brought to self-awareness, call forth the complex internal behavior called "conscience," a term literally meaning "shared knowledge." If this "conscience," that is our general other, passes in review all the particular role enactments, there is, as it were, an internal court which will let "the left hand know what the right is doing." Compartmentalization of roles and of role demands will work so long as the generalized other is *not* concerned, that is, so long as no ethical universals are involved. The Sunday Christian who professes to be an honest dealer may no longer be able to jab his business partner, without discarding or trying to cheat his own conscience. The same goes for the "high minded citizen" who may vote for higher taxes—for others, but not for him, to pay. If he has internalized the professed values of his Christian community or of his nation, his generalized other is bound to saddle him with guilt for whatever acts fall short of the professed demand level.

What is expedient for the purpose at hand is not necessarily high-minded, law abiding, or moral, however successful we may be in deceiving ourselves and others, and however intense and widespread the tacit consensus of a group. Uncertainty continues to exist so long as there are critical out-groups that are ready and capable of pointing to disparities between expedient practice and ethical professions. Victorian cant is painfully transparent to everyone—in retrospect; for Karl Marx, for example, it was plainly obvious at the time. When what is done cannot be undone, self-expurgating behavior is a ritual; the motto "now it can be told" usually prefaces such retrospective and harmless exercise. It is the sequel to twentieth-century cant which H. Nicolson has defined as the tribute vice pays to virtue.

The speed with which decision makers, in their sixties today, have repeatedly written off presumably universal principles produces mass skepticism and cynicism and the increasing realization that ours is indeed a secular age in which the exploitation of moral values for expedient interests is quite standard. The motto, wrought on the gate of the Dachau concentration camp—"Labor Means Liberty"—dramatically highlights the condition of "moral man" who in malaise, drifts in "immoral society."

4. Awareness of Motives

Two experiences lead us to believe that there are motives which operate but of which the individual himself is not aware:

I. We may arrange a special type of interview with another person and decide about real and sham motivations on the basis of this interview. This interview may be a variant of a highly personal or intimate situation; but in addition to privacy it may contain the authority of both scientist and physician—the psychiatrist. By systematic and skillful questioning, the psychiatrist may so arrange and conduct the interview that the person will confess motives which he comes to believe are his real motives yet of which he was previously unaware. In the interview he loosens up the set vocabularies which he has typically used and which he had come to ascribe to others. He may now use this new vocabulary in the presence of self; he may also publicize it to chosen others, or to a wider public.

The new motives thus emerging from the psychiatric interview may come to approximate more closely the true state of the psychic structure, and they may, in time, be used in resocializing this psychic structure. Such interviews do not occur only in psychiatric work. Rather sudden shifts in motivations may occur in intimate life situations, as well as in the police interview, where regular techniques have been worked out to detect the lie or sham. Of a Gestapo agent, Anna Seghers has written: "He arranged the slips of paper, looked over his notes, sorted them, underscored words, and connected various items by a certain system of lines. . . . His notes for an examination were comparable only to intricate musical scores." [9]

II. The phenomenon of motives which operate, yet of which the person is not aware, appears even more convincingly in hypnotic situations. If several persons are hypnotized and while in this state it is suggested to them that they breathe faster while reading every other page of a book, they will do so in the posthypnotic period, without being aware of doing so or of the planted motives which impel them. [10]

[9] *The Seventh Cross*, J. A. Galston, tr. (Boston: Little, Brown, 1942), p. 156.
[10] See E. R. Kellogg, "The Duration and Effects of Posthypnotic Suggestion," *Journal of Experimental Psychology* (1929), Vol. XII, pp. 502-514. Compare

On the basis of the psychiatric interview and the hypnotic experience, one must suppose that many motives operating in social life are outside the awareness of persons. We may approach this fact by asking: What conditions favor the operation of motives of which the person is unaware, even when he is alone?

If an act can be typically construed by the actor in such a way as to have others and himself ascribe it to an acceptable motive, then a premium has been placed upon the act. Other feelings and actions are typically tabooed by virtue of the motives to which they are usually ascribed. Tabooed actions and the impulses and emotions associated with them may be restricted to private occasions by the actor, or he may seek to represent them in terms of some more favorable vocabulary of motives. But there is another way in which such motives may be handled: the conduct, feeling, and discussion of them in a tabooed vocabulary of motives may be repressed, which simply means that they cannot be recalled by a simple act of attention.

There are topics and feelings for which vocabularies exist and are used in *all* public situations, just as there are feelings and impulses, which can be discussed openly in *most* conversations. Other topics and feelings are restricted to intimate occasions, and still others which may be available only to the person when alone. Finally, there are topics and feelings which the person will not discuss even with himself. These situations, in brief, range from those in which a vocabulary of motives is quite socialized to those in which given topics or feelings are not verbalized even by the person when alone.

As we descend this scale of conventionally premiumed to permissible topics and to those which are conventionally tabooed, we also descend into those spheres which are most likely to be "unconscious." For the prime meaning of "unconscious" is that which is unverbalized, or sometimes even, unverbalizable.

Just as a man who is writing a note for his own future reference may abbreviate it so that only he can understand its meaning, so our internal speech follows a grammar of its own, in which symbol condensations and images may call forth whole streams of thought. This inner speech may be very important in the person's self-

Erich Fromm's discussion of motives planted during hypnosis: *Escape from Freedom* (New York: Farrar & Rinehart, 1941).

understanding. To communicate our inner speech to others we have to translate it into discursive, outer speech, and it is this explaining to others which gives rise to "objectivity." The terms which the person uses to refer to his own feelings are socially confirmed by their use by other persons. Self-knowledge that is not socially confirmed, not yet disciplined by interaction with others, is not secure knowledge.[11]

If we do not publicize the vocabularies we use for our motives and feelings, we may develop little areas of private speech which we use only with very intimate friends or perhaps only in introspection and soliloquy. Sometimes two persons who are very intimate will share such patterns, although no one else can understand the meanings which these two use privately. In this way, the unconscious may be made articulate and partially shared with a few selected others "who understand." For sometimes in these intimate conversations, using very private cues and innuendos of motive, a person will suddenly become aware of motives which he did not know as his own. Then what was unconscious is no longer unconscious but privately conscious.

The becoming aware of previously unconscious feelings and impulses proceeds by just such socialization. But the social area in which these elements of the psychic structure are socialized may still be restricted. From the standpoint of the urbane character structure, only the yokel or the fool will give away his "private" motives in "public." Urbane "maturity" involves a specialization of displayed motives in varying degrees and according to private and public appearances.

Those topics which are excluded from public conversation with others will more likely be part of the private world of the individual, and if the taboos are strong and morally enforced by significant others, they will tend to become unconscious. Then the person will not discuss them even with intimate others, and he will not be able to discuss them with himself.

That which the person is unaware of is related to that which is

[11] George H. Mead has done much with the question of the social character of objectivity in his *Mind, Self and Society* (Chicago: Univ. of Chicago Press, 1934). See also C. S. Pierce, "How to Fix Belief," Vol. V, of *Collected Papers* (Cambridge, Mass.: Harvard Univ. Press, 1934). Vigotsky has systematized this matter and has introduced the distinction between inner and outer speech. See his essay "Language," *Psychiatry*, 1940-41.

tabooed in his society. The approved motives which are typically ascribed to conduct are sanctions which reinforce that conduct. Disapproved motives are sanctions which discourage the conduct to which they are typically applied. Vocabularies of motives are thus a special class of premium or taboo.[12]

When we are motivated by impulses that are disapproved, we sometimes cannot stand the image of ourselves, and so we keep these motives out of our awareness. Various impulses which we thus "repress" pop up in our daydreams, or in our dreams at night. But we do not face them when we are alert; the mechanisms of awareness exclude them in the interests of self-security; they catch us only when we are alone and our level of consciousness is lowered.

The subjective is what the person presents only to himself. When he communicates it to another it is no longer subjective, but objective, no longer private but socialized. We may communicate such private feelings, moods, and motives in intimate relations, or even sometimes among perfect strangers. And as we do so we are learning about ourselves. As we tell our motives to others, we become aware of new aspects of ourselves. For by telling them even to one significant other, we may justify our having them or seek relief from them. We are developing or using a vocabulary of motives with this particular other, and on the basis of this vocabulary we understand our own motives in a more socially acceptable way.

We can integrate these motives and moods into our own self by socializing them to others, even to a few others, who understand. Thus making others understand us, we can understand ourselves and reconstruct our image of self. If we faced our motives alone, our sense of unity and identity of self might be threatened. Just as we repress a motive, an act, a mood, a feeling from public display, we may also repress it to the point where we ourselves are not aware of it. It may be that we cannot by an act of attention recall some motive or some feeling until it is put into a vocabulary of motives which we *might* use before some others without loss of self-esteem and security. The vocabulary in terms of which our motives are thus phrased may not be approved by many others, indeed it may be a vocabulary which we can accept only because of the authority of the one psychiatrist who gives us the words, tells us that it is all right since at times "others" feel the same way.

[12] See Chapter VII: Institutions and Persons, Section 3: The Theory of Premiums and Traits of Character.

Motivation may be discussed in terms of the organism, the psychic structure and the person. Although we have paid attention to each of these, we have approached the problem primarily from the standpoint of the person. So approached, motives are viewed as social justifications for one's own conduct, and as means of persuading others to accept and to further one's conduct. Such statements of motive arise when we are faced with alternatives, with unexpected choices, or when there is opposition to one's role, for in routine conduct our motives are often not questioned.

When there are many vocabularies of motives, it becomes difficult to know the "real motives" of persons. The more closely integrated our vocabulary of motives with our person and our psychic structure, the greater the chance that it contains our real motives. Such integration is most often present when we use the same motives in public, in private and when alone. In some societies this is generally the case; in others it is not. And when it is not, when various institutions and roles compete with each other, there is a confusion of motives, as we have shown by contrasting the problem of motivation in a preindustrial village and an industrialized metropolis.

All this does not mean that there are not motives which affect conduct but of which the person involved is not aware. We have suggested, with due regard to individual complications, that these unconscious motives may be explained primarily in terms of unverbalized areas of feeling and conduct.

CHAPTER

VI

Biography and Types of Childhood

SOMATIC development refers to the growth of the organism; maturation, as we shall use the term, to changes of the psychic structure; biographical development, to the development of the person, to changes in the roles that are taken up and cast off in the passage from one age group to another.

These three lines of somatic, psychic, and biographical development proceed together and each is involved in the course of the others. Yet, in their interplay there is no universal pattern or sequence. Changes in the vegetative system and the use of the motor mechanisms of the body require an appropriate integration of sensory organs and psychic components. The person cannot perform certain roles without properly developed psychic and organic functions and prerequisite dispositions. The emotions of the psychic structure are timed and shaped in their expressions according to the roles required of the person.

Thus one sequence of these three lines of development *limits* and *facilitates* another, but no one of them *determines* what occurs in the other two.

Development of any sort involves differentiation and integration. The unco-ordinated and "mass activity" of the infant becomes differentiated into specialized verbal responses and motor skills, and these specializations—of organism, psychic structure, and person—are integrated with various kinds of human character and conduct.

1. The Organism

Everyone begins life as part of another; birth is a biological separation: the infant is ejected and cut off from the mother. Then it begins its slow movement through infancy, childhood, preadolescence, adolescence, and adulthood. Soon after adulthood, the organism begins to decline, it passes through middle age and begins its senescence, until finally, it dies. If birth is a biological separation, death is a social separation. After we are biologically dead we "live" only in the memory or ancestor worship or imagination, or—if we were important enough—in the legends of others.

The history of the human organism is one of very rapid growth during the first year of life, of more gradual growth up to maturity, and then a gradual decline in vigor, alertness, and capacity. From conception until birth the weight of the organism increases about a billionfold; during the rest of the entire lifetime it increases only about twentyfold, a great deal of it during the first three years after birth.[1]

Regardless of race or creed, the biological history of every man is limited by his animal ancestry. During the first year after birth, it is scarcely proper to distinguish organic from psychic maturation, and it is unknowledgeable to speak of personal development, although other persons and their activities do, of course, influence the maturation of the organism and the psychic structure. Even while it is in the uterus, the organism does not unfold according to an unalterable pattern. It interacts with the uterine environment which thus facilitates or retards its growth. Moreover, the economic environment, as registered in the family's class position, vitally influences the fetus and the birth of the child, with or without professional service. In typical United States cities, in the 1930's, the infant's chances to stay alive immediately after birth were three times as great if its family earned $1,250 a year than if they earned under $450 a year.[2] Thus, even though there is as yet no person, social-historical influences bear vitally upon even the prenatal organism.

[1] B. T. Baldwin, *The Physical Growth of Children from Birth to Maturity* (Iowa City: The University, 1921).

[2] Robert Woodbury, "Infant Mortality in the United States," *Annals of the American Academy of Political and Social Science* (November, 1936).

Some eight weeks after conception, the unborn child responds to external stimulation; the skin around the areas that will become its nose and mouth being sensitive to tactile stimulation. Later, definite reflexes appear and other skin areas become sensitive. By six or seven months, all the reflexes needed for postnatal life have appeared.[3] The birth of the infant may occur as early as twenty-four weeks and as late as forty-eight weeks, and a variation of some three lunar months is quite frequent. Yet the pattern of organic maturation proceeds irrespective of such irregularities of birth.[4]

As a little animal, the child is equipped with certain invariable responses which occur when given stimulations are presented. These reflexes, as we have already seen, may be transferred in such a way that they will occur as reaction to stimulations other than the ones which at first evoke them. Such conditioning is perhaps the bottom level of what may be called development in the infant. Habits, once learned, may become quasi-automatic. The stereotyping and restereotyping of reflexes and of habits enable the infant to meet situations which recur; they do not enable him to meet new situations. Conditioning, and the learning of habits, are subject to conscious modification by others, and, in time, even by the child's own will.

The infant does not at first distinguish persons from inanimate objects, and even for children, physical things often seem to be animated—as the content of fairy tales, nursery stories, and movie cartoons witness. But by continually doing things to him, other persons stimulate the infant more and more; they elicit more responses and more changes of bodily feelings than do the objects of the inanimate environment.[5] Soon they become identified as

[3] Based on D. Hooker, "Reflex Activities in the Human Fetus," Chapter 2 of *Child Behavior and Development*, R. G. Barker, J. S. Kounin, and H. F. Wright, eds. (New York: McGraw-Hill, 1943).

[4] Arnold Gesell, "Maturation and Infant Behavior Pattern," *Psychological Review* (1929), 36, pp. 308-19.

[5] See the precise studies of Orvis C. Irwin, "The Amount and Nature of Activities of New Born Infants Under Constant External Stimulating Conditions During the First Ten Days of Life," *Genetic Psychology Monograph No. 1*, 1930, pp.1-92. See also M. A. Ribble, "Clinical Studies of Instinctive Reactions in New Born Babies," *American Journal of Psychiatry* (1938), 95, p. 149; and F. Peterson, "The Beginnings of Mind in the New Born," *Bulletin of the Lying In Hospital of the City of New York* (1910), 7, p. 99.

sources of food and warmth, the first image of the mother probably centering about the feel of the breast. The fact that persons are a source of vital stimulations, and the fact that persons are active and move by themselves, form the basis of their being distinguished from mere things.

2. The Psychic Structure

As the child matures he engages in a greater variety of behavior, of motor skills, of displayed feelings and interests, of psychic abilities. As the "mass activity" of the infant develops into segmental activities and functionally segregated acts, his psychic elements are linked with them. So perception, touch, and grasp come to form the child's total image of given objects; he links the sight with the taste with the feel of these objects. The normal adult can wiggle his big toe without waving his entire foot; the infant is not so able; he has less poise, less "distance" from internal stimulation as well as from environmental influences. An impulse is directly and quickly translated into activity; a simple frustration is likely to affect the whole inner condition and external activity of the infant.

The feelings of the newborn infant seem to be undifferentiated At first, they may be described simply as "excitability," but gradually this capacity becomes differentiated and, as it is linked to bodily movements, two "emotions" may be socially distinguished: distress and delight—terms which may describe slight visceral differences in the infant, but, more importantly, indicate differences in the provoking situations and in observable behavior and gesture. Whether they indicate a distinct awareness of feeling on the part of the infant is an open question. As differentiation continues, what may later become fear and anger arise from a sort of generalized distress: fear at sudden shock, anger at interference. Delight, in due course, becomes joy and affection.[6]

Any "marked interference" with the normal functioning of the infant's organism seems to lead to "unpleasant emotions" which appear to be a reaction to the restraining of the child's free action —as John Watson observed—of infantile rage.

During early phases of development, the clinging and sucking

[6] For this vocabulary of infant emotion, see K. M. B. Bridges, "A Genetic Theory of Emotions," *Journal of Genetic Psychology* (1930), 37, pp. 514-26.

reflexes of the infant are linked; later the act of clinging becomes more purposive, more deliberately aimed at support. In fact, clinging for support occurs when the child experiences his own bodily weight as a challenge and, as Paul Schilder puts it, "strives to make himself independent of others in preserving his equilibrium."[7]

The motor actions of the child move him toward the world of objects around him, which is full of danger and the possibility of physical trouble. His fear of danger is a response to what happens to him when he reaches and falls. He may also fear loss of food, or of bodily support, or even of the stroking of his skin by another.

Parents may, of course, play upon these fears in a great variety of ways. "The Kaffirs terrorize their children with tales of horrid monsters. The Manus try to evoke evil bush demons, but the children, trained to self-reliance, physical bravery, and the experimentation necessary for effective physical adjustment to their pile-dwelling life, take very little stock in these bogey-men. As adults, they are the only Oceanic people I know of who are not afraid of the dark."[8]

The contents of fear, as well as of other emotions, undergo change as the psychic structure matures. The infant exhibits what may be taken to be fear in response to intense or sudden stimuli, to unexpected or unfamiliar events. During their first year after birth, one group of children belonging to urban, upper-income American families experienced fear in response to noises and events associated with noises, to falling or sudden, unexpected movements, and to persons or objects associated with pain. From between two to six years of age, the fear of noise, of falling, and of strange persons tends to decline.

As their spheres of social activity are enlarged, the fears of children involve more complex and wider circumstances. They no longer fear some of the things they previously feared, but they become afraid at *signs* of danger, and they experience imagined fears. Signs of fear seem to appear when the child knows enough to recognize possible danger, but cannot understand nor control it. The proportion of their fears in response to being left alone—especially in the dark—of imaginary creatures, and dreamed of

[7] "The Relation Between Clinging and Equilibrium," *International Journal of Psychoanalysis,* Vol. 20 (1939), p. 62.

[8] Margaret Mead, "The Primitive Child," *Handbook of Child Psychology,* Carl Murchison, ed. (2d ed. rev.; Worcester: Clark Univ. Press, 1933), p. 682.

events tend to increase. With his enrollment in school, the American child meets competitive situations and is subject to many achievement ratings. At about this age, he also experiences fear relating to personal prestige and achievement, as shown by his fear of social exclusion and personal inadequacy. And as he grows older, the proportion of such fears increases.

The immature psychic structure does not yet have organized and effective outlets. A temper tantrum—in which the child bursts into disorganized mass behavior, kicking the floor and screaming—may be the only way in which he can let out his anger or aggression against adults. Later, as the psychic structure is more integrated and disciplined by foresight of consequences, the style of rage and of aggression usually becomes more pointed and effective. In this respect, there are differences in children's psychic development according to the class position of their parents. In New York City, as L. B. Murphy has shown, the chance for children to display and express such traits as affection and helpfulness is apparently freer and greater in lower economic groups than in children from professional families with higher incomes.[9]

3. Learning

The development of habits requires a chance to practice them. Boys who grow up on a flat desert do not develop so readily as mountain boys the network of habits, the postural swing and the leg work, required in skiing. And what is true of motor skills is also true of psychic traits and social conduct. Many traits which are often thought of as "inborn" may be traced back to the simple fact of ample and early opportunity for practice.

We may thus ask of the total situation of a child—his home and school and the play space provided—what opportunities are given for the practice of this or that skill or trait? Opportunity for practice is a very important feature of the child's development. The more the child can practice some skill or trait, the more will opportunities for further practice be given him. Whereas children who have had less practice and so less skill will often be afforded still less practice. The structures which we build up facilitate and limit the functions we can later learn to perform. Other people

[9] *Social Behavior and Child Personality* (New York: Columbia Univ. Press, 1937).

often let us put our best foot forward; that is why the worst foot often fails to develop.

"The Samoan child is taught to sit cross-legged almost as soon as it can sit at all. . . . The baby's hands are clapped to the dance rhythm while it is an infant in arms, and as soon as it can stand it is taught to dance. Ten-year-old Samoan children are so set in their postural and rhythmic patterns of their conventions that I found it impossible to teach them so simple an activity as skipping, and sitting upon a chair for any length of time is torture to them. Manus children, however, taught physical skill and agility rather than any formal set of postures, could adapt themselves to new physical activities with ease." [10]

In modern Western societies there is not so heavy a weighting of early successes and failures. Premiums and taboos are often relaxed in recognition of the child's immaturity. Yet premiums and taboos are used to facilitate and retard certain lines of development. If crying and whining are "rewarded" by social attention and fondling, crying and whining will become more and more used as infantile tools. But if whining goes unrewarded it will not be as likely to develop into a stable bid for attention.

Such techniques and traits as are successful in the cradle and home may become firmly integrated and used in the school. When some such pattern as whining is established and linked with satisfaction, this habit may prove an obstacle to further and more independent learning. We do not readily undo patterns of behavior which achieve satisfactions. Habituation enables the child effectively to meet certain situations, but it narrows the versatility of response to these situations. Training may thus incapacitate one for further learning, as well as provide a basis for it.

The repeated performance of identical tasks leads to routine practice. With the security which habits lend the individual in these situations, the attention and feelings at first involved are now minimized; they become available for an expanding area of new, not yet routinized, experiences. The novice at handball is painfully aware of the way he holds his hands and body; the expert can keep his eye on the ball.

The young child finds few fields for early triumphs of learning in the mastery of self-chosen tasks. But as his attention and feelings

[10] See Margaret Mead, *op. cit.*

are freed by the automatic service of habit, he can then strive further to "stand on his own feet." Development is more an achievement than an unfolding, but the general direction of conscious learning shifts as the integration and organization of automatic activities proceed.

4. Language and Person

The first vocal sounds of the baby are aspects of a more generalized "mass activity" involving almost all portions of the organism. This mass activity and crying modifies the baby's social environment: persons are stimulated to do things for and to the infant. At first, the infant's movements are "an amorphous mass of activity"; later, specific or segmental activities are articulated, which involve only local parts of the organism. Although both generalized and segmental movements may be consequences of internal physiological stimulation, from an early period the responses of other persons are likely to be differentiated according to the infant's movements. These different responses of others help the infant to articulate segmental movements; in time, he learns to use his movements and cries as instruments for the control of others.

The growth of language in the child is undoubtedly the most important single feature of his development as a person.[11] Language becomes his most important tool in dealing with others and with himself. The infant's cries, signaling others to attend to it, are components of mass actions in response to internal or environmental discomforts; later the child babbles, thus engaging in segmental action—the use of the voice. Sometimes babbling seems like an outlet of exuberant energies, at other times like a response to irritations, and at all times it is rhythmic. Thus babies play with their voices, if we may call babbling vocal play.

The first spontaneous cries of the infant and child are not socially meaningful, but others respond to certain of these noises, thus

[11] On the language development of the child, see Frank Lorimer, *The Growth of Reason* (New York: Harcourt, Brace, 1929); G. H. Mead, *Mind, Self, and Society* (Chicago: Univ. of Chicago Press, 1934); J. Markey, *The Symbolic Process and Its Integration in Children* (New York: Harcourt, Brace, 1928); Jean Piaget, *The Language and Thought of the Child* (New York: Harcourt, Brace, 1926); and especially D. McCarthy, *Language Development of the Preschool Child*, Institute of Child Welfare, Monograph series, No. 4 (Minneapolis: Univ. of Minnesota, 1930).

socially confirming them. In time, the sounds become fixed units calling forth adult actions which bring the child bodily comfort and social attention. The baby who cries ends up with a comfortable diaper.

The babblings of the child become socialized speech when he addresses his hearers in an expressive effort to influence them, when he becomes aware that a given sound which he makes is going to call forth a certain response in another. As the talking experience of the child increases, his speech becomes more socialized and comprehensible to others. The early incomprehensible babbling is split into "internal speech" and comprehensible "outer speech." The vocal sounds of American children of both sexes at one and one-half years are only about one-fourth comprehensible; but comprehensibility increases until at four years practically all that the child says is understandable. What begins as a component of mass activity in response to organic discomforts becomes, after three or four years, a chief feature of a little person, who has several hundred words with which to ask naïvely simple and penetratingly disarming questions about himself and the world.

There are, of course, differences in the rate and type of children's linguistic developments, and these differences often correspond to the social and economic position of their families. Thus an early study asserts that "the child of the rich understands more words and less actions, and the child of the poor less words and more actions." More recent studies have indicated that the "expansion of a child's environment . . . tends to increase nouns relatively to other parts of speech. Conversely, with a constant or relatively constant environment, the other parts of speech will increase relatively to the nouns." Upper-class children tend to do better than lower-class children on tests which involve linguistic ability, the differences between the educated and the working class sometimes being the equivalent of about eight months in linguistic development. These differences in linguistic development, corresponding to economic and educational level of family, are not to be attributed to differences in "intelligence." [12]

[12] Summary of results obtained by Chamberlain, Drever, and Descoeudres, Stern and Markey, *Handbook of Child Psychology*, D. McCarthy, pp. 303-04. Cf. also Frank J. Kobler, "Cultural Differences in Intelligence," *The Journal of Social Psychology* (1943), Vol. 18, pp. 279-303.

Some time, usually rather late in childhood, the child appears to need persons who are on his level, who have similar attitudes and feelings toward the adult world. He is no longer content to live with more or less authoritarian adults, and more or less complaisant toys and pets. He requires an environment of persons significantly *like* himself, and with these equals he learns to compete, co-operate, and compromise.

As the child becomes a person—acquires language and begins to enact roles—these social acquisitions interact with the maturing features of the organism and the psychic structure. Emotion, perception, and impulse are caught up in the integration of his childish roles, and these roles pattern his impressions into focused perceptions, elicit and style his gestures and feelings, discipline his impulses into purposes.

The manner in which perception is socially stereotyped ranges from admonitions in specific situations ("look this way," "pay attention to this") to a more subtle building up of sensitivities by means of vocabularies for color or social relations. The perceptions thus socially directed are accompanied by feeling tones of pleasure or displeasure with which they are integrated.

The impulses of the psychic structure tend to be disciplined into those activities which are socially held to be "proper" conduct. By assuming roles under the guidance of others, we form and re-form the elements of our psychic structures: some are shaped by our sensitivity to what others think, as well as by the tribulations caused by our own impulses. "When a young man," E. M. Forster once remarked, "is untroubled by passions and sincerely indifferent to public opinion his outlook is necessarily limited." [13] It is necessary, although sometimes difficult, to link our passions with the opinions of others, and during early adolescence the stress and strain of the attempt may become quite acute.

5. Four Theories of Biography

There are at least four general conceptions of "the crucial stage" of the human biography. They include: I, the cross-sectional view of functional autonomy; and the polar opposite: II, the genetic view, which emphasizes infanthood. Between these two are III,

[13] *Howard's End* (New York: Knopf, 1921), p. 24.

the autonomous hierarchal view and IV, the theory of the adolescent upheaval.

I. According to the strictly cross-section view, the motives and
traits of the adult character structure are "self-sustaining." To understand them we have only to examine the contemporary position of the person, and the function of traits and motives within
his total character. For although these traits and motives may have
"grown out of antecedent systems," they are at any given moment
viewed as "functionally independent of them." The tie between
earlier experiences and the present character is thus seen as strictly
"historical, not functional." Although contemporary features of
character are continuous with earlier experiences, they do not in
any sense depend upon them. To understand a given character
and its traits, we must study its present structure and position.[14]

II. At the other extreme, the adult character structure is viewed
longitudinally or genetically. Everything, no doubt, has a history,
and it may be thought that everything about a character structure
is present in seed-form at birth. Maturation is then conceived as
a more or less mechanical unfolding of what was already there.
To understand a character structure and its traits, according to
this view, we must grasp it in its beginnings. This view tends to
place great weight upon biological factors, and it conceives of
the experiences of infancy and childhood as the most important
features of the biography of a character structure.[15]

III. Between the attempt to understand all features of a character in terms of its contemporary structure and situation, and the
attempt to know all contemporary features in terms of its genetic
development, there is the position that at each of several age
levels of experience a system of traits, feelings, and experiences
develop. The experiences belonging to adult life are then understood as occupying a position higher than those assumed by the

[14] This position has been taken by Gordon W. Allport with reference to
motives; he terms it the theory of "functional autonomy" in his *Personality: A
Psychological Interpretation* (New York: Holt, 1937), pp. 190-212, especially
p. 194.
[15] This position, of course, owes much to the work of Freud; although it
is a position which many nonfreudians share with Freud. See below, this
section.

experiences of youth, and these, in turn, stand above the experiences of childhood. The more recently acquired experiences are assumed to control the experiences of earlier phases of the biography. Each such level is thus a "storehouse" of the experiences of each phase of the biography, and each of these levels "preserves in its mode of action the characteristics of the mentality in which it had its origin." When we dream of infantile experiences or feelings, the later levels have temporarily lost their controlling function and we regress to re-experience the earlier formations. Just as we may lose control of our motor habits as when the skilled craftsman ruins his carving by a clumsy slip of the chisel, so may we let infantile or adolescent feelings or self-appraisals slip into awareness when the control of a later level of experience and integration of the psychic structure or person lapses. What is normally controlled becomes for an instant controlling.[16]

IV. Another theory of development holds that the leading characteristics of the adult character structure arise and are set at the adolescent juncture of the biography. Adolescence is viewed as a new birth, or, in G. Stanley Hall's words, as "the infancy of man's higher nature." [17] Although the child may be father to the man, in adolescence a new child is created. The individual, Hall continues, is "reduced back to a state of nature, so far as some of the highest faculties are concerned, again helpless . . . The floodgates of heredity are thrown open again somewhat as in infancy." Childhood unity and integrations are "broken up" and "powers and faculties, essentially nonexistent before, are now born." Some older impulses are reinforced and greatly developed; others are subordinated and lost. The self finds a new center. "Love," according to Hall, "is born with all its attendant passions—jealousy, rivalry . . ." The "old level" of childhood is "left forever." Like milk teeth juvenile interests fade away, and the "well matured . . . [have] utterly lost all traces and perturbations of the storm and stress period, because they are so contradictory and mutually destructive, and because feelings themselves cannot be well remembered."

[16] This position has been set forth by W. H. R. Rivers in "Freud's Concept of the Censorship," reprinted in *Psychology and Ethnology* (New York: Harcourt, Brace, 1926), pp. 21-35.
[17] The view summarized in this paragraph is that of G. Stanley Hall. See his *Adolescence* (New York, D. Appleton, 1904), Vol. 2, especially pp. 70-73.

The strictly *cross-sectional* view treats experience and character as functionally autonomous at any given moment of the biography. The relations of past experience to present character are simply historical, and not connected in any functional way.

The extreme *genetic* view treats the present traits of character as simply unfolded features of what was given at birth in seed-form, or alternatively, as experiences which in later life operate as precedents or models structuring new experiences in their terms.

The third view which we may call the theory of biography as an *autonomous hierarchy* accepts the genetic emphasis upon childhood and the identity between early experiences and later regressive traits, but also accepts the cross-sectional view of each age level of experience as autonomous in its respective action. To these acceptances, it adds the autonomy and retention of earlier systems of experience and the view that these earlier systems may be re-experienced when the controlling function of later systems relaxes, as in dreams and various phenomena of the unconscious.

In the fourth view—the theory of *adolescent origins*—we see the adult orientation and the leading features of a character structure as arising from an adolescent upheaval. We take this period in the life history as the most important for the formation of adult character.[18]

What shall we make of these theories? How can we best realize the truth, if any, in each of them?

6. *The Theory of Adolescent Upheaval*

The theory that adult character is "born" in adolescent upheaval is open to two major criticisms, one of principle and one of adequate fact.

I. The principle is that of selective and cumulative development. Although it is not feasible to telescope all contemporary trends and traits of a character structure into its past, it is necessary to see past organizations of conduct, feeling, and attitude as setting a limit within which later developments may occur. In this sense, our past does limit and select our present, and in turn these selec-

---

[18] Our brief statement of these four views is an intentional simplification of Allport, Freud, Rivers, and Hall, respectively. We are not writing a history or a systematic account of positions held by various scholars. Hence, we select and stress basic ideas without qualifications in order to set forth sharp contrasts.

tions become part of the total selective structure. Development is thus cumulative. To be sure, there are rapid accelerations and sudden conversions and traumatic reverses, but these, too, are explainable in terms of diverse, often inadequate, integrations and selectivities in the line of biographical development.

II. The most telling criticism of the theory of adolescent upheaval, however, has to do with fact. The theory assumes that adolescence is always an upheaval, and of course this is not the case. It takes as universal the rather extreme experience of adolescence in the modern West, and more specifically the middle-class experience with its prolonged gap between organic capacity for and actual assumption of the adult roles of marriage and of the job. From the standpoint of an adequate comparative sociology, we see at once that ours is merely one possible way in which a society may handle the changes of puberty. Some societies are so organized that these organic changes are passed through with no upheaval at all.

Biologically, adolescence extends from puberty to physiological maturity. Chronologically, it may begin as early as eight years and last until as late as twenty-five. The individual's growth is accelerated and, sometimes to a lesser degree, his co-ordination improved. Some organs, such as the heart and the organs of reproduction, grow in size very rapidly, while others, such as the brain, do not perceptibly increase. During puberty the voice tends to fluctuate, "changing" before it settles down.

Since "the further one moves from birth," as Sullivan has written, "the less relevant an absolute physiological chronology becomes, the epoch of adolescence is the least fixed in terms of bodily changes. Adolescence varies from culture to culture, and its actual time of appearance in young people among us is very widely varied." Interactions with significant others "are the predominating factors in bringing about delays . . . and accelerations . . . in the later stages of personality development." [19]

The "quiet miracle of preadolescence" in American society usually occurs between the ages of nine to twelve. It is not a sudden happening but the continuation of a trend toward a fuller social integration. Early adolescence is marked by the fact that "the

[19] Harry Stack Sullivan, "Conceptions of Modern Psychiatry," *Psychiatry* (February 1949), Vol. III, No. 1.

satisfactions and the security which are being experienced by someone else, some particular other, begin to be as significant to the person as are his own satisfactions and security." Indeed, one's own satisfactions and security are facilitated by the satisfactions and securities of the loved one. Perhaps at this point the approval of a significant other takes on its sharpest significance. This fact goes far to explain the usual and much discussed social behavior of adolescence in American society. The social upheaval of adolescence—especially typical of the middle-class young man or woman —results in large part from this intensified need and awareness of the approval of others.

But why this awareness and this need? The roles played by the American adolescent approximate adult roles, yet the adolescent seems only to *play* them. In two key roles in particular, the boy is not yet fully adult: he is not integrated with a durable mate by marriage, and he does not fulfill a regular occupational role. Economically and emotionally he is still a dependent, and because of this he often strives all the harder to be accepted as an adult. He shaves the downy cheek, and plays the man with girls, older girls if possible, to the fullest extent of his abilities and opportunities, and for want of sexual gratification he masturbates.

In American society, adolescence is a juncture at which childhood roles are abandoned and adult ones not yet fully available or internalized. Adolescence is a major point of social reorientation and since the person is in this transition, previous integrations of person and psychic structure are likely to be loosened. Often these integrations undergo such extreme modification that it is no wonder some students view it as a social rebirth.

Among the typical features of adolescence in modern Western societies, especially among middle-class children, are an increase of inner absorptions and reverie, of self-criticism and sometimes a drastic tightening up of scruples; there is frequently an extreme assertion of individuality, a susceptibility to poses, mannerisms, affectations; there are all-absorbing friendships.

These general characteristics may be summed up by the statement that imitation [20] and identification [21] as processes of develop-

[20] Imitation is the conscious patterning of behavior upon a model afforded by other persons. It is learning by example.

[21] Identification is the unconscious taking on of traits which another displays. It refers to a development, without awareness, in the direction of another person.

ment and learning are often at their height during adolescence, or at least they are more open to our observation.

Conceivably, one could coast through childhood under guard and guidance without ever being *absorbed* in one's self. But at adolescence one must make decisions on one's own, and face many models which would guide one in these self-scrutinies of development. The rest of one's life as a person will consist largely of getting in and being accepted and getting out of voluntary associations, and such decisions must now be faced in some earnest. The middle-class adolescent, in deciding the general directions that this cumulatively selective process of his social career will take, wants to find out what kind of man he seems really to be. And so he will usually experiment with the models and self-stylizations available to him.

In ancient Sparta and in many preliterate societies definite tests of fitness for adult roles were specified and known to adolescents. In the modern West the very standards of adulthood are often contradictory, various, and not readily accessible to youth. During the teen age, the requirements for adult roles are often temporarily lowered. This allows the psychic structure an increased opportunity: One can be inebriated without the use of intoxicants, as sensitivities and emotionalisms expand and hot and cold feelings may alternately flood the adolescent. So he is the more easily carried away by total euphoria or equally total despair.

It is characteristic of modern Western societies not to have a generally understood and clearly demarcated "threshold" between childhood and adulthood. Religious rites such as "confirmation" remain segmental, as they do not coincide with the transition from school years to employment and marriage. As we have noted, two major choices are expected of the individual, the choice of occupation—more and more closely connected with problems of education—and the choice of a mate. Having the "freedom" to make these choices for himself, the individual also takes on the responsibility for his choices, that is, "he has no one to blame but himself." During times of mass unemployment it is difficult to say who feels more at a loss for advice, the parents or their grown-up children.

The pressure on adolescents to commit themselves to vocational choices varies according to the social and economic status of the parents; the higher the class position of the youth's home, the longer time he has to make up his mind. The social elevator of higher education carries the youngster past entire fields of inferior occupational choices, up to vantage points from which he may assess opportunities which otherwise would not be concretely visible, much less available. Thus, the well provided student "can wait." Similar differences in the time of waiting have been shown to differentiate lower- and upper-class youth with regard to sexual conduct. Whereas the lower-class youth comes to consummate normal sexual activity at the biologically adequate age, middle-class youth waits until presumably the attainment of the coveted social and occupational status position permit things "which can come later." In the meantime, there are the widespread substitute gratifications of adolescence—masturbation and necking—and the accompanying frustrations incited further by the imageries of eroticism that are ubiquitous in advertising, the pulps, and slick celluloid. One result of all this is often an inarticulate giggle pattern among middle-class youngsters, especially the girls.[22]

[22] Cf. Alfred C. Kinsey, Wardell B. Pomeroy, and Clyde E. Martin, *Sexual Behavior in the Human Male* (Philadelphia and London: Saunders, 1948), which contains data on the sexual behavior of 5,300 white American men, who co-operated in interviews. Regardless of allowances that may have to be made with regard to precise details and small differences in proportions, Dr. Kinsey's major findings concerning the differences between lower- and higher-class members are so great that we do not believe more precise and rigorously controlled studies are likely to change their direction and therewith their significance. The following facts are from "The Kinsey Report":

The working class adolescent engages in sexual intercourse earlier, although frequently more promiscuously than the middle- and upper-class youth, who more frequently seek substitute gratifications through masturbation, homosexual activities, petting, or involuntary although experienced nocturnal emissions. Youths between sixteen and twenty years of age with grade school educations find less than 30 per cent of their "sexual outlet" in masturbation and 57 per cent in intercourse; college men, however, find 66 per cent of their outlet in masturbation, and 10 per cent in intercourse. High school boys of the same age stand midway between the two groups. Among college men up to twenty-five years of age, petting to a climax accounts for nearly half as much of the total outlet as does intercourse. Such petting is the compromise which allows the college girl to preserve technical chastity and at the same time to be helpful in granting her lover substitute gratification. College men rank lowest in homosexuality, with 2.4 per cent of their sexual outlet in this form; grade school and high school boys find 6.9 and 10.8 per cent of their total outlet in homosexual activities.

Such figures indicate that different values and attitudes prevail among lower and higher classes in matters of sex which in turn reflect broader

Biological adolescence is over with the completion of puberty. Social adolescence is over when the person is regularly expected to enact, and does enact with greater or lesser conformity, the roles which adults of his social position typically perform. But when is "psychological" adolescence over and full adulthood established? The psychiatrist Stack Sullivan held that the adult is one who has established "durable situations of intimacy such that all the major integrating tendencies are freely manifested within awareness in the series of one's interpersonal relations." [23] This is an adequate definition of adulthood. It is also an expression of a philosophy of life for free men and women living in modern society.

7. The Relevance of Childhood

We must reject the philosophical assumption of the extreme genetic theory that a biography is simply, or even primarily, a mechanical unrolling of traits already present at birth in seed-form. This mechanical theory of growth must be rejected even for the organic features of character; and we have already seen that both the person and the psychic structure are formed, developed, and integrated very largely through the mediation of other persons. The maturation of character structure is not *determined* by inner features of development, just as it is not shaped altogether by the

characterological differences. Eli Ginzberg has stressed that "these essential differences between the two classes" revolve around the fact that the entire environment of the poor boy operates to place a premium on current gratification, for the future is not propitious, at least no more so than the present. There is little or no rational basis for his "delaying gratification." But the college boy's "entire existence is in the nature of a postponement. He is using up parental capital rather than adding to it; he is studying today in order to profit tomorrow. He has been trained to accept postponement in gratification and he has also been encouraged to seek gratification from other experiences—his studies, his sports, his extracurricular activities. By recourse to masturbation and petting, he manages to reach a tolerable, if not a desirable, equilibrium. He can wait: for him the future is propitious." See Eli Ginzberg, "Sex and Class Behavior" in *About the Kinsey Report, Observations by 11 Experts on "Sexual Behavior in the Human Male,"* Donald Porter Geddes and Enid Curie, eds. (New York: Signet Special, 1948), p. 136; cf. also: Morris L. Ernst and David Loth, *American Sexual Behavior and the Kinsey Report* (New York: Bantam, 1948). The detailed tabulations are taken from the Kinsey Report, pp. 374-83, 417-48, 488-93.

[23] "Conceptions of Modern Psychiatry," *op. cit.*

external forces of the environment. The human biography results from the interplay of inner features of character previously given and acquired, with the external world of man and nature, and with hopes and fears, demands and expectations of the future. We call this interplay "experience," and we know that it continues, although at different pace and with differing intensity, throughout the individual's biography.

In our attempt to answer the question of how much weight we should assign infant and childhood experiences in the adult character, we must pay attention to two questions:

I. What types of infant and childhood experiences are most likely to be important in influencing the formation of an adult character structure? .

II. *How* do these experiences "influence" adult character? Or, what are the mechanisms that connect earlier experiences with later traits of the character formation?

I. Two general and interrelated types of infant and childhood experience may be especially important in forming the structure of childhood character: (a) The impact of the social constellations of the family and the child's reactions to them; and, (b) the sanctions and regulations of such organic functions as feeding, excretion, and the sensations of sex.[24]

All experiences of the infant and of child are socially limited, or even determined, by the kinship structure, for it is the personnel of this structure who administer to the organic needs of the young member, and it is their relations to one another and to the child that are his first social contacts. The infant must be covered and warmed and cooled, lest he die from inappropriate temperatures; he must breathe air through his own mouth and nose; others must feed him. Biologically, the child is helplessly dependent upon others, and particularly upon those who have most to do with his creature comforts, as well as his privations and discomforts.

The infant-mother relationship is often intimate to the point of

[24] For an excellent summary and critique of the literature on "infant care and personality" see Harold Orlansky's article of that title, *Psychological Bulletin*, Vol. 46, No. 1, pp. 1-48. His conclusion is generally negative. See also W. H. Sewell, "Infant Training and the Personality of the Child," *Amer. Journ. of Sociology*, Vol. LVIII, No. 2, September 1952, pp. 150-59.

forming an emotional communion. If the mother did not want the child, or is frightened or disturbed about something, there are often endless feeding difficulties. And if the child is breast-fed, the slightest indigestion on the part of the mother will be "chemically communicated" to the infant. Long before any explicit understanding between mother and child could emerge, Sullivan has noted, there seems to be an emotional contagion between them.[25]

The very biological dependency of the infant and child upon some adult is of great aid to the infant's becoming a full-fledged human being. He becomes a person because others are indispensable to him as an organism; his helplessness qualifies him for great modifications and vast learning. His helplessness is due to the fact that the human animal is singularly devoid of rigid, innate, instinctive patterns of behavior. "Instinct," wrote Paul Schilder, "is a diminishing, if not a disappearing category in higher animal forms, especially in the human." [26]

The mother is a social instrument of the infant's organic satisfactions: she is also a source of insecurities and anxieties. The satisfactions of such privations as hunger depend upon significant adults, who usually want the child to develop those traits they think well of and to avoid those patterns which they taboo. If he does not meet their expectations, the adults may deprive him of organic satisfactions as well as social attention. Since the child, according to L. L. Bernard, "does not think that deprivation may occur in the natural course of events, but is rather the result of ill-will," deprivation seems "equivalent to aggression and violence" and often the child will react with counteraggressions.[27]

Child clinicians, psychiatrists, and nursery students have taught the social psychologist the important role childhood experiences may play in the early formations of emotional life. In this connection, of course, one overlooks the contributions of Freud only at the risk of serious omission. Whereas pre-Freudian psychologists saw early childhood as a psychological state of paradisaical innocence, Freud taught us to view this stage as problematic and crucial for the formation of character. What Freud did, in brief, was to con-

[25] Cf. Harry Stack Sullivan, *op. cit.*, pp. 7, 8.
[26] See Paul Schilder, *Goals and Desires of Man* (New York: Columbia Univ. Press, 1942), p. 79.
[27] *Instinct* (New York: Holt, 1924), p. 509.

nect the formation of character with the structure of authority in the family.

Within the kinship structure, there is an interplay between deprivations and satisfactions, between the organic needs of the child and the authoritative agency of socialization which provides for these needs. The family upon which the child is dependent is thus the early context of his insecurities and of his gratifications. The child's experience of the organs of his body and his recognition of what he can and what he should not do with them is guided by adults, who try to regulate the rhythm of such functions as excretion and sexual sensations as well as his attitude toward them.

The regulations of organic functions and the social impact of family roles upon the child are closely related experiences. For what Freud called the Oedipus and Electra complexes—attraction for the parent of the opposite sex and jealousy toward the other—is, as Karen Horney notes, simply "engendered by the parent's care of the physical needs of the child," [28] and by the child's dependency upon the parent for this care.

The decisive childhood drama of man's psychic life was schematized by Freud in terms of the identification of the male child with the father of the family who establishes for his boys his model of primary aspiration. As the father loves the mother so does the son, who thus becomes, as did Oedipus, the father's competitor for the exclusive love of the mother. For the female child a similar early triangle is supposed to be repeated, which Freud called the Electra complex. These complexes may originate from the end of the first year up to the age of four or five: however, the critical age, according to most psychoanalysts, is between three and five.

Schemes of this sort have the great merit of showing early character formations in the social context of the family. By knitting together such strong motives and mechanisms as love, identification, and authority, they provide useful explanatory models. It is, however, a model that is open to much abuse—even in the hands of its originator.

One of Freud's greatest shortcomings is that he understood this process as at least quasi-biologically set, and hence a universal occurrence; but this is a universalization of a partial observation, for it overgeneralizes the psychic impact of a particular type of

[28] *New Ways in Psychoanalysis* (New York: Norton, 1939), p. 791.

kinship organization—that of the occidental patriarchal family. Freud, as a sociological thinker, was thus handicapped by Freud, as a medical man. His formulation pointed toward an important sociological phenomenon, but it was not itself sociologically informed. Yet the internalization of a family constellation by the character structure of its youngest member was an important point to observe.

Preliterate as well as historical societies show a great variety of kinship structures, of which the patriarchal organization represents only one. In the absence of the patriarchal family one cannot very readily expect the Oedipus complex to develop in the child's character, much less exert an influence upon the later adult. And even within patriarchal families, this complex is probably not universal. "Restrictive discipline and companionship," Meyer Nimkoff has shown, "are two . . . factors of importance in determining the child's relations to his parents. In general . . . that parent will be preferred who offers more in the way of companionship and exacts less in the way of discipline." [29] The preference for the mother may thus be connected with that type of patriarchal family in which the mother is a source of maternal tenderness and care and the father is the more severe disciplinarian. The development of an equalitarian family in which the parents are equally responsible for discipline and for companionship leads to the child's equal preference for, or equal independence from, both parents. The connection of types of child preference and identification with types of family structure is not, of course, completely uniform.

The Hopi child shows no marked preference for either parent, having agreeable relations with both. The Samoan child, who like the upper-class English child does not typically reside with his parents, has a minimum relation with, and is usually emotionally independent of, them. Marquesan children of both sexes prefer their fathers, who are their adult companions; their mothers, being specialized as courtesans to the limited number of males, neglect or even abuse them. In the Marquesan situation there are

[29] "The Child's Preference for Father or Mother," *American Sociological Review*, August 1942, pp. 517-25. Several of the cases which are given below in the text are taken from citations in this excellent summary article. Others are from Margaret Mead's article, *op. cit.*, and her *Coming of Age in Samoa* (New York: Morrow, 1928); and from Wayne Dennis, *The Hopi Child* (New York: D. Appleton-Century, 1940).

more males than females, a definite maternal neglect, few restrictive regulations on the sex life of the child, and no punishments. There does not occur in this society any Oedipus complex, and females are usually represented in a hostile manner rather than as inflated images of maternal tenderness.[30]

In Freud's formulation, the father is the child's sexual rival and has the most potent authority. Yet these functions are, after all, determined by a particular kinship structure.

The peasant father often exploits his sons in work, whereas the prosperous middle-class fathers may treat theirs as sources of pleasure and display. In some societies, family relations locate family jealousies between brothers, rather than between father and son; in other societies in which there are strong brother-sister taboos, jealousies are likely to occur between brothers over their sisters, rather than over their mother.

Authority certainly does not stop with the father; the authoritarian regulation of impulse and of conduct may begin in the family and with the father, but they are continued in later epochs of the biography by sanctions of the school, church, and job, and ultimately by the state.

Bronislaw Malinowski has compared the Oedipus complex of European patriarchal society with the situation among the Trobriand Islanders. In the latter case, the husband of the mother is not the authoritative male in the life of the child. The mother's brother, or the child's maternal uncle, is the authoritative male, while the child's father is merely a kindly counselor, a helper and companion. The Trobriand father does not support his wife and child, but rather his sister and her children. The wife, therefore, is economically dependent upon her own brother, who, as a maternal uncle, is the arbiter and disciplinarian of the child.[31]

In United States society, the child's dependence upon the mother is used by her to enforce certain regulations upon the child. Among the Marquesans, such dependence is frustrated by the absence of the mother's care, but no restrictive regulations of organic and social activity are imposed. Children are more independent at an

[30] Abram Kardiner, *The Individual and His Society* (New York: Columbia Univ. Press, 1939), p. 248.

[31] See *Sex and Repression in Savage Society* (New York: Harcourt, Brace, 1927) and H. D. Lasswell's critique of Malinowski's work in *Methods in Social Science*, S. H. Rice, ed. (Chicago, 1931), pp. 480 ff.

earlier age than in the United States and acquire a self-confidence which contrasts sharply with the lack of confidence in similar age groups in Western societies.

The Oedipus constellation, with its close blend of dependence upon and craving for the mother, occurs most frequently, according to A. Kardiner, "in societies where the sexual goal is interfered with in childhood. In societies where Oedipus attachment does occur, it should be viewed as the result of kinship organization and restrictive regulations on childhood sexual tendencies which tend to prolong and complicate the dependency of the child." [32]

The imprint of family roles upon the child's character thus varies with the kinship arrangement. The social conditions which the child experiences and his psychic reactions to them must be carefully reconstructed if we are to understand his early character formation.

II. To the individual himself, the most obvious manner in which any earlier phase of his biography may influence later phases is memory. Memory seems to be an inner connection between events and experiences along the biographical line. It also seems to be closely connected with language. Memory is past experience regained by an act of attention.

The young child lives in the immediate present, and probably does not have much conception of the past or of the future. His impulses demand immediate gratification and he cannot delay and wait upon the future to satisfy them. He cries. For the adult, experience is a conjunction of past memories, present situations, and anticipations of the future. To recapture the past by memory, surmount the immediate present, and anticipate the future by imagination, requires the guidance and use of signs. "In studying infantile situations and infantile experiences," Paul Schilder has written, "we should not forget that it is difficult to come to clear conclusions transcending the mere observational, since language—the most reliable sign system—is either absent or not developed in the child." [33]

[32] Op. cit., pp. 481-82.

[33] Goals and Desires of Man (New York, 1942), p. 129. For a wonderfully sensitive account of memory—which unfortunately we came upon only after this book was in press—see Ernest G. Schachtel, "On Memory and Childhood Amnesia," reprinted in A Study of Interpersonal Relations, P. Mullahy, ed. (New York: Hermitage Press, 1949).

Language gives us the pegs upon which memories as well as future anticipations may be fixed. Stenographic reports of the two- to three-year-old child indicate this connection of memory with symbols and verbal processes. Once linked to organic habits, psychic feelings, or segments of experience, symbols may be constantly reorganized in memory and imagination.

We remember others from whom we have been separated according to our desires and fantasies, and the same is true of our memories of our own past selves. The photographs and the stories told us by others limit this work of reconstructive fantasy, but not altogether, for the act of perception is also a construction that is often influenced by our fantasies and anticipations, and the stories our mother and other relatives tell us, to which we listen, and which we remember, are not usually the whole story. Mothers are not notable as scientific observers of their children.

Although patterns formed by the impressionable experiences of the childhood epoch may be difficult to dissolve by subsequent experiences, their influences upon the adult do not seem to be primarily transmitted by explicit memory. Those experiences, actual or imaginary, which were not explicitly nor adequately symbolized are more likely to be the bearers of our past which influences our present and future. But just how do these early formations influence later formations of character?

The conditioning of reflexes and the development of habits during the childhood phase of the organism may carry over into later life. It is doubtful that they persist in identical form, though they may persist in newer integrations and they do limit the later habits that can be acquired. There is continuity and development, not mere repetition; there is a cumulative selection exerted by previously organized habits. Habits, developed in one phase of the biography, are thus often unconscious determinants of later habits. We may be quite unaware of them, until they get us into trouble or limit our learning of new ways. Habits are among the persistent heritages from the training and history of our bodies.

It is the psychic structure that is perhaps most crucial in this question of the adult burden of childhood experiences. Given societies, for example, do not conventionally symbolize many phases of emotional experiences. Sexual interests and sensations may thus remain outside the verbalized areas of the character, and yet determine conscious conduct and psychic life. For the childhood feel-

ings and imagination that are not socialized and anchored by verbalization may nevertheless exert an influence upon later psychic
life. In fact, the influence of such unconscious elements and linkages
may be all the more controlling because they are not normally
remembered and brought to awareness. No symbolic organization
is socially provided for them. And, like the mass activities of the
infant, such elements may avalanche upon the person during
severe crises or strains.[34]

Fears which the child experiences with reference to sex may be
tabooed in conversation and hence remain unverbalized, unana-
lyzed, and subject to the constructions and modifications of imagination. Because of the conventional taboos and inadequate vocabularies on the part of the parents, a *verbal lag*—as far as the psychic
structure is concerned—is typical in Western societies. It has been
noted, by Norman Cameron,[35] that among some strata in Western
civilization "sexual attitudes enter relatively seldom into social
communication. The ratio of sexual attitudes functioning in private
to those freely and genuinely shared with the community is dis-
proportionately high when compared with most other commonly
held attitudes." That is why the imagery, motives, the day and
night dreams, and uncontrolled verbalization in the authoritatively
controlled yet intimate interview, are likely to reveal a large percentage of sexual content. And yet, as we have already noted, the
ready availability of sexual imagery and themes in public life—
in magazines and movies, as well as in "unwritten literature," in
highly informal channels—naturally attracts the child's attention
and concern. It is fair to assume that most children of any given age
are more "knowing" than most parents (and teachers) think they
are.

The verbal lag is facilitated by conventional suppression and
lack of a happy rapport with parents during later epochs of the
biography. The experience and the imagination of the child and
later of the adolescent continue to interplay with, reinforce, or
repress these emotional cravings and impulsive squirmings of the
psychic structure, which show up in the giggles of girls and the

[34] See A. Kardiner, *The Traumatic Neuroses of War* (London: Hoeber,
1941). See also the acute remarks on verbal organization in Lorimer, *op. cit.*,
pp. 185 ff.

[35] See "The Paranoid Pseudo-Community," *American Journal of Sociology*,
July 1943, p. 36.

whistles of boys. They may therefore be unintegrated aspects of the adult character, and may be *repeated* in the adult character in a form identical with their childhood shape. More typically, however, they are modified and fulfill some contemporary function within the adult's integration. Yet they may not be adequately integrated, and hence may be in conflict. In trying fully to understand the adult character, as Karen Horney has held, we must grasp these so-called infantile elements as they function contemporaneously.

To think of infantile trends of the psychic structure as being repeated in identical form in the adult is to assume that they remained "isolated and unaltered" by subsequent developments. Observations—such as the child's tendency to repeat previous experiences, the re-experience of traumatic incidents in similar or identical detail, the practice recall of past experiences under conditions of the psychoanalytic interview—these observations can be adequately explained on grounds other than that of a supposed persistence in the adult of childhood experiences.[36] Moreover, the undue genetic emphasis is open to the criticism that it does not explain *why* the childhood trends and traits persist. Normally, the person "grows out of them," or at least they do not seem to operate within the adult character. But why do they persist in certain cases?

To answer this we have to examine the whole adult psychic and character structure and find out what role they perform in their contemporary setting. In the adult character supposedly childish emotions and techniques of conduct may have a meaning and fulfill a function quite different than in the child. A woman may cry like a child, but her crying after all may not be very childish.

The influence of children's experience upon their adult characters may leave a residue which can be directly discerned. Thus, we "spontaneously" like or dislike a person because this person is linked with early memories of people whom as a child we experienced pleasantly or unsatisfactorily. More importantly, the influence of the childhood experience may be due to the simple fact that the adult character structure develops from the one formed in childhood. It is in childhood that the character is first formed

---

[36] This position is taken by Karen Horney, see *op. cit.*, Chapters 4, 8, and 9, especially pp. 136-38 and 158.

and the adult one is thereby started. Although one may not often draw a straight and isolated line from an adult trait back to a specific childhood experience, one can see that the experiences which formed the adult character include the childhood structures and developed from them. If early traits fit in with, and reinforce present trends of character, they are all the more likely to exert an influence upon the adult's conduct and experience.

The general direction and the degree of this development depend upon the adult functions which traits acquired in childhood may come to have. And as we shall now see, the answer to this psychological question also depends upon distinctively sociological factors.

8. *The Social Relativity of Childhood Influences*

To answer the questions of how much weight we should assign to the childhood phase of the biography, and what adult features of character are most likely to be infantile in origin, we have to know something about the full biography and something about the society in which it is lived out. We have to consider entire biographical patterns, not only as they are lived out but as they are laid down in different social structures. Let us first discuss several types of societies which permit very different answers to our general question.

If the pace of social change is rapid, then the world of youth is more likely to be different from the adult world. Historical tempo is not of course the only condition leading to such differences between child and adult. Even if the rate of social change is slow, the age stratification of the society may be very rigid and the things expected of the child very different from those expected of the adult. Still another factor favoring differences in roles played by the youthful and by the mature is the extent of the societies' complexity. For this means that there may be complicated roles which take time to learn to enact in an acceptable and mature manner.

Yet this need not be the case, for a complex society may be specialized in such a way that any one person need only learn his specialty: the child may have to develop beyond the youthful roles only in one or two respects—such as the job; the remainder of his roles may not be so very different from those he learned in childhood; these roles may continue to work quite well throughout the person's biography.

An extreme division of labor and specialization may block the development by practice of features other than those held suitable to childhood. Only in the skills required for the specialty will development occur. Thus the theoretical expert may be relatively undeveloped in manual skills, not knowing how to use a snow shovel or lathe, or he may be "deficient" in the capacity for mature love and affection, experiencing throughout his life an adolescent embarrassment in front of all women.

If in a society there are many large differences between the roles expected of the child and the roles of the adult world, then patterns acquired during childhood are less likely to be successful if they persist in the adult. Accordingly we may ask of any given society, how many psychic or character traits which "worked" in childhood continue to secure satisfactions and security in adult life?

A narrow gap between the child and the adult world may be due to a lack of complexity, the intrinsic difficulties and diversities of the roles in the adult society, or to the fact that the expectations for adults are from a very early period focused upon the child.

Societies differ greatly in the degrees to which childhood roles approximate those of adults. Thus, among the Chuckchees, childhood seems "largely an imitation of the life of elders." [37] "The plains Indians constructed for their children miniature camps, encouraged them to enact the scenes of adult life; the Samoans banish children from even imitating adult conditions and give them small tasks graded to their skill; the Kaffirs give their children unpleasant jobs and lie about the facts of life, and the children retaliate by developing a small outlaw state with a secret language and spy system of its own. The Manus use play only to develop physical proficiency, no attempt to instill the cultural conventions or the industrial techniques is made." [38]

To view anxiety in an adult as an infantile attitude is "to confuse two different things, to mistake for an infantile attitude an attitude merely generated in childhood. With at least as much justification as calling anxiety an infantile reaction one might call it a

[37] See Abram Kardiner, op. cit., p. 121.
[38] See Margaret Mead, "The Primitive Child," Handbook . . . p. 680.

precocious attitude in a child." [39] It is, in large part, a question of the size of the social gap between child and adult with reference to specific traits and roles.

Infant or childhood patterns which are successful in satisfying the infant or child are less likely to be modified or dropped. If many childhood patterns are not agreeable to an adolescent's peers, he will cling to them only at the risk of losing prestige. In America the modifications and rejections of childhood patterns are accompanied by a good deal of the pose of toughness and the mannerisms taken to be the adult swagger. A society that not only contains a large gap between the expectations on various age groups but which is also very rapidly changing, thus accentuating this gap, will typically require many changes of trait and mannerism in the course of the biography.

If the early adolescent cannot find new alternative patterns which can replace the gratifications of the older patterns he is more likely to cling to childhood ones. If the sequence of life experiences permits gratifications to accrue from these early patterns, repeated in adolescent and adult worlds without much modification, we may speak, not of repetition, but of *social lines of facilitation.*

These lines are just as important in understanding the persistence of childhood or adolescent traits as are the original experiences of childhood or adolescence during which the traits were acquired. Indeed they may be more important, and they are certainly more immediately relevant to the understanding of the function of the trait within the adult character structure.

The conception of social lines of facilitation permits us to individualize our discussion of the differing bearings of such social factors as age stratification upon the adult persistence of traits acquired during childhood. Of any given person and his society we may ask: Has this person found adult roles which permit or even encourage the continued use of traits acquired during childhood?

There are certain types of marriage, for instance, the success of which rests upon tacit agreement to allow the husband or the wife, or both, to play the child or adolescent in certain roles and aspects of personality. Housewives may thus successfully employ

[39] K. Horney, *The Neurotic Personality of Our Time* (New York: Norton, 1937), p. 78.

the infantile tear, or the temper-tantrum, or the form of hysteria known as the crying-jag, in order to achieve their ends. In popular songs, phrases like "sugar daddy"—social expressions and facilitations of infantilism—are explicitly revealed: "O! Daddy!" one such "incest song" runs, "You ought to get the best for me!" And another: "While knocking off, a game of golf, I may make a play for the caddy; but when I do, I don't follow through, 'cause my heart belongs to daddy."

The weight of childhood in adult character is conditioned by regression under traumatic experience, the adult function of traits within the adult character, the spread of the age-structure of a society, and by the availability and use of social lines of facilitation for given character traits and formations.

Character structure, as we have seen throughout Part Two, refers to the unique individual. It stands for the individual variations of the types of persons usual in given societies or strata within given societies. These variations arise because of different constitutions and because of the different ways in which the psychic structure is integrated with the person. The uniqueness of the individual—the particular composition and unity which he achieves—arises from his differing experiences and from his cumulative ordering of these experiences. Although the roles which two persons play and have played may seem identical, the way in which they have each played them and the different sequence in their respective biographies means that very different character structures are formed.

Yet all of the uniqueness and unity of a character structure may not be telescoped into the past. Experience and its effects involve an interplay of past, present, and future. Unique traits may arise from differences in life goals and anticipations, as well as from past experience and present situation. The future as well as the past and the present need to be taken into account in explaining a given character structure.

We do not simply remember isolated events in our past. We remember events fitted into a framework. This framework is given us by our society, and that which fits into it and fills it out may be remembered better than what we cannot thus locate. It is reported by Bartlett that after several members of a Zulu tribe visited London the one thing which stood out vividly in their memories was the image of an English policeman standing in traffic with uplifted arm. This gesture happens to be the sign of greeting among members of their tribes; it was one of the few images that fitted immediately into the social framework of their memories and was retained.[40]

In similar manner, the life plan of the individual, his philosophy of life, and his expectations and specific goals, normally fit into a large social framework, which is typical of members of his social position, and which limits the scope of his construction of a possible future. To limit, however, is not to determine. The structure of a man's future as he sees it is subject to marked individual modification from the life plan suggested by his social position in a particular society at a given time.

Problems occur and decisions must be formulated which involve anticipations of the future as well as habits of the past. Conflicting expectations exacted of us by others do not necessarily end in a deadlock or in mere drifting, but often in a redirecting of our conduct and sometimes of our life plan. Some major goal of our life plan may be the rallying point of present conduct. This selection of goal and the arrangement of present activities as means to its realizations are, of course, a distinctive form of the conscious and intelligent character. In varying degrees we control our present conduct by the future which we anticipate and desire, and just as we respond to the cut of the knife before we are cut by it, so we take roles in anticipation of the reactions of others, in order to avoid anxieties or to gain ends wanted.

By anticipation, the future operates in the present; we act now in terms of that future. These anticipations are the conditions of our present conduct and stylizations of self. All experience probably has such elements of the anticipated future in it, for we respond to the present signs of future objects: we run when there is smoke, although we have not seen fire. And when we are frustrated, we seek out such signs, items available in the present which indicate the future. By selecting these signs and changing our behavior in terms of them, we use future consequences as guides for present conduct.

Were we fully to trace out the biographies typical of a society's

[40] F. C. Bartlett, *Remembering* (Cambridge: Cambridge Univ. Press, 1932), p. 248.

members, from before birth until after death, we would also have to study a great deal about the roles and institutions of the society. For the biography of a person consists of the transformations in character which result from abandoning roles and taking on new ones.

PART THREE

SOCIAL STRUCTURE

C H A P T E R

V I I

Institutions and Persons

IN the present chapter, we shall elaborate some of the ways in which persons and institutions may be related, thus attempting to make clear the psychology of institutions and the sociology of persons. For we believe that the psychological results of social relations often provide the necessary and sufficient motivations for personal conduct, and since social relations occur within societies, if we are to understand the single human being, we must develop a general view of institutions and of social structures. In terms of our model of man and society, then, what are the more or less direct ways in which character and social structure are related?

1. The Institutional Selection of Persons

Institutions select and eject their members in accordance with a wide variety of formal rules and informal codes. Formal prerequisites for assuming and relinquishing roles may be specific criteria of age, sex, health (as in recruitment for the United States armed forces); they may involve elaborate examinations of specialized skills or aptitudes or tests of "personality traits" (as in the civil service or in many larger corporations). Churches may recruit their members hereditarily, by infant baptism, or they may demand self-conscious choice and personal commitment, indicated by "conversion experiences," as necessary qualifications for adult baptism. Such formal rules may be supplemented by informal codes of entrance; in fact, it is quite usual for both formal and informal types of qualifications to operate in the institutional selection of persons.

Birth is a necessary, but not always a sufficient, condition for the assumption of institutional roles. The ancient Greeks and Romans, for example, practiced infanticide. The Spartan magistrate surveyed the newly born and selected those fit to survive; infants which this eugenic-minded military man thought unfit were condemned to death by exposure. The Roman *paterfamilias* considered the newly born "his child" only after having ceremoniously acknowledged it to be such; without this religious act the unwanted progeny was subject to infanticide. Thus, in pre-Christian antiquity, the child neither had a "right to be born" nor a "birth right" to be reared. Only after religious induction by the father did it become a "person" endowed with "rights." Similarly in certain regions of India there are strikingly imbalanced ratios of male and female children because high castes practice female infanticide, leaving it to lower castes to rear brides for their sons.

Birth alone, then, does not guarantee that the newly born will be incorporated into a family, and if he is, he may be only a provisional member of the household. Should he prove to be handicapped, physically or mentally, to a degree unsatisfactory to the relevant institutional orders, the authorities of these orders may "institutionalize" him in another order.

Birth also places the Western infant in a particular social stratum and milieu of a national state, and, where "infant baptism" exists, into a religious institution. All of this, in Western societies, is understood to be part of "the accident of birth." In the United States, whether one is "born with a silver spoon in one's mouth" or is the descendant of a Negro slave is considered to be a matter of blind fate. But in India, where the child is born into a caste society and there is belief in the "transmigration of souls," no such "accident of birth" exists. The highborn and the lowborn are believed to have "merited," in compensation for a previous life, their respective fates at birth.

The more a society gauges people in terms of their "backgrounds," the more fateful for them as individuals will be their descent or "birth right." Thus, the child does not enter social life as an "original man." The stage is set for him; with his birth cry he announces merely his claim to be admitted to a drama that has long been underway. During his life cycle he learns to assume and to discard roles, and each phase of his life offers role opportunities of its own.

Age often determines what we may and may not do. What the child plays in earnest, the adult may play for fun; what the adult plays in earnest is beyond the child's ability and understanding. As adults we become "too old" for some roles; as children we are "still too young" for others.

The same is true for sexual differences. In most societies girls and boys, women and men play certain widely different roles. Among adults we speak of the "sexual division of labor." We speak of the "housewife" (but not of the "househusband"), and when we speak of the "provider" we are usually thinking of the male rather than the female. Of course, the interchanging of role does occur, as during the depression of the thirties. Then quite a few women learned to earn money after their husbands had given up any hope of finding gainful employment. Again, in the forties, many a young woman was gainfully employed—she, "the provider," and he, her "dependent"—in order to see her G.I. husband through college.

Before World War II, when men spoke of "women in arms" they thought of ancient Amazons or of goddesses like Pallas Athena with lance and shield, or of Diana with bow and arrow. So when Russian women made their appearance as tank-riding soldiers in the Finnish-Russian war of 1939, the Western world was taken by surprise. But the incorporation of women into the United States armed forces, as Wacs or Waves, may be only the beginning of "equality in arms." Once it was held that women had to be silent in church, but they fought for and gained the right of prophesying. Once it was held that woman's place was in the home, that she had no right to higher education and professional employment; but she "emancipated" herself from such restrictions and gained such rights. By the end of World War I, throughout the Western world (with the exception of France) women had gained the right to vote, although they still receive less compensation for the same work than men receive. Social differences between men and women, it is clear, are due less to "natural differences" than to differences in institutional opportunities.

Man's weakness in childhood, and again in old age, binds him close to the household. He begins by learning to play his roles in a few "primary groups," in the family, the play group, the neighborhood. When he is enrolled in kindergarten and grammar school, in Sunday school and youth associations, he is introduced into "secondary groups." He learns to compete for grades, to struggle for impersonal standards of achievement, to abide by the "rules of the game," to "take his defeat," to be a "good loser," and to enjoy his triumphs. He acquires physical and symbolic skills; and he learns to identify with Our Classmates, Our School, Our Town, Our Religion, Our Nation.

To grow up, as we have said, means to discard specific childhood roles and to assume an expanding range of adult roles. These roles make up the social content of our mature personalities.

Men assuming identical roles are variously esteemed for the ways in which they play them. Thus, we speak of great presidents and of weak ones, of eminent and of not-so-eminent teachers and scholars. We rate persons who are assuming provisional roles, as promising or not so promising, in anticipation of their future contributions. These estimates of the ways men play their roles should be distinguished from our estimations of the roles themselves—whether these roles are more or less important, of central or of peripheral significance; whether in terms of social visibility they allow the actor a conspicuous or an inconspicuous position. When focusing upon such aspects of the role as such, we often refer to "status position," which we shall later discuss in its psychological aspect.[1]

Individuals often experience the roles they assume as a series of tasks, according to the demands and expectations which others address to them. They may completely identify themselves with certain roles, and so "put their hearts into" enacting them. This is likely to happen when they have deliberately chosen their roles, say as lover and spouse of this particular partner, or as militant fighter for this cause and for no other: "Here I stand, I can do no other, so help me God," said Luther at the end of his speech before the Reichstag at Worms. Similar postures may occur when men are born into their roles, as members of nations, churches, language communities—and so take them for granted—or when they take authoritative roles assigned them by superiors, much as children in patriarchal families will "honor" their parents by accepting the marriage partner or occupation chosen by them.

But in a society which expects its youthful members to choose their roles "freely," that is, at their own risk and accountability, the internalization of roles will vary greatly in depth. This is especially so in a dynamic context of competitive values and controversial ideas, for then some people may become confused and dis-

[1] See Chapter XI: Stratification and Institutional Orders, Section 3: The Status Sphere.

cover that they lack the capacity to "make up their minds." Others may discover that it does not pay to identify themselves with their roles too closely or too intensely, and that a relatively loose fitting of the role—while on the look-out for the next chance—rather than fixed attention to the task at hand is more rewarding and offers more "bargaining power."

Where their skills are scarce and in demand, persons may seek to drive home their "indispensability" by constantly threatening to cease enacting the roles involved. Where many workers or staff members actually do come and go, we speak of a high turnover of labor or of staff. At some given point such turnover may prove wasteful, since those who leave take with them their experience and those who come have to be "broken in on the job." Thus, when the distribution of skills is unmanaged, labor shortages may exist side by side with unemployment.

It is in such contexts that men learn to see themselves "distanced" from any particular occupational role. They face their occupational life in terms of a multiplicity of opportunities, with only segmental involvement in any one of them. They are ready to take up different jobs, finding fulfillment in all and in none, that is, allowing none to take firm hold of their entire personalities. German humanists of the Napoleonic age protested, in the name of universal man, against vocational specialization. And economically secure nobilities may consider aloofness from any special occupational role their privilege, and so busy themselves only with occasional political, administrative, or military tasks, never allowing any single pursuit to fix them into an enduring role.

On the other hand, the old-world peasant and artisan, as well as the modern professional career-man—the teacher, army officer, artist, minister, doctor, or lawyer—is more likely to identify himself with his vocational role intensely and for life.

Roles in voluntary associations are often stratified as permanent, provisional, or transient. Where there is a premium on "seniority," those with permanent roles may successfully claim prestige. In political parties such claims are usually raised by the "old vanguard," "Fascisti of the first hour," "Old fighter of the Nazi party," "Charter member," and the like. In local communities, the corresponding phrases are: "old families," the "pioneers," "old settlers," or "old timers," in contrast with "newcomers," "new residents," or "new members." Transient members of communities and organizations are frequently called "footloose" or "floaters"; in political parties, they are frequently called "fly-by-nights" or "driftwood." In the family we speak of "the newly married" and we honor long marital companionship by celebrating a "silver" and a "golden" wedding anniversary. In the economic order, honorific distinctions are made in favor of "old wealth," in contrast to recently acquired wealth. In most modern societies, inherited wealth ranks higher than newly accumulated wealth; the heir or the heiress of the economic royalist ranks higher than the "self-made man" who, at least in some circles, is made to feel a parvenu by those having more exalted "backgrounds." In this, as in many other respects, the countries of the New World no longer differ from those of Old Europe.

Man's resignation from institutions is variously patterned. Some organizations, such as churches, monastic orders, or totalitarian parties, acknowledge death as the sole legitimate exit for their members. The formal act through which an individual is eliminated from his role in an economic institution usually takes the form of a "notice" or a "nonrenewal" of contract, or a retirement from business or assignment to the status of the temporarily unemployed or permanently unemployable. In the religious order, loss of membership may be voluntary or may occur against the will of the member. In the latter case, in the Catholic church, we speak of "excommunication," or in certain Protestant churches and sects, of "being dropped from membership." In the political order, especially the state itself, the person may be deprived of "civic rights"; if naturalized he may be "denaturalized," and if an immigrant, he may be "deported" to his country of origin, or banned as an "outlaw."

In a world of national states, to be expelled from one state for political or religious reasons often makes admission to the territory of another quite a problem. Leon Trotsky, after his expulsion from the Soviet Union, for instance, found himself in "a world without visa"; many other earlier fugitives from Bolshevism found themselves "stateless" and received a special status through the League of Nations' "Nansen Pass." Since the advent of Hitlerism, no comparable instrument has been created. Jews driven from Germany to the East found themselves for months in a no-man's-land, for Poland refused to admit them. The age-old right of the political fugitive to asylum in another country is no longer honored. Nowadays in Europe, eight years after "the shooting war," there are still millions of "displaced persons," that is, "stateless persons," without civic rights, who have found no country willing to accept them as "new citizens."

In the kinship order we speak of the "divorcée" and of the "lost son." In the military order, of the "veteran" or the "reservist" who has received his "honorable discharge," or of the man who has been tried by "court martial," of the man who absentees himself without permission as "having gone AWOL," and finally of the "deserter." If such men escape court jurisdiction, we speak of "fugitives from justice." The disloyal party member is called a "renegade"; the disloyal religious believer an "apostate." Hitler was ruled out of Christendom by President Roosevelt, although the Pope—an expert in divine matters—did not declare him an "apostate," however sinful a Christian he may have been considered.

So, during their active lives, do men enter, play, and leave roles.

During their declining years they see their friends drop out of their lives; then opportunities to mourn become more frequent and opportunities to continue their roles with their age peers diminish. In time, they "retire" from vocational life; and as the range of their active roles shrinks, they become housebound, and finally they die. For although in industrialized nations more people live longer than formerly, we shall all have to die although no one knows when he personally will have to go. This knowledge is biographically acquired, and like all thoughts of "unpleasant facts" it is not always fully accepted.

In one of his most ingenious, although as usual problematical, papers,[2] Freud has interpreted the heroic valor of the soldier who "goes over the top" as a regression to an archaic psychic state in which the individual acts as if nothing could ever happen to him, that is, a state in which he is basically convinced of his own immortality. Freud's "hero" is thus a soldier who has "forgotten" that he is mortal, risks his life in combat, and so unwittingly loses his life. This may well be an oversimplification: some soldiers may *knowingly* seek death in combat. For example, the "crusader" who knows what he fights for and fights for what he knows may minimize his fear of personal death to the zero point, and accept his death as inevitable and near. The image of the last stand of the

[2] Sigmund Freud, "Thoughts for the Times on War and Death," *Collected Papers*, Vol. IV (London, 1946), especially pp. 307 ff.

Spartan warriors at Thermopylae also comes to mind, and we should remember that the Romans summed up their military morale by the saying: "It is sweet and becoming to die for one's country," which would seem to characterize men who realize that they are mortal yet are willing to risk and, if need be, lose their lives in combat. And there is the ideal image of the Christian martyr, who, though he died for a different cause, was in general agreement with this Roman view. The same holds for pioneers of modern ideas, such as Giordano Bruno, who was burned at the stake, or for Communists such as Levine, court martialed at Munich in 1918, who referred to himself, in the language of expressionism, as a "corpse on vacation."

At any rate, we do not experience our death: it is the end of all experience. Yet whatever we experience just before death can be known to us only if the decline of our life does not end in death but in recovery. Man's knowledge of death does sometimes add a component of fear to his image of death, but even after the loss of consciousness—since anesthesia—man may "fight death" and recover. On the other hand, men may reconcile themselves to death and die as Abraham did, "full of days"; and some may even seek death in suicide. Yet what testimony we have concerning the alleged "experience of death" is the testimony of those who, like Dostoevski before the firing squad, were "close to death" but somehow continued to live. They did not experience death itself, and so they report their attitude toward death, not their experience of it.

Though death is man's final exit from all worldly roles, his corpse remains to his relatives, and to a variety of experts. In funeral rites and in sanitary services, funeral directors, cemetery wardens, gravediggers or cremators, are in charge. The mummification of ancient Egyptian pharaohs and, in our time, of Lenin; the royal tombs in the form of Egytian pyramids or the mausoleum in Moscow's Red Square, the Christian cross and its alleged remains in the form of relics, the organized care of soldiers' cemeteries, the memorial rites for the Unknown Soldier of World War I at the Cenotaph in London, the Arc de Triomphe of Paris, and the Arlington Cemetery in Washington—all these serve to "immemorialize" the memories of men who are felt to have cast long shadows through history. Religious and filial piety, biographical interest and secular hero worship, thus monumentalize the memory image of the deceased after men cease to play any live role.

2. *The Institutional Formation of Persons*

Institutions not only select persons and eject them; institutions also form them. In our discussion of the biography, we have indicated some of the ways in which this occurs. Institutions in the several orders, as we shall see, may also have special educational spheres by means of which people are socially trained to enact the roles of the institution;[3] and, of course, in the informal context of any institution, education—even to the point of a social transformation of the person—may proceed. Impulse and sensitivity are channeled and transformed into standard motives joined to standard goals and gratifications. Thus, institutions imprint their stamps upon the individual, modifying his external conduct as well as his inner life. For one aspect of learning a role consists of acquiring motives which guarantee its performance.[4]

But the key mechanism by which institutions form persons involves the circle of significant others which the institution establishes.[5] This is important because it in due course leads, for full institutional members, to changes in the generalized other. By internalizing the expectations of institutional heads, as particular others, the persons who enact the institutional role, come to control themselves—to pattern and to enact their roles in accordance with the constraints thus built into their characters. As they develop as institutional members, these constraints are often generalized, and are thus linked psychologically with particular institutions.

There are two general ways in which persons may be attached to institutions, and only one of them involves the generalized other, socially anchored in the institution and internalized by persons who are its members.

(I) Institutional heads may appeal to their members in terms of the generalized other, and so make it a religious or moral duty for them to develop sentiments of attachment to the institution. So Jews and Christians teach their children "Honor thy father and

---

[3] See Chapter IX: Institutional Orders and Social Controls, II, Section 4: The Educational Sphere.

[4] See Chapter V: The Sociology of Motivation.

[5] See Chapter IV: The Person.

thy mother: that thy days may be long upon the land which the Lord thy God giveth thee." Christian parents are unlikely to teach Jesus's words "Follow me; and let the dead bury their dead," or "I am come to set a man at variance against his father and the daughter against her mother." Thus is institutional solidarity explicitly trained and upheld. (II) Those in control of an institution, or acting within it, may appeal to the sense of expediency of the members. Affiliation with or adherence to the institution is then regarded as a rationally calculated advantage.

In the first case, where the generalized other is trained, the individual is expected to maintain membership "for better or for worse"; in the second, where rational calculation is the rule, the maintenance of the individual's membership is dependent upon his advantage in the maintenance of the institution, or upon the mutual advantage of the several members. Accordingly, the nature of solidarity and of its sentimentalization differs, which is what Ferdinand Tönnies had in mind when he spoke of the differences between "communal relations" with their moral sentiment, and "societal relations," with their expedient calculations of interest.

Different institutional orders seem typically to vary as to which type of attachment prevails: communities of actual or alleged common descent—such as the family, clan, sib, tribe, nation—are characterized by solidarity sentiments making it a magical, sacred, or moral obligation of the members to give such sentiments priority over all considerations of expediency. Nationalism, to be sure, is a modern mass sentiment of great complexity and variation, but the slogan, "My country, right or wrong" places the attachment to one's nation "beyond good and evil," and thus corresponds to the valuation of the king as the head of the nation who "can do no wrong." [6]

The intensity of such solidarity is based upon its foundation in the superego of persons, combined with rationalizations of power

[6] Since the end of World War I this evaluation of the heads of states has been widely renounced. In articles 227-30 of the Versailles Peace Treaty, the allied powers placed Wilhelm II under public accusation because of infractions of "the international moral law and the sanctity of treaties." After World War II a new international law was proclaimed which is based upon "natural law" and introduces the principles of retroactivity and guilt by association. It does not define "aggression," and so, given the present power constellation, one can only conclude that among modern nations, "the victor can do no wrong."

and prestige which enlist a variety of private interests—economic, military, and bureaucratic. Hitler summed it up in the phrase "Right is what benefits the German people," which may be said to mark one end of all universalist standards, whether religious, moral, or legal. The intensity of such loyalty sentiments is relevant for the degree to which a social structure is politically cohesive; and the scope of the values which institutional leaders can successfully attach to such loyalty patterns—by holding their particular institutions to be the depository of all possible values—is of course relevant for social cohesion, because the individual who is confronted with such claims may be too weak to define his own value position in the face of such a "total opposition." Accordingly, such loyalties are decisive for the sacrifices which individual members are expected to be ready to make for the common cause.

Totalitarian societies and regimes seek to build up such total loyalties by their programs of "cadre training." Hitler, however, despite the aid of his "German Christians," never succeeded in breaking Christian universalism. Stalin, on the other hand, after having made his peace with the Eastern church, has been more successful: the juxtaposition of a "dialectical science of nature" (as against, for example, "bourgeois genetics"), of "proletarian or socialist realism" in the fine arts and in literature (as against "bourgeois formalism" and other deviations), and of "Soviet Man" (against all other types of man—feudal, bourgeois, cosmopolitan, or petty-bourgeois) divides sharply the value preferences and thoughtways of the communist ingroup from all those on the outside. Universalist criteria of the true, the good, and the beautiful are thus discarded, and in fact considered quite unavailable.

One of the features of this new orthodoxy is that no institutional order is permitted to develop prestigeful roles on its own ground. For all loyalties, and thus for all prestige and for all authority, there must be one fountainhead. Success in any field may thus be ascribed to the head of the state, who in turn distributes all honor. So there are medals for warriors and for workers, for artists and for the mothers who bear many children. All achievement is preconditioned by the correct course of the totalitarian leadership, and hence all achievement is credited to its wise and infallible course. Criticism may be made only of its inadequate means, not— once they are officially promulgated—of its ends. And no one can deviate from whatever "line" has been defined for each field of endeavor.

The modern totalitarian leader thus resurrects the image of the ancient patriarch who was supreme judge, chief provider, military leader, and head religious functionary, all in one. The individual member of his family had no alternative orientation, and functionally specialized motives met on the common basis of all obligation, defined in terms of filial piety. Such obligations included the obligation to honor one's father and mother, to provide for them to the end of their days, to be devoted to their memories and to care for their burial and their grave, to obey their expressed wishes with regard to the disposition of the inheritance, to take over the blood feud as a right and an obligation of successorship, never to depart from the God of the fathers and His ways, and to respect one's wife, chosen by one's father.

If the private integration of persons and the public cohesion of institutions may be achieved by (a) personal leadership, (b) by eliciting co-operation in common tasks, or (c) by joint utilization of things—such as the house and its contents—then we may say that the patriarchal family of old, as well as the totalitarian society of the Soviet Union today, is "integrated" on all three levels. For such societies make all the instruments of production, administration, and warfare a "common property," develop a cult of the leader, and define common tasks for all in terms of the "quota fulfillments" set forth in the "plans" promulgated from on high.

3. The Theory of Premiums and Traits of Character

The chief mechanism by which persons are formed by institutions has to do with the way types of persons are "built" by the combinations of various roles which compose them, and by their cumulative reactions to these roles. In Chapter IV, as well as in the present chapter, we have discussed some of the relevant mechanisms as they involve images of the self and the generalized other. In this section, we want to display a further way by which individual phenomena—specific "traits" of the individual's character— may be linked with institutional contexts.

Traits of the individual may usefully be classified according to the scope of the occasions on which the trait appears, and the zone or zones of the character structure in which the trait is integrated. These two points of observation may be related. For example, if a trait is a feature of the organism, the scope of its appearance may coincide with the appearance of the individual, and it may in one way or another, become integrated with all zones of the character structure. Thus the roles available to a man born with a hunched back will be restricted, and the way he combines and reacts to these roles, as well as the self-images reflected from them, will be modified. These facts about his roles and his self may in turn affect the opportunities of given components of the psychic structure to be socialized, in which case the organic trait of his hunchback may be integrated with traits in all zones of his character structure. Such traits may thus cue a pattern of other traits in other zones of character, restricting and shaping whatever traits are to become part of the total character.

There is no general principle of character structure in terms of which any one trait always leads to the selection of other traits. The reason for this is that character traits are presented by and through the medium of interpersonal relations and most traits are relative to the institutional and other interpersonal contexts in which they are presented. The traits of a person should not, therefore, be ascribed merely to that one person, as if he were a turkey into which different traits were stuffed. What is "selfishness" to one circle of persons may to another circle be "initiative," or to either circle the trait may be selfishness *or* initiative according to when, how, and where it is revealed.

There are two considerations involved: first, the context of the trait's occurrence, and second, the different way or ways in which it may be evaluated by different persons. Those traits which appear in the enactment of a limited number of roles we may call *specific traits;* those which are presented in a wide variety of roles enacted by the person we may call *general traits.* If a trait is evaluated positively by significant others, we may say that a *premium* is placed upon its development and presentation. If the trait is evaluated negatively, or if the person is in any way restrained from presenting it, we may say that the trait is *tabooed.*

A premium or a taboo may itself be used generally or specifically. Thus, if selfishness is generally tabooed, it means that all its appearances are interpreted as selfishness and are tabooed. If it is specifically tabooed, only in certain roles will its presentation be tabooed.

In like manner, a trait may be generally or specifically "premi-umed," that is, a premium may be placed upon it no matter when, where, or by whom it is displayed, or, a premium may be applied only when the trait is displayed by certain persons enacting certain roles on certain occasions.

Taboos or premiums may be applied by coercion—by actual re-straint of the bodily movements which are involved in presenting the trait; by co-operating socially with the performance or failing to do so; by the use of gestures—the smile, the frown, the flicker of an eyelid—to encourage or to restrain the presentation of the trait; or by using words which designate the trait in question in a positive or in a negative manner. Systems of premiums and taboos need not be verbalized, but if they do become fixed in the language, this fact may stabilize the system and facilitate its diffusion from specific to generalized application. An eulogistic term for some trait may thus increase the chances that people will approve it.

There are no general psychological traits which exist as universals in the character structure, irrespective of specific contexts. The only meaning we can usefully give "general trait" is: used in all or most contexts. We can then ask: What are the sociological con-ditions which favor the development in persons of general traits? And, conversely, what are the conditions under which we may expect specific traits to be developed?

We must emphasize this specialization of character traits, because a nonsociological psychology and an idealistic emphasis upon the "harmony" of the human personality have caused some students to underestimate, if not overlook, it. Character traits are not universals within a character structure; they must always be seen and under-stood by the social psychologist as tied to given ranges of social situations.

The controversy as to whether or not a person has "general traits" or only "particular traits" may be resolved with the aid of the con-cepts we have presented. Generalized traits are likely to develop if the roles a person incorporates are all similar. And the fact of such similarity is, of course, dependent on the kind of society in which the person lives, as well as upon his choice of roles, from all those available, at any given time.

Where a majority of the institutional roles making up a society follow a similar principle, the character traits formed in one context have a chance to operate in another. To this extent, the opportunity for general traits to develop in persons is maximized.[7] In many contexts, however, such a generalization of traits is not socially possible. Perhaps it is true that a man who has acquired control over his body in dangerous sports is likely to be more sure of his bodily control in dangerous physical work or in warfare, whereas a man who lacks this readiness to risk his body may the more readily ascribe "courage" to those who do have it. Yet, the "courage" of the artist to brave for years the scorn of outraged critics is different from the "courage" of the soldier. In fact, the courageous man of the typewriter need not at all be the courageous man of the machine gun—yet both may be "courageous," willing to face risks.

When the roles composing a social structure are specialized into more or less autonomous institutions, the traits of men are likely to be segregated and specific. A man may cheat his wife but not his business partner, or vice versa. On the field of sport the football player may be a ruthless tackler, but on the dance floor an awkward partner and timid competitor. The political courage of a local leader may or may not carry over to the courage of a national leader, the dimensions and requirements of the latter role being enormously enlarged. Lenin is a case in point; Kerensky represents the reverse. An American may be enraged at earlier British treatment of the Burmese, but not upset at American treatment of Southern Negroes.

Because of such facts, no general discussion of allegedly universal traits in terms of the isolated person is apt to be fruitful. In any society, and with reference to given types of character structure, it is a matter for empirical research to determine how far traits are generalized or how far they are segregated according to contexts. We may, however, contribute to the tools useful for such work by considering various kinds of individual traits as they are presented and evaluated by others:

I. A general trait that is generally premiumed has a high chance to continue to be presented by the person and to be firmly organized into his character. A person predominantly composed of such

[7] The so-called "problem of transfer of training" has been given relatively fruitless answers by many psychologists because they fail to consider the sociological conditions that are involved. Experimental studies, in U.S. society and laboratories, have usually indicated very little transfer.

traits in a society of harmonious premiums is apt to be unified—and static.

II. A specific trait that is generally premiumed will tend to spread, to become a general trait. A person predominantly composed of such traits in a society of high and ready premiums is apt to be an expanding person, although perhaps suffering the tensions of his growth. Suppose a general premium is placed upon the specific trait of kindness; we would then expect that kindness would tend to become general. Yet the general premium on kindness may continue to be restricted to kindness toward certain kinds of persons, for no premium is absolutely general: to be kind to Negroes may continue to be tabooed in many contexts of Negro-white relations. General premiums of specific traits may even be turned into specific taboos: during a war, to be kind to one of the enemy may be tabooed, indeed, it may be treason.

Premiums thus have a life of their own, a dynamic by which they become less general and turn into specific premiums, or even change into specific or general taboos. Skill at welding may be highly premiumed by everyone when it is done in the shop, but the welder's wife may taboo it in the kitchen: it is a specific trait generally premiumed but it is not likely to become a general trait.

III. A general trait that is specifically premiumed will tend to become a specific trait, or, if kept general, to be modified or camouflaged in all contexts except the one in which it is specifically premiumed. If a person presents traits that are evaluated as selfish or grasping in all his roles, the lack of general premiums on these traits may make him restrict their presentation to one or two roles, such as occur in small business conduct, where there is a chance that they will be specifically premiumed.

A person who is predominantly composed of general traits that are specifically premiumed is like "a bull in a china shop." He has not yet learned to segregate the display of traits according to appropriate contexts; he is making too much of what, in its proper place, might be a good thing.

IV. A specific trait that is specifically premiumed will tend to be stabilized; a person predominantly composed of such traits will be a compartmentalized specialist.

A similar scheme of the social tendencies of personal traits is possible in terms of taboos: I. The chances for a general trait that is generally tabooed to develop in the person are very low, but if developed, its chances to disappear are very high. II. A specific trait that is generally tabooed will tend to be given up in its specific context and not to spread to other contexts. III. A general trait that is specifically tabooed will tend to become less general or even to become a specific trait. IV. A specific trait that is specifically tabooed will tend to be repressed in the specifically tabooed context. If it is firmly integrated in the person, he may try to realize it in other contexts.

So far, in our discussion of the sociology of individual traits, we have written in terms of the person, intentionally omitting consideration of other zones of the character. We have stated several general propositions on the assumption that "other things were equal." We must now probe behind these "other things," for in reality, economists not withstanding, other things are not "equal."

Omitting traits that are visible features of the organic constitution, there seem to be three general factors which select and refract traits in any given character structure. To understand how a given trait comes to be part of the character structure requires that we pay attention to these factors:

I. Social premiums and taboos are applied to traits by currently significant others, who by thus responding to them, determine their meaning, and, as it were, *socially refract* the traits. The premiums and taboos that are applied by these significant others may be stable or they may be unstable, and they may be in conflict or they may be in harmony.

Where the unity of a social structure is disintegrating, the grip of institutions upon men relaxes, which means that no general, harmonious, and stable system of premiums and taboos operates. The responses and traits of men are accordingly less predictable, for then a greater range is open for traits to develop, and experimental types of character may arise. Some of these types may later set up a new system of premiums and taboos which will, in turn, select and refract the development and presentations of traits in other persons.

II. The premiums and taboos applied by currently significant others are not the only ones which must be taken into account in explaining the histories of various traits. For societies have histories, and persons have biographies. We must pay attention to the specific premiums and taboos to which persons have been exposed by previous others during the course of their biographies. These previously internalized taboos and premiums select and refract those which may be currently effective. We point to this fact by terming it the *biographical refraction of traits,* for it introduces a certain depth into our considerations, the depth of the person's biography.

III. There is another depth factor, which involves the maturation of the psychic structure and its integration with the person. In the interplay of social career and psychic maturation certain traits which have been premiumed, and others which have been tabooed, form a more or less stable configuration. The psychic structure may also have a certain dynamic of its own which is involved in the selection and refraction of traits. And at any rate, the premiums and taboos which have been applied to a person select and accentuate certain components of his psychic structure as well as of his person. So we must consider the *psychic* as well as the *social* and the *biographical* refraction of traits. Analyzing a specific character structure, the social psychologist tries to understand its formation in terms of the acquisition of various traits in their different institutional contexts, and to trace what happens to these traits as they are integrated in this particular character structure.

If in educational institutions there is a premium upon competitive examinations as a means of selecting and evaluating students, then competitive and individualistic traits may be developed in the student. But if group and team work prevail and premiums are placed upon such traits as co-operativeness, the student will be encouraged to be helpful to his fellow students. Educational institutions may thus encourage individual competitiveness or co-operative teamwork. Such premiums and taboos need not be verbalized as explicit rules, yet successful adjustment to the rules of the game will necessitate traits of the type required by the objective institutional arrangements and its operating premiums and taboos.

In internalizing the going premiums and taboos, a person may not be aware of the impact they are making upon his personal and psychic structure. He may be a very self-conscious competitor while not being aware of how he got that way or indeed that he is. Intensified competition is apt to call forth anxieties in the persons exposed to it. Then premiums upon such traits as generosity, light-heartedness, and the ever-ready smile may be lessened in the scope of their application, and even transformed by some anxiety-ridden persons into taboos. Thus do premiums stabilize traits into the person and into the dynamic trends of his character.

In order to understand what happens to a socially available trait during its internalization and integration in the character structure, we must grasp its angle of refraction, in terms of the biography of given persons and in terms of their psychic structures, for these modify the traits that are socially offered. The autonomous dynamics of both psychic structure and person may thus select from and then organize what is socially premiumed.

4. Anxiety and Social Structure

We have been discussing some general ways in which institutions select and form persons by means of the roles persons enact and the traits they internalize. Persons are linked with social structures and with particular institutional orders in another way having to do with what we have called the symbol spheres—or more generally, the communication processes as a whole.

We shall now examine one type of emotion—anxiety and fear—in order to illustrate how psychological states involving the psychic structure as well as the person cannot be understood without reference to the institutional framework in which they go on, and in particular, the communicational processes which often define them.

Freud has taught us to speak of anxiety rather than of fear when the fear is out of proportion to the object or occasion which arouses it. In pathologically extreme instances, psychologists speak of "phobias," which are classified by object or occasion. Thus, claustrophobia refers to an inordinate fear of closed-in places. Where there is no concrete object or occasion discernible, one may speak of "free-floating anxieties."

Public communications can be seen as psychologically relevant to anxiety by means of the shifting definitions of loyalties and of definitions of social reality itself which they provide. The level of anxiety and of fear nowadays existing among American populations, for example, due to Soviet-United States tensions, is in some part due to the great definitional shift in military perspectives: the old categories of "land power" versus "sea power" have become partially obsolete—due to developments of air power, atom bombs, and snorkel submarines. Accordingly, there is a loss of firm definitions of military reality, and for many people this is a source of anxiety or fear.

So far as persons are concerned, we may classify their psychological state of security in terms of the institutional areas it involves and the intervals during which it occurs. The areas of a person's life in which he is secure are wide if he is secure in all his roles, if he "knows where he is going" and what his situation is. They are narrow if he has an adequate definition of his situation and its wider context only in a few of his roles. Similarly, the interval of security may be longer or shorter. The person may be secure all the time, or such security as he experiences may be intermittent.

If we cross-classify these areas and intervals of security, we come out with four possibilities:

Fully secure people are secure in all their roles all the time, or at least for long periods of time. At the opposite end of the scale are those whose area of security is narrow and even then, intermittent—which, we might suppose, is the psychological counterpart of Hobbes's state of nature, where life is "nasty, brutish and short." There are also persons whose security rests on some narrow range of roles played, but within this range their security endures. ("At least I don't have to worry about that.") And, in the opposite situation, there are persons who are secure in all relations but only for short intervals.

This simple classification of types of security seems useful to us, but of course it does not in itself establish any links between security or anxiety and social structure. When we begin to examine more closely what we mean by "areas of security," and to discuss explicitly the emotion itself, we find that we cannot very well do so without closely linking our discussion with given institutional contexts. Emotions such as fear cannot usefully be divorced from their objects—from *what* is feared; and these objects, involved in the shifting anxieties of men, are historically given and socially learned. "Man's fear," as Kurt Riezler has put it, "is fear *of* something or *for* something; *of* illness, loss of money, dishonor; *for* his health, family, social status." [8]

I. In the kinship order there may be fear of illegitimate children, or of the marriage of daughters to class and status inferiors.

[8] *American Journal of Sociology*, May 1944, p. 489.

But whether there is or there is not fear of illegitimate pregnancy of course depends on the institutional definition of pregnancy as illegitimate, the severity of social sanctions against the illegitimate child and its mother, or against the *mésalliance* as defined by a more or less rigid status code. The worries of fathers and mothers thus depend on the existence of a status system and the competitive craving for family respectability.

II. In the military order, there may be fear of death and fear of defeat. But even the fear of death can be reduced, virtually to zero, by intensive cowardice-courage programs of morale building. Since Napoleon, courage has been "taken for granted" in all patriots, but in the twentieth century cowardice and courage have become part of the manipulative technology of morale building. Surely there are great differences in the anxieties which surrounded mercantilist warfare, for which Voltaire depreciated courage, and those which surround warfare in the hills of Korea.

III. In the economic order, the laissez-faire entrepreneur may fear bankruptcy, and hence loss of respectability, as well as loss of money. The employee may fear unemployment. But in the corporate economy, the risk of big business is often largely taken over by the state. The fears thus become political rather than focused on the laissez-faire market. As the old inscrutable market and the business firm itself are rationalized so as to reduce entrepreneurial anxiety, new anxieties about whether the corporation has a political "in" give business fears a new focus and shape.

IV. In the political order, the politician may fear loss of office in an election; the citizen may fear the loss of prestige of the state with which he is patriotically identified, among the prestige strivings of the great powers. But for the politician, the party machine's fear may be the basis of his discipline. And "the citizen" who knows anxiety from national loss of prestige is likely to be of the upper-class gentry whose evaluation of self is closely joined with the prestige of the nation, which he represents to representative men of other nations.

V. Some sociologists—Herbert Spencer, for example—define religion as fear of the dead. Other thinkers, Freud for example, have stressed fear of guilty conscience and of death itself. The symbol spheres of some religions, however, seem to have to do with hope as well as with fear, indeed the two are frequently interrelated in religious symbols and institutional life. If religious institutions form a dominant order in the social structure, and if the people are devout, all their fears and anxieties—no matter what their social source—may feed into the religious order and its symbols.

Agents of a religious hierarchy may fear demotion or reassignment to less desirable parishes, and, like any office holder, they may relieve their anxieties by knowing the ropes and pulling the strings. What religious laities fear varies with the religion in which they believe, and the demands raised by the religious leaders in the name of its God. The level of anxiety—for example, consciousness of sin—will vary with the level of demand that prevails.

Thus, typical fears and anxieties may be located sociologically in each institutional order and sphere. Although some men may feel that we have nothing to fear but fear itself, most men, in the long history of mankind, have had better reasons to fear. In preindustrial times, when nature was still unconquered, many fears were primarily based upon the calamitous consequences of that fact. In modern societies, anxieties are more likely to have their sources in the opaque and unpredictable drift of the social structure and the similarly unstable dynamics of interpersonal relations.

Fifty years ago, "nervousness" was most frequently discussed in connection with Victorian problems of love, prudery, and hysteria; nowadays—after two world wars and a vast depression—insecurities and anxieties are more likely to be seen as connected with social, economic, and military securities, or their prevailing absence from the life of men.

Just as sociological conditions lead to anxieties, so do they channel the compensations which relieve anxieties. A number of typical mechanisms for such relief, which Karen Horney has called "cravings," may be distinguished: [9] A person may compensate his anxieties by becoming a *perfectionist*, eager to perform his roles in such a way as never to lay himself open to criticism; accordingly,

[9] For an extended discussion of anxiety, love, affection, and power see Karen Horney, *The Neurotic Personality of Our Time* (New York, 1937), Chapters 3, 6, and 10.

he may develop the traits of the exaggerated punctilio. Anxiety may also be personally refracted by an increased craving for love and affection and the development of the traits of the overly *affectionate person*. In this craving, the person may allow himself to be exploited "for love's sake" and thereby actually damage his self in other roles. He may crave *affection* at all costs, in order to gain protection, his motto being "If you love me, you will not hurt me."

Closely allied to this type is the person who may be compulsively submissive and comply with every wish of the other, "self-less" as it were, lest he risk being hurt. The person *withdraws* from involvement in the roles of an institutional order, giving up all psychic commitments. Again, the person may crave *power*, lest he have to fear anything from anybody. In extreme cases, we refer to megalomania, but ordinary job anxiety may lead to an inordinate development of striving for family power, and accompanying traits may be developed and premiumed by the person.

These compensatory mechanisms may of course be combined in various ways. For example, inordinate cravings for power and the accompanying traits, as a way out of anxiety, may be closely related to inordinate cravings for love: in love, one lays himself open to the powers of another; in power, one strives to dominate the submissive other. An individual who oscillates between such opposite tendencies, and their accompanying traits, is generally called ambivalent. What is logically exclusive need not be psychologically exclusive.[10]

[10] "Genuine love" differs from the raw impulse of sex in that the loved partner is incorporated in the devoted lover's circle of significant others and hence, self. The lover is eager to "give" and to "surrender" his best to the person he cherishes, and is far from considering his loving partner an "object to be gotten" for he wishes to "give." Love and death are the great equalizers of men. By loving the weak, the strong learn to be tender and to control rather than to exploit their strength lest they brutalize their weaker partner. For love's sake, the more intelligent will not use their superior intelligence to show up their beloved partner, lest they shame them, or are themselves shamed. The rich who are in love with poor partners will eagerly seek to prove that "money does not matter." So love leaps over all differences that divide men, and if the work of art has been called "a promise of happiness," the art of "making love" in the Western World has served as an intimate reminder of the prophetic promise of a psychological state in which the lion shall rest beside the lamb, and swords shall be made into plowshares.

In order briefly to demonstrate some of these compensatory mechanisms, and especially to show how they may be combined in specific types of character, we shall briefly discuss, as types of men, the classic Puritan, the Confucian mandarin, and the nobleman of France's *ancien régime*.

I. As we have already shown, the vocabulary of motives need not coincide with the actual operation of the psychic structure.[11] The heroic Puritan of seventeenth-century England could methodically pursue his quest for salvation by disciplining himself for hard work and thriftiness, and thus by his success assure his religious worth and his salvation in the hereafter. He could, in short, relieve his anxieties by hard work, by work for work's sake, and, under the appropriate premiums, take great pains to develop a new "contract morality" in business relationships. Thus perfectionism and moral rigor, punctiliousness, and pleasure-denying work, along with humility and the craving for his neighbor's love all combined to shape the character structure of the classical Puritan who sought to master the world rather than adjust to it.[12]

II. As an organization, the bureaucracy of gentlemanly literati in ancient China was stable and weathered great political crises, but as an individual the Confucian mandarin was highly insecure. In his career, there existed no socially transparent link between skill and merit and rewards for success. Pull and bribery, the arbitrary favors and disfavors of superiors, and "luck" dominated his bureaucratic climb. He was exposed to great reversals of personal fate in a highly competitive context where many aspirants pressed upon each office holder. The individual official was a stranger in his administrative bailiwick, was subject to reassignments to other provinces, and had to rely upon an unofficial adviser who, in fact, made decisions for which the mandarin was held accountable.

These conditions, as well as others, produced an intensive and lasting sense of insecurity and anxiety. And these anxieties, in turn, were compensated by a great emphasis upon a rigid code of etiquette and ceremony of great polish and finesse. The magical significance attributed to the Confucian code or rules of propriety seems to indicate its compensatory function in relieving anxiety

---

[11] See Chapter V: The Sociology of Motivation.
[12] For further comments on the Puritan, see pp. 234-36 ff. and 360-63 ff.

states. In passing, we may mention that Confucius himself had lost his office by the arbitrary act of his prince, and that he had developed his teachings in a highly competitive context of itinerant political intellectuals striving for power positions at the courts of rival princes.

Alongside perfectionist, ritualistic tendencies, we observe the intense power cravings of the competitive careerists who, after all, were without specialized training for administration. These administrators were saddled with the responsibility for anything that went wrong in their bailiwicks, whether it was a harvest failure due to flood or drought, a tribal invasion, or sheer administrative negligence. For Confucian thought made no distinction between nature and society—between the "acts of God" and the responsibilities of men. And the mandarin, partaking of the supposedly magical power of the "Son of Heaven" was accountable for more than what men can control. Naturally this maximized his pompous sense of megalomaniacal power and his stylized conceit—as well as his underlying state of anxiety. Given ancestor worship as part of the unwritten constitution of Chinese despotism, the disturbances of social order—cosmic or human—were ascribed to the unrest of the ancestral spirits, for which the mandarin bureaucrats—ultimately the Son of Heaven himself—were blamed.

Thus, perfectionism in rigid ceremonial deportment was supplemented by intense cravings for power which emerged in an opaque context of career striving. These two tendencies were further supplemented by compulsive conformism with Confucian orthodoxy, a system of "organized thought" based upon the hallowed classical writings of ancient authors. This conformism was enforced by the ubiquitous ideological agents of a powerful board of censors. However efficient this spy system may have been in guaranteeing the disciplined cohesion of the bureaucracy as a whole, for the individual bureaucrat it meant an additional source of great insecurity, and the resultant anxiety was compensated for by the discouragement of independent thought, intellectual initiative, and any direct confrontation of the problems at hand. Whatever was thought about or came up for decision was stated and elaborated in terms of the sanctioned body of classical writings.[13]

[13] On the Chinese literati, see Max Weber, *The Religion of China*, H. H. Gerth, tr. (Glencoe, Ill.: Free Press, 1951).

III. The nobleman of the *ancien régime* stood on the shaky ground of prerevolutionary France. Middle-class intellectuals had debunked the justification of the divine right of kings as a mere sanction of despotism, and the authority of the priesthood had not gone unquestioned. Despotic coercion had forced the nobility to become a leisured class, living as absentee owners and *rentiers* divorced from all productive functions. The competition for the king's favors—for offices and for politically profitable marriages—was intense and led to great anxieties.

These anxiety states were heightened through the breakdown of the dividing line between marriage and extramarital relations with mistresses, between legitimate and illegitimate children of kings and nobles. Since the king with his Christian and royal mistress set the tone and established the model for all courtly behavior, the mistress became politically and socially indispensable for the court noble. Good relations with mistresses were important for getting the news behind the news.

Machiavellian attitudes and practices permeated the ruling strata. Efficiency in dueling and cautious self-discipline at meals—where poison cup and dagger might threaten and the lap dog as a pre-tester of food was not always reliable—were needed. As in Chinese mandarin society, a polished ritualism of conventional behavior emerged, and froze into a rigid code of court etiquette.

The competition of cavaliers under the watchful eyes of hostesses blurred the lines between influence and love, and made genuine love a tool in the quest for power and influence, and influence an opportunity for exploitative love. Love-making became a technology of psychic manipulation and seduction a fine art. Men could never know whether love meant devotion or unwilling vassalage. The *Liaisons Dangereuses* by Laclos may be mentioned as the great document of the perversion of love into power.

Intense craving for power and a ritualist etiquette in personal relations which barred "genuine love"; the craving for love and popularity as means for the furtherance of personal careers; flattery, conformist attitudes, and posturing to win the favors of the absolute and always suspicious despot—all these were so many compensations for the basic anxieties of a class whose spokesmen on the eve of revolution proclaimed: "Après nous le déluge." [14]

[14] See, for a good account of the old regime, Frantz Funck-Brentano, *The Old Regime in France*, Herbert Wilson, tr. (London: E. Arnold, 1929). See

In a comparable context, the Tsarist nobility was subject to intense competition for the office appointments on which the noble rank of the family in the social hierarchy depended. Some responded by an attitude of withdrawal which was implemented by a mystic Eastern Christianity. Especially during the nineteenth century, many Russian "repentant noblemen" went abroad, even preferring to be expropriated by the government than to return. This attitude has found a profound elaboration in the figure of Goncharov's "Oblomov," who withdraws from competition with his erotical competitor, dreams nostalgically of the patriarchal relations of old, and hence accomplishes nothing. In Russia, this state of apathetic withdrawal and soulful quietism has been known as "Oblomovism."

In this chapter, we have discussed some of the major ways in which man and society—character and social structure—are linked. We have seen that institutions select persons by formal and informal rules of recruitment and ejection, and form them by explicit training and by means of the particular and generalized other, which the person—in internalizing instituted roles—comes in time to acquire. We have also explained how the traits of the person may be socially premiumed, and thus reinforced, or socially tabooed, and thus weakened, by various institutional contexts.

We have suggested that the symbol sphere of institutional orders, by socially defining situations that the person confronts, is often a cue to his fears and anxiety as well as other psychic elements, and we have illustrated this by examples from the kinship and military, the economic, the political and the religious order. Finally, we have discussed certain compensatory mechanisms as revealed in the Puritan, the mandarin and the nobleman.

also L. Ducros, *La Société Française au Dix-huitième Siècle* (Paris: Haties, 1933).

CHAPTER

VIII

Institutional Orders
and Social Controls, I

WE wish, in the present and in the next chapter, to elaborate our conceptions of institutional orders and spheres, as well as to raise certain questions appropriate to each of these units of our model of social structure.[1] It is certainly not our intention to exhaust the topics which we discuss: even an attempt to do so would require a many-volumed universal history of mankind. What we do want to do is to define certain useful conceptions; to lay out the range of institutions available to sociological observation; and to describe certain pivotal types of institutions that have at various times characterized political and economic, military and religious, kinship and educational endeavors. In doing so, we shall pay particular attention to the social controls that often prevail in each of these institutional orders or spheres and the types of persons that they tend to select and form.[2]

1. The Political Order [3]

The political order, we have said, consists of those institutions within which men acquire, wield, or influence distributions of

[1] For preliminary definitions of these orders and spheres, see Chapter II: Character and Social Structure, Section 2: Components of Social Structure.

[2] For further statement of our guiding questions for such work, see Chapter II: Character and Social Structure, Section 3: The Tasks of Social Psychology.

[3] The student will find the following readings of signal importance: Max Weber, "Politics as a Vocation," *From Max Weber: Essays in Sociology*, H. H. Gerth and C. Wright Mills, trs. and eds. (New York: Oxford, 1946), pp. 77-128; H. D. Lasswell and A. Kaplan, *Power and Society* (New Haven:

power. We ascribe "power" to those who can influence the conduct of others even against their will.

Where everyone is equal there is no politics, for politics involves subordinates and superiors. All institutional conduct, of course, involves distributions of power, but such distributions are the essence of politics. In so far as it has to do with "the state," the political order is the "final authority"; in it is instituted the use of final sanctions, involving physical force, over a given territorial domain. This trait marks off political institutions, such as the state, from other institutional orders.

Since power implies that an actor can carry out his will, power involves obedience. The general problem of politics accordingly is the explanation of varying distributions of power and obedience, and one basic problem of political psychology is why men by their obedience accept others as the powerful. Why do they obey?

A straightforward, although inadequate, answer is given by those who see men in the large as herd animals who must be led by a strong man who stays out in front. The explanation of power and obedience in terms of the strong man may hold in some primitive contexts in which only the strong fighter has a chance to become a military and political chieftain; [4] it may also hold in the "gang," where awe of the strongest holds the others to obedience, and contests over power are decided by fist fights. Beyond such situations, however, the problem of power cannot be reduced to a problem of simple physical might.

In Bernard Shaw's *Saint Joan,* the dauphin dryly remarks that he lacked a great deal in almost everything because his ancestors had used it all up. Yet, despite such personal weaknesses, other men looked up to the dauphin and obeyed him. Physical and mental weaklings are often found ruling proud and strong men. We cannot therefore always explain authority and obedience in terms of the characteristics of the power holder. Although Bismarck once said that you can do all sorts of things with bayonets except sit on them, obviously power and obedience involve more than dif-

Yale Univ. Press, 1950); H. E. Barnes, *Sociology and Political Theory* (New York: Knopf, 1924); G. Mosca, *The Ruling Class,* H. D. Kahn, tr. (New York: McGraw-Hill, 1939).

[4] "And when Saul stood among the people, he was higher than any of the people from his shoulders and upward" (I Sam., 10:23).

ferences in the biological means and the physical implements of violence.[5]

The incongruity of strong men willingly obeying physical weaklings leads us to ask: Why are there stable power relations which are *not* based on the direct and physical force of the stronger? The question has been answered by political scientists and philosophers in terms of a consensus between the subordinates and the powerful. This consensus has been rationally formulated in theories of "contract," "natural law," or "public sentiment."[6] For the social psychologist, such approaches are valuable in that they emphasize the question of voluntary obedience, for from a psychological point of view the crux of the problem of power rests in understanding the origin, constitution, and maintenance of voluntary obedience.

There is an element of truth in Laud's assertation: "There can be no firmness without law; and no laws can be binding if there is no conscience to obey them; penalty alone could never, can never do it."[7] In any given political order, we may expect to find both "conscience" and "coercion," and it is the element of conscience, of voluntary obedience, that engages our attention, even though we keep in mind the fact that regardless of the type and extent of conscience, all states practice coercion.

An adequate understanding of power relations thus involves a knowledge of the grounds on which a power holder claims obedience, and the terms in which the obedient feels an obligation to obey. The problem of the grounds of obedience is not a suprahistorical question; we are concerned rather with reconstructing those central ideas which in given institutional structures in fact operate as grounds for obedience. Often such ideas are directly stated and theoretically elaborated; often they are merely implied, left inarticulate and taken for granted. But, in either case, different reasons for obedience prevail in different political institutions.

[5] The extent of violence in political orders varies. Thus thirteen out of fourteen nineteenth-century presidents of Bolivia died by violence, but only four out of thirty-three presidents of the United States. Cf. P. A. Sorokin, "Monarchs and Rulers," *Social Forces*, March 1926.

[6] See Chapter X: Symbol Spheres, especially Section 1: Symbol Spheres in Six Contexts.

[7] Cited by John N. Figgis, *The Divine Right of Kings* (rev. ed.; Cambridge: University Press, 1934), p. 265.

In terms of the publicly recognized reasons for obedience—"legitimations" or symbols of justification [8]—the core of the problem of politics consists in understanding "authority." For it is authority that characterizes enduring political orders. The power of one animal over another may occur in terms of brute coercion, accompanied by grunts and growls, but man, as Susanne Langer has written, can "control [his] inferiors by setting up symbols of [his] power, and the mere idea that words or images convey stands there to hold our fellows in subjection even when we cannot lay our hands on them. . . . Men . . . oppress each other by symbols of might." [9]

Power is simply the probability that men will act as another man wishes. This action may rest upon fear, rational calculation of advantage, lack of energy to do otherwise, loyal devotion, indifference, or a dozen other individual motives. *Authority*, or legitimated power, involves voluntary obedience based on some idea which the obedient holds of the powerful or of his position. "The strongest," wrote Rousseau, "is never strong enough to be always master, unless he transforms his strength into right, and obedience into duty." [10]

Most political analysts have thus come to distinguish between those acts of power which, for various reasons, are considered to be "legitimate," and those which are not. We speak of "naked power" as, for instance, during warfare, after which the successful tries to gain "authority" over the defeated; and we speak of "authority" in cases of legitimate acts of power, and thus, of "public authorities," or "ecclesiastic" or "court authority" and so on. In order to become "duly authorized," power needs to clothe itself with attributes of "justice," "morality," "religion," and other cultural values which define acceptable "ends" as well as the "responsibilities" of those who wield power. Since power is seen as a means, men ask: "Whose power and for what ends?" And most supreme power holders seek to give some sort of answer, to clothe their power in terms of other ends than power for power's sake.

Machiavelli, to be sure, formulated a rationale of power for its own sake, relegating all the alleged and professed purposes of

[8] See Chapter X: Symbol Spheres.

[9] *Fortune,* January 1944, p. 150. See also her *Philosophy in a New Key* (Cambridge: Harvard Univ. Press, 1942), pp. 286-87.

[10] J. J. Rousseau, *Social Contract*, rev. tr. by Charles Frankel (New York: Hafner, 1947).

power to instrumental positions.[11] He did this in an effort to analyze the necessary and sufficient means for getting and for holding power. His name accordingly became despised and to this day "Machiavellian" carries an infamous connotation, although it has rightly been said that perhaps Machiavelli was the one honest man of his age. His debunking of the moral purposes of rulers, and his principled distrust of "power" as such, is carried on by the often quoted dictum of Lord Acton that "Power corrupts and absolute power corrupts absolutely." This statement, however, seems to us quite one-sided; we might assert with equal justice that "Power ennobles and absolute power ennobles absolutely." We need merely substitute "responsibility" for power to make the point obvious. Persons in positions of authority are expected to make "responsible decisions," and some men do grow with the tasks which they take up. If men choose tasks, tasks make men; high or exalted position sometimes provides more opportunities for a man to become "high minded" and to act accordingly. As Ralph Waldo Emerson, writing of the English nobility, put it,

"You cannot wield great agencies without lending yourself to them, and when it happens that the spirit of the earl meets his rank and duties, we have the best examples of behavior. Power of any kind readily appears in the manners; and beneficit *le talent de bien faire*, gives a majesty which cannot be concealed or resisted." [12]

Decision-making groups in our time—with increasingly powerful machines and far-flung organizations—necessarily hold more power and more authority than ever before; accordingly, their corruption seems more hideous, and their ennoblement more grandiose, than in previous times.

In his *Anthropology* of 1789, Kant emphasized liberty and law —which restricts liberty—as the two pivots around which civil legislation turns. But he added that force has to be included as a mediating element in order to make effective legislation according to the principles of liberty and law. Kant imagined several combi-

---

[11] Niccolò Machiavelli, *The Prince; and The Discourses* (New York: Modern Library, 1940).

[12] *English Traits*, Chapter One, cited in *The Writings of Ralph Waldo Emerson* (New York: Modern Library, 1940), p. 622.

nations of force, liberty, and law: thus, law and liberty without force would seem to be anarchy. Law and force without liberty are despotism. Force without liberty or law is simply barbarism. Force with freedom and law are the bases of a republic. Only this last condition, according to Kant, deserves the title of a "true civil constitution," although he did not mean by republic that form of state we call democratic, but any constitutional state.[13]

2. Nation and State [14]

The term "state" first became popular in sixteenth-century Italy. There the Italian city-states first organized bureaucratic administrations, professional bodies of diplomats, and armies of citizens who were ready if need be to forego the salvation of their souls—as Machiavelli says in honor of the Florentine citizenry—in order to preserve the liberties of their city.

A state is a political institution which successfully claims supreme power over a defined territory. This claim can be realized when the state effectively monopolizes the use of legitimate violence against external and internal enemies, however the state-leaders may define "enemy."

A state capable of conducting wars against competing states and of monopolizing legitimate violence within its own territory is sociologically one state, even though legally it may be a confederacy of substates. That the United States of America is one state, for example, was decisively established by the American Civil War. And it is the fact of a monopoly of legitimate violence that makes the difference between the United States and such interstate creations as the late "League of Nations," or the prevailing "United Nations."

A *nation* is a body of people which by cultural traditions and common historical memories is capable of organizing a state, or at least which raises the claim for such an autonomous organization with some chance of success.

[13] Paraphrased from Immanuel Kant, *Anthropologies in pragmatischer Hinsicht* (5th ed.; Leipzig: Karl Vorlander, 1912), pp. 286 ff.

[14] The most informative volume on nationalism is probably Hans Kohn, *The Idea of Nationalism* (New York: Macmillan, 1951). See also Max Weber, *op. cit.*, pp. 159-79.

The symbols by which claims to statehood, to the state-organized cohesiveness of a nation are advanced and justified may be called *nationalism*. After a state is organized, these nationalist symbols may prevail as legitimations. Nationalism is thus the justifying ideology of a nation-state or of a nation aspiring to become a state. Nationalism expresses loyalties and aspirations, and tends to involve the feeling that the typical features of one nation may be used as a yardstick of traits alleged to characterize other nations.

We have to distinguish between "patriotism" and "nationalism" as complex sentiments differently related to the political order of a society. National sentiment incorporates patriotism, but, because of its power reference to the nation-state, it involves more.

Patriotism refers to "love of one's country and people" without necessarily involving emotional investment in the political order and its institutional peculiarity. Patriotism is a pride in the culture heritage of the nation devoid of aspirations to win "glory" (the prestige of power) in international competition. In fact, to stay out of international power contests, and to be left alone by others, is the core of this sentiment, which is often most intense among the smallest nations, such as Norway or Switzerland.

Nationalism is a specifically modern sentiment which binds the mass of the citizenry to the political order in a common aspiration to hold their own in power competition with other nations by organizing all institutional orders in the framework of a sovereign state. Nationalism claims the right of the nation to determine its own fate, that is to organize itself without intervention from the outside. To the people, nationalist spokesmen address specific expectations "in the name of the nation," and they define conduct patterns and symbolic behavior normatively as "national," that is, as conduct to be ascribed to the nation as a whole, and against what is "alien." Nowadays such appeals are made to diverse aggregates and organized publics by power holders in all institutional orders. Thus, commercial advertising campaigns demand "Buy American" or "Buy British." Purists may crusade against the borrowing of foreign words and ideas. Nationalist Christians tend to conceive of Almighty God as having distinct national preferences, especially during world wars. Protestantism, particularly, has always had an intimate relationship to nationalism. Publishers and literati, of course, promote "national literature" and "national art," and historians write "national history."

As the symbols of justification for the acts of a state, nationalism promotes loyalty and obedience to state authority. Nationalist symbols, however, may be highly elaborated. And in intellectual circles they may be thought of as the very ground or embodiment of the nation-state, rather than merely symbols justifying state power. Thus Montesquieu's "national genius" and Herder's *Volksgeist* have been used and abused in state propaganda for increasing internal loyalty and external aggression.

Chauvinism is nationalism carried to the extreme of exclusive, and hence fanatical, assertion of a nation's mission, and the studious devaluation of all other nations. The term was put into circulation because of Napoleon's political aide, M. Chauvin's, rather extravagant glorifications of France.

Nation and state need not, of course, be identical, either in territory or in political domination. The belief that national unity *should* be the basis of state unity is, of course, a political choice and not a universal historical fact. The existence of cultural and national minorities in many states, the absorption of national communities by larger, imperial states, and the existence of nationals outside the state's dominion—these are facts which run counter to the ideology of national self-determination. Indeed, the *idea* of national self-determination is modern, involving liberal democratic conceptions quite foreign to early dynastic states. During the nineteenth century, the Polish nation was organized by three states: partly by the Russian Tsar, partly by the German Reich, and partly by the Austro-Hungarian monarchy. The latter state, indeed, organized several nations under one state. On the other hand, pre-Bismarckian Germany was one nation organized in a plurality of states. The principle of nationality (namely, that each nation should correspond to an autonomous state) was propagated by such men as Mazzini and Napoleon III; it was given grandiose influence by President Wilson's late "self-determination" program for Europe, and Lenin's for the colonial peoples.

In the first half of the nineteenth century, nationalism was the sister creed of liberalism and defended one liberal goal: the release of peoples from the rule of alien states. Positively, nationalists sought to establish constitutions. But of course, nationalism had repeatedly passed from defense to aggression and back again: rather than the release of aspiring political communities from alien state rule, nationalism came, in the nineteenth century especially, to involve the attempt to subjugate other peoples to its rule. In many places "National Unity" superseded "The Consent of the Governed." Thus nineteenth-century nationalism closed with a flowering of imperialism.[15]

When loyalty to a ruling house is replaced by loyalty to a national state, national symbols are propagated by means of public educational systems. Concentrating upon the masses of the population, magazine and novel, newspaper and radio and motion picture all help to disseminate favorable images and stereotypes of the nation. Scholarly writings are organized in terms of national histories. As the territory dominated by the nation is typically larger than that dominated by, say, the tribe, and as the population is not necessarily connected even distantly by blood or religion, modern nationalism has had to rely more on mass education and propaganda. The development of compulsory education, cheap printing, and recently of radio and motion pictures may thus conveniently be viewed in connection with nationalism.[16] It is clear that the state of communication facilities affects the extent and penetration of nationalism within the territory of the state. When communication facilities are not universal in their coverage, the sensitive spots will be the frontier or border zones and the national capital, the intervening areas remaining less affected.

Lack of correspondence between the territory dominated by a state and the population composing a nation has stimulated the search for other possible bases of nationhood. "Nation" has thus been used to refer to feelings of loyalty among a population having language, literature, folk heroes, historical tradition, culture, race, or religious denomination in common. All of these factors, in various combinations, may indeed be elements in the situation of a nation, which is to say that they may increase the chance that aspirations for national self-determination, for the setting up of an

[15] See William A. Dunnigan, "Fundamental Conceptions of 19th Century Politics," *Congress of Arts and Sciences, St. Louis, 1904* (New York, 1906), Vol. VII, pp. 279-92.

[16] See Chapter IX: Institutional Orders and Social Controls, II, Section 4: The Educational Sphere.

autonomous state, will be realized. The actual reasons, however, for belief in the existence of a national community vary enormously, and may change during the course of national history.

Rather vague ideas of common descent are often at the bottom of nationality feelings. But such feeling need not exist at all, and frequently does not. Nor do "races" by any means correspond with nations. The population of modern Germany, for example, is composed of diverse ethnic groups, and in such nations as the United States, Brazil, and the Soviet Union practically all the major strains can be found among the citizenry. "Race," used in reference to Turks, Germans, or English, is, as Franz Boas put it, "only a disguise of the idea of nationality."[17]

Most nation-states have been ready, willing, and eager to declare themselves "a God-fearing people." The denominational varieties of Christianity have been conveniently accommodated to this eagerness. Religious and national differences and conflicts may be very closely intermingled, as in the conflict of the Irish and the English, and national heroes may be treated as saints, as among the Serbs and other Greek orthodox nations. That Joan of Arc was canonized by the Catholic church—after the Franco-Prussian war of 1870-71—is a fact relevant to French nationalism.[18]

A specific language, given its practical incompatibility with other languages, is perhaps the most important common "social" feature of a nation. Yet a national community organized under a state may have several languages—as in the case of modern Switzerland. In terms of feeling, the national identity means a specific kind of pathos, which is more likely to develop where there is a common language and religion, conventions and style of life, history and destiny.

All these communal factors, as components of a national situation, tend to increase the idea of an autonomous power organization or state, which may already exist or be ardently longed for. The more this power or state aspect is emphasized, the more specific is the nation. To understand differences between nations, one must examine the components of the national situation for every empirical case, yet two general and closely related factors are

[17] Franz Boas, "Race and Nationality," *Bulletin of the American Association for International Conciliation*, January 1915, p. 8.

[18] See Max Hildebert Boehm, "Nationalism," *Encyclopaedia of the Social Sciences*, Vol. XI, p. 236.

essential to the social psychologist who would understand "national differences":

I. It is important to understand the institutional composition of the national social structure, and especially the relations of the state to the several institutional orders. We shall in due course specify the procedures which we think most useful for this task.

II. It is also important to understand the types of persons who within a given national social structure are held up as models of imitation and aspiration. These national types—the Prussian *Junker*,[19] the Japanese *Samurai*,[20] the British gentleman,[21] the French *honnête homme*, the American self-made man, the Russian Soviet man—serve to unify national images and may become the stereotyped image of the nation itself.[22]

The image of the nation, and the entire conception of nationality, will vary from one stratum to another within the national social structure. In the United States, for example, such status groups as the D.A.R. and "Pilgrim societies" may stress Anglo-Saxon descent, while industrial workers, liberal intellectuals, and immigrants think rather of the American Dream or "the melting pot." Various images of the nation may be seized upon by vested interests or movements. Thus "Americanism" and "the American way of life" may be identified with laissez-faire economics and a free competition for workers (no trade unions) by capitalist groups.

The initial claim of a people to nationhood is typically advanced by an intellectual vanguard who out of material and ideal interests tend to sentimentalize their native language and to develop it into

[19] See Max Weber, "Capitalism and Rural Society in Germany" and "National Character and the Junkers," *op. cit.*, pp. 363-95; E. Kohn-Bramstedt, *Aristocracy and the Middle Classes in Germany* (London: King, 1937); and Paul Kosok, *Modern Germany* (Chicago: Univ. of Chicago Press, 1933).

[20] See G. B. Sansom, *Japan: A Short Cultural History* (rev. ed.; New York: Appleton-Century, 1943); and Hillis Lory, *Japan's Military Masters* (New York: Viking, 1943). For a sensible statement of difficulties, see John F. Embrose, "Standardized Error and Japanese Character," *World Politics*, Vol. II (1948-50), pp. 439 ff.

[21] See Wilhelm Dibelius, *England*, M. A. Hamilton, tr. (New York: Harper, 1930); G. J. Renier, *The English: Are They Human?* (New York: P. Smith, 1931); and Karl H. Abshagen, *King, Lords and Gentlemen*, E. W. Dickes, tr. (London: Heinemann, 1939).

[22] Walter Bagehot has laid stress upon the social selection and diffusion of such types in his penetrating discussion of "Nation-making"; see *Physics and Politics* (New York, 1912), Chapters 3 and 4.

a medium for a national literary expression. In this creative process the peculiarities of the language are discovered, elaborated, and defended as superior or at least equal to any other. In these nationalist endeavors intellectual prestige and the business interests of publishers may clash or fuse with the interests of politicians. Once it becomes the official language of educational, scientific, and jurisdictional institutions, the national tongue acquires additional prestige. A national literature as an art form is apt to emerge and be democratized. As long as this literature sentimentalizes prominent features of the territory, prominent folkways, and memories of the people, we may speak of "cultural patriotism." From this it is but a short step to modern nationalism, which embodies a specific political pathos for the community at large. Symbols of the people's martyrdom—national heroes and founding fathers—in the face of aggression stand opposite symbols of forthcoming liberation, that is to say, autonomous statehood.

In the twentieth century, these processes of nation-building are being repeated in dependent political areas in the Middle and Far East, in the Caribbean, and in various British Dominions. Nationals educated as clerks, lawyers, journalists, for purposes of working in the domination structure of the Western powers, usually form the vanguard of these movements, which are typically viewed by the dominant country's leaders as "a handful of agitators" rather than a revival or creation of a national community. In modern nations, the middle classes usually become the most ardent followers of the nationalist intelligentsia, although, especially during wars, nationalist enthusiasm tends to be universal among all classes of the political community.[23]

Once a national community is fully a state, it monopolizes the use of legitimate violence within its domain, defends its domain against other states, and may attempt to expand it. The combat range of modern armed forces and the range of communications and transportation are important factors in determining the size of the political territory of a state. Although, as Butler remarked, the "sphere of action of . . . the greater part of mankind is much

---

[23] See, for example, Rupert Emerson, Lennox A. Mills and Virginia Thompson, *Government and Nationalism in Southeast Asia* (New York: Institute of Pacific Relations, 1942); and D. H. Buchanan, *The Development of Capitalist Enterprise in India* (New York: Macmillan, 1934).

narrower than the government they live under," [24] the sphere of action of the great power state is typically larger than its own pacified domain. Pride in one's nation, as we have noted, often involves an ethnocentric affirmation of the nation's peculiarities. This sense of superiority typically feeds on the notion of the exemplary significance of one's own nation-state for other nations, if not for "the rest of the world." This sense may exist without any ambition to do more than propagate this prestigeful image. Any nationalist expansion of power may thus be rejected by "isolationist" sentiments and policies.

On the other hand, nationalism may inspire ambitions territorially to expand the political influence of the nation so as to make its actual or potential policies count heavily in international affairs. Usually various spokesmen for the nation attribute a specific "honor" to their nation, which forbids them to tolerate or "to take" one thing or another from various other nations. Their policies of expansion may take several forms:

I. When a state holds out diplomatic and, if need be, military or naval protection to its businessmen, religious missionaries, and so forth, who are living or working in a foreign territory, and when the foreign political unit has no means of asserting its sovereignty over these foreigners, we characterize the foreign territory as a "sphere of influence" of the superior power.

II. When a weaker power relies upon the military protection of a superior power against third powers, and accordingly is compelled or willing to co-ordinate its foreign policies and their internal institutional prerequisites with the demands of the superior power, we speak of a "protectorate."

III. When a nation-state extends political protection to the trading areas of its businessmen we speak of "imperialism." [25] The most explicit types of imperialism involve the acquisition of a colonial empire by purchase, or conquest, or both. There are many reasons for such expansion, and many techniques of accomplishing

[24] Samuel Butler, "Sermons," *Works* (London, 1874), II, p. 154.

[25] See J. A. Hobson's classic work, *Imperialism* (London, 1902); Nikolai Lenin, *Imperialism* (New York: International Publications, 1939); Rosa Luxemburg, *The Accumulation of Capital*, A. Schwarzchild, tr. (New Haven: Yale Univ. Press, 1951); and Fritz Sternberg, *Capitalism and Socialism on Trial* (New York: Day, 1952); and J. A. Schumpeter, *Imperialism and Social Classes*, H. Narden, tr. (New York: Kelley, 1951).

it. A country may seek colonies in order to settle "surplus populations," that is, people who cannot readily be absorbed in various institutional orders. It may seek colonies in order to expand its politically guaranteed market area; or in order to win and establish a politically guaranteed monopoly over resources, raw materials, and labor, or it may merely wish to deny access to such resources to other powers. Again, and this is more modern, one power may seek to expand its military area of control by establishing naval and air bases abroad without assuming overt political responsibilities in the face of foreign political bodies. It may prefer other nations to adjust to whatever implications ensue from its establishment of such bases. These nations, in turn, find it difficult to acquire those "rights" which colonials in the long run have acquired, as the history of the British Empire—now the British Commonwealth of Nations—shows.

The political process is thus a struggle for power and prestige, for authoritative positions within each nation-state and among various nation-states. Since the French Revolution, this competitive system of sovereign states has led to the unification of Italy and Germany; and since World War I, to the dissolution of the feudal multinationality state of the Hapsburg empire into small nation-states. In the nineteenth century, the several major states were sufficiently equal to block the possibility of one of them violently upsetting the entire balance of power competitors. In addition, each of them was interested in maintaining this balance of power; they seemed "saturated," as Bismarck remarked of the Germany he unified. The "family of nations" was thus more or less self-balancing, and the balance as a whole was guaranteed by the power competition between the British and the Tsarist empires.

With rapid, although uneven industrialization, urbanization, and population growth, the differences between the various European nations widened. The universal revival of imperialist tendencies after the 1890's eventuated in World War I, which America entered at the side of Great Britain and Russia. But after that war, the United States abstained from the League of Nations, while at the same time actively intervening in European affairs through the Dawes and Young plan, thus combining active economic intervention with minimal political responsibilities. All this, along with the peacemakers' work at Versailles and the exclusion of the Soviet

Union from the League of Nations proved abortive and short-sighted. The period between the two World Wars has aptly been referred to as The Twenty Years' Crisis, When There Was No Peace.[26]

3. Democracies and Dictatorships

Since Aristotle, states have been classified into six types: Monarchy and tyranny, the good and evil types of one-man rule; aristocracy and oligarchy, the good and evil types of the-rule-of-the-few; and polity and extreme democracy, the good and evil types of the-rule-of-the-many. In order to classify modern states, however, we must take into account the nature of their territory, the terms in which they enlist the loyalties of the organizations and people they would control, the type of political organizations managing the integration of society with the power of the state, and the nature and composition of their ruling groups.

When we examine the *territorial base,* we are able to distinguish between the great river-states of the ancient Middle and Far East, the "coastal states" of the Mediterranean polis—such as Athens, Phoenicia, or Carthage—the states of the plains like the U.S.S.R. or the U.S.A., and the "oasis state" of the Middle East. When we examine the *loyalty structure,* we may address ourselves to political formulae or legitimations such as "in the name of the King," "the divine right of Kings," the "sovereignty of the people," or "in the name of the law," or the alleged charism of totalitarian leadership states under *Duce, Führer,* or *Caudillo.* When we examine the *integrative political organizations* we may speak of the totalitarian one-party state, or of a multiparty parliamentary democracy. When we examine the *nature and composition of ruling groups* we may find a capitalist oligarchy supreme, as in France before the storm of 1848; or a semifeudal group of agrarian capitalists, militarists, and high bureaucrats, as in the Junkerdom under the Kaiser; or a nobility, as in Russia under the Tsar, or party bureaucrats, as after Lenin.

[26] E. H. Carr, *The Twenty Years' Crisis* (London: Macmillan, 1949), is well worth reading as a retrospective debunking of the diplomatic phraseology of vain, frightened, short-sighted, and popularity-craving statesmen. H. F. Armstrong, in *When There Is No Peace* (New York: Macmillan, 1939), gives an astute account of the war preceding the latest "shooting war."

The most diverse "social contents" may exist under the same "political form." The term "democracy," especially as used in modern propaganda contests, has literally come to mean all things to all men. The Soviet use of "People's Democracy" is characteristic —literally it means "people's people's rule," which would seem one too many. Dictatorships, as well as democracies, are ways of organizing political orders. They mean quite different things for men in different social structures and in different historical eras. And in particular, since the middle of the nineteenth century, political choices have become inextricably involved with various economic alternatives.

The civic sources of modern democracies are found, first, in ancient Athens, where for the qualified citizens there was direct democracy. The "town meeting" was possible, for no city was larger than perhaps 50,000. The affairs of the town were run directly, foreign ambassadors, for example, reporting directly to the open assembly. And there was no specialized staff of professionals.

The second source of democracy was the indirect democracy of the medieval cities or guild communes. Decisions were made by delegates from the guilds, in a manner not unlike UN delegates today. These delegates had no real leeway and the organizations they represented were very unstable. Some guilds were much wealthier and stronger than others and accordingly tried to become the bases of hereditary offices. Then minor guilds might make urban revolutions, and as in ancient city tyrannies, dictatorships arise. The history of the Italian city-states dramatizes these developments.

The medieval form of indirect democracy evolved finally into modern constitutional democracy. The parliamentary deputy, however, unlike the medieval guildsman, became a free agent, being restricted only by his fear of not being re-elected and by the "pressures" that are exerted upon his decisions.

And as the rule of law replaced the rule of men, loyalties were attached to the authority of the constitution as the supreme law of the land. Wherever kingship survived the middle-class revolutions of the seventeenth and eighteenth centuries, it was reduced to "representation." The king was a figurehead, and the "kingdom of prerogative" was reduced to a "kingdom of influence."

Regardless of constitutional forms, the modern state in an industrial society is always an essentially bureaucratic state. This simply means that its army, its executive departments, and its judiciary consist of centralized offices that are arranged in a hierarchy, each level having specified jurisdictions. To understand such states we must understand how other political bureaucracies, the party machines for example, are integrated with the officials at the heads of the state's various civil and military hierarchies. We must examine the party structure and its linkages to pressure groups and the major strata of the social structure, and that we pay particular attention to the integration within the political order of parties with state machine.

I. Arthur Rosenberg has taught us to understand *liberal democracy* as that phase of Western parliamentary government during which the propertied and the educated shared political decisions, the franchise being restricted by census qualifications and effectively denied to the mass of workers as well as to women.

II. *Imperialist democracy* refers to parliamentary governments which rule an empire consisting of such diverse units as dominions, colonies, dependencies and protectorates, radiating finally into spheres of influence. "Colonial democracy" refers to a territory under a parliamentary government which is in fact dependent upon the decisions of a great power. Such democracies are often debtor states dependent upon the good will of the creditor country.

III. *Totalitarian democracy* refers to the absence of a division between private and public life. Ancient Athens and the city-states of the Italian Renaissance exemplify this absence of division, as do the heroic episodes of democracies establishing themselves in warfare, during which there is no private retreat for the citizen. Nontotalitarianism means that the political order permits its members to keep part of their lives private, and to practice politics only intermittently. A minority of the United States electorate elect the president, although his legitimation is in terms of "majority rule." For many people voting thus would seem to make little difference in many decisions of national consequence.[27] Insofar as democracy exists in such a situation, it is expressed mainly by com-

[27] See W. E. Binkley, *The Powers of the President* (Garden City, N. Y.: Doubleday, 1937) and Harold Laski, *The American Presidency, An Interpretation* (New York: Harper, 1940).

peting pressure groups and parties. As a type, totalitarian democracy enables us to take into account the fact that in constitutionally democratic states there has been a tendency, implemented by the emergencies of war and peace, for controls to become increasingly total.[28] The United States has been spared many controls, even during World War II, for there was no mass evacuation of children, no total civilian defense, and no intensive control of the kitchen.

IV. *Socialist democracy* refers to a parliamentary regime with a democratic-minded labor party at the helm, engaged in socializing strategic industries and extending welfare services and housing facilities to lower classes. Pursuing a policy of "full employment," socialists would displace capitalism's "anarchy of production" by a policy of public planning. Such a regime would contain a strong judiciary with legal guarantees, as well as parties which compete but which are not strong enough to overrule juridical decisions. Democratically accountable planners and managerial boards would, according to this view of democracy, debate what products should be made: there would be production planning on the basis of consumer demands, explicitly linked with mass organizations. How many television sets or houses should be made would thus be a public decision, and consumption and production of the nation would be considered as in one big household. Under such a socialized and planned economy—which would involve the confiscation of private property—co-ops would own some industries, and various public authorities—local, regional and national—would own others. These bodies would appoint managers, and hold them accountable. Inheritance would have nothing to do with who was in charge. Co-ops and trade unions would have voices in the places of decision, and at least a veto right over managers. Unions would also propose, as well as veto, managerial decisions. Democracy would thus involve both the political and the economic order.

In distinguishing various types of despotism, it seems convenient to classify them, first, as Oriental or Western. The Oriental variety superseded feudalism by establishing a bureaucracy—of Confucian gentlemen, as in China; or of priestly scribes, as in ancient Egypt and Mesopotamia. These bureaucracies controlled,

[28] See Franz Neumann, *Behemoth; The Structure and Practice of National Socialism* (New York: Oxford, 1942); and Arthur Rosenberg, *The Birth of the German Republic,* I. F. D. Morrow, tr. (London: Oxford, 1931).

among other means of life, the rivers, with which they managed irrigation systems. Two types should be mentioned:

I. The *Caesarism* of Rome's empire was based upon an imperial bureaucracy of army officers and tax farmers. The Diocletian Empire is the clearest example of an imperial bureacracy led by hereditary dynasties and punctuated by military usurpers. It was a theocracy with Caesar as god. The military order was important, as a chronic state of war was necessary to provide slaves for the economy. Public financing was shifted from taxes to services in kind. A money economy broke down as the area of domination spread, so the center of gravity shifted inland. The rich, who provided the liturgies, fled from the cities and, going to country estates, rusticated.

II. *Sultanism* operates with a harem: the despot, by prudent choice of women, attached various sibs to his own ruling household. Within the harem, however, sib rivalry may be implemented, as ambitious women join an opposition. The harem thus added an additional element of unmanageability. The Chinese dynasties, for example, went through cycles which regularly ended in the un-Confucian rule of empress-dowagers and eunuchs, the so-called "petticoat government." At any rate, in the typical cycle, the decision-making center resolves into factions, and then a charismatic peasant builds up an army and goes against the court. In his rise to power, he gets training for the despotic role that he will later play.

In Western civilization, the following historical types of despotism have widely prevailed:

III. The *feudal monarchy* of the European Middle Ages, with its permanent tensions between Pope and Emperor, was a loose set of principalities, castled and self-equipped warriors, of fortified semiautonomous city republics, and corporate church and monastic bodies. The emperor had no adequate administrative and technological means of enforcing sovereign rights from on high, and accordingly had to bargain with variously privileged estates, which however were held together by a common faith in Christianity.

IV. The *absolutist regimes* of European kings and petty princes, from the sixteenth to the eighteenth centuries, introduced bureaucratic administrations which co-ordinated military and fiscal policies. Within this framework, territories have contested for prestige and power through warfare and dynastic marriages. As the mercenary army displaced the self-equipped feudal knighthood, princely absolutism, based upon the "Divine Right of Kings," undermined the various feudal estates having varying degrees of political and legal power. This absolutism centralized the scattered prerogatives of feudal Europe, reduced the nobility to office nobles and army officers; with cannon fire, it broke up their strongholds and castles. It reduced the status of quasi-autonomous cities, and leveled men into subjects inhabiting the territory which it had pacified. With the exception of the priesthood and the privileged nobles, the subjects of princely absolutism were held to regular taxes, which in the *ancien régime* of France, for example, were collected by 30,000 privileged entrepreneurs, or, as in Prussia, by a tax-collecting machine of military bureaucrats.

Princely absolutism was a type of police state which sought to establish totalitarian control. It sought to increase its population by having ministers exhort the people to "be fruitful and multiply," and by attracting privileged immigrant groups. It sought to steer the economy by investing tax-income in schemes for technological and industrial improvement. It sought to hoard precious metals as a war chest, and to promote agricultural settlement schemes for the sake of increasing the tax yield. It sought also to inculcate loyalties to the state and to its prince. Thus Colbert had his standing army of mercenary soldiers dig canals during peacetime—an early modern case of public works performed by "forced labor."

Yet with all this, given the level of preindustrial technology and communications, princely absolutism was overthrown or reduced by the industrial middle classes, who strove for democracy and constitutional government, for a secure and calculable legal order guaranteeing "due process of law," and thus for the opportunity to orient themselves in a predictable way to competitive markets, and other matters of income and property.

V. The middle-class revolutions of England and France brought forth *Bonapartism*—a Cromwell and a Napoleon—to stabilize their revolutionary attainments. Kemal Atatürk, regarded as the creator of modern Turkey, might be compared with Napoleon. The military juntas of Spanish-American countries, or Pilsudski's regime of colonels in Poland between the wars, are different forms of dictatorship in largely agrarian and debtor countries. "Bonapartism" means a one-man rule on the basis of acclamation. Yet we should remember that these despotisms are not totalitarianism: they are not based on one single mass party, they do not manage the complexities of a corporate capitalist economy in terms of a planned economy set up for a chronic state of war.

VI. None of the pre-twentieth-century types of despotism has, in fact, much in common with the *totalitarian dictatorship* of the Soviet Union, or the Fascist regimes of Italy and Spain, or the Nazi dictatorship. These modern despots mobilize industrialized countries for imperialist wars in an attempt to redivide the world. Modern dictators are revolutionary usurpers, usually going against a center which is faction-ridden. Their usurpation is usually preceded by a condition in which there is a plurality of pressure groups and parties, and no chance to establish a stable government. The individual experiences fully his inability to meet the public crises which intensify his anxieties. He longs for a center of management. Nobody seems to do anything, although everybody is busy. Both the right and the left may unite against the middle, but they cannot form a stable government. So, the dictator—the conspicuous man thrown up by crisis and eager to assume emergency powers and responsibility for all public affairs—arises on the basis of a party and establishes a one-party state.

The social content, the ruling elites, the justifying symbols and ideologies—these vary with the social setting and the political aims at hand. For example, where Hitler's regime sought to strengthen the individual peasant farm as well as *Junker* landlordism by organizing agrarian society into a compulsory cartel for purposes of autarchy, the Bolshevists, after some detours, abolished individual holdings and organized agriculture in a network of tractor stations and state farms. They thus reduced the peasantry to wage workers and so guaranteed greater efficiency of production and a higher tax income from the land than would have been available under private property.

Totalitarian states go beyond the bureaucratization of democratic states by subjecting all organized channels of communication, including concert hall and exhibition of art work, as well as radio, print, and film to their control. This requires that various skill groups—journalists, cameramen, film directors, artists, radio men—be organized into quasi-bureaucracies, that is, transformed into "officials" who have all the responsibilities of regular state officials but not their decision-making functions, their rights of tenure, their pensions, or their anonymity. Such skill groups must then define and promulgate official images of the world and what is happening in it, official "definitions of the situation."

Public opinion, as Hans Speier puts it,[29] involves the right of the citizenry publicly to engage in critical communications to and about the government and its policy decisions. Such public opinion does not exist in totalitarian societies. There is only the precarious role of the small-audience satirist, who, like the old court jester or official fool, may speak the truth—within limits and so long as no one takes him seriously.

4. Economic Institutions [30]

Economic orders are composed of institutions by which men organize labor for the peaceful production and distribution of goods and services. The dominant economic organizations as well as their integration vary according to the particular economic ends sought, of which there are generally two types: one may produce for one's own household and thus belong to a "subsistence economy"; or one may produce for profits to be gained through indirect exchange in a "money economy." Accordingly, we speak of the "subsistence farmer," such as the old-time European peasant, and of the "cash crop farmer," such as, predominantly, the American farm operator. Modern industrial economies may also be classified as composed of competing "private enterprises"; of "mixed" enterprises, in which public authorities and private enterprisers join forces; or of "public enterprises."

Georg Simmel identified "rationality" with money exchange because money is a common denominator of qualitatively different

[29] Paraphrased from Hans Speier, *Social Order and the Risks of War* (New York: Stewart, 1952), p. 323.

[30] The reader will find the following to be important: Max Weber, *General Economic History,* Frank Knight, tr. (Glencoe, Illinois: Free Press, 1950); Karl Marx, *Selected Works in 2 Vols.* (Prepared at the Marx Institute, Moscow, by V. Adoratsky, edited in English by C. P. Dutt, New York); Thorstein Veblen, *The Theory of Business Enterprise* (New York, 1935); Georg Simmel, *The Sociology of Georg Simmel,* K. Wolff, ed. and tr. (Glencoe, Illinois: Free Press, 1950); Werner Sombart, "Capitalism," *Encyclopaedia of the Social Sciences,* Vol. III, pp. 195-208, and *The Quintessence of Capitalism* (London, 1915); J. A. Hobson, *The Evolution of Modern Capitalism* (London, 1926); and J. A. Schumpeter, *Capitalism, Socialism, and Democracy* (New York: Harper, 1950).

goods. Money allows for the quantification of all qualities, and this quantification, in turn, allows the analytic breaking down of qualities into equal units, as well as for the translatability of one quality into another—and hence for calculation. For Simmel, capitalism is therefore seen as a diffusion of the exchange medium, money, and the concomitant mental attitudes of (1) rational calculation, and (2) the objectification of personal properties and belongings.

In prepecuniary eras, all goods and artifacts were identified with their owner; they extended the range of his personality, they embodied his personality traits. But in pecuniary eras this intimate psychic linkage of persons with the goods they own is broken, and goods become objects circulating or ready to circulate among different persons. Hence economic goods become abstracted from the personal work invested in them. Simmel thus defines capitalism in terms of the money economy.

Werner Sombart, in contrast, emphasizes the rational calculation of profits, costs, and income as the constitutive element of modern capitalism. Hence, for Sombart the emergence of modern capitalism dates from the invention of double entry bookkeeping by an Italian monk in the Italian city economy of early Renaissance days.

For both Simmel and Sombart the sphere of distribution—the market—is the decisive anchorage of capitalism. The ramifications of technological changes implementing novel modes of production are not of primary significance to them. Capitalism is the use of the pecuniary principle in different fields of economic pursuits; this principle gradually engulfs the economic orders of whole nations and cultural areas, and in due course perhaps, permeates the entire world.

For Karl Marx and Max Weber, in contrast to both Simmel and Sombart, "modern capitalism" is anchored in the sphere of production. Accordingly, the historical emergence of modern capitalism is not seen as a quantitative expansion of markets, but as the emergence of the factory as the productive unit or, in Weber's terms, of a rational organization of formally free labor for the continuous acquisition of profits. Because of his emphasis upon production, Marx focused upon the labor supply and the exploitability of the "reserve army of labor." Weber was more interested in the origin and psychology of a stratum of middle-class entrepreneurs.

Marx believed that fraud and violence implemented the initial phase of the primary accumulation required for capitalism. Yeomen, small propertied groups, and artisans were brutally dislocated from their traditional pursuits.

Weber also placed great emphasis upon noneconomic factors, but his central problem became a psychological one: how is it possible that strata of enterprisers and workers emerge that are willing to engage in methodically persistent, hard work and thereby gain a competitive advantage over less principled, more traditionalist economic agents? These men forego the traditional enjoyments of wealth—the expansion of their consumption, or the investment of wealth in ostentatious ways. How is it, then, that men arise who work hard, despite the fact that in the value terms of their economic tradition and epoch they have no understandable motives for doing so? Weber's answer lies in his reconstruction of the religiously motivated asceticism, the inner-worldly or this-worldly asceticism, of the heroic puritan.[31]

In his causal analysis, Weber thus specializes in the problem of *modern* capitalism. For him industrial capitalism is not sufficiently defined by profit-making, because profits are made by Chinese traders as well as by Armenian middlemen. Nor is capitalism a matter of acquisitive instincts, which are revealed by all sorts and conditions of men in contexts which lack the specific character of capitalism—modern industry. In contrast to Sombart, Weber was not interested in how profits are counted, but in the fact that they are made.

For both Marx and for Weber, modern capitalism, therefore, does not exist in the Italian Renaissance cities, or in the Roman empire, or the Tokugawa epoch of Japan. In its modern sense, capitalism is a specifically Occidental or Western economic order, beginning primarily in England during the sixteenth and seventeenth centuries.

5. Types of Capitalism

It is within the realm of comparative economics, however, that Weber developed his "types of capitalism" which in reality constitute a panorama of economies existing prior to distinctively mod-

[31] See Chapter IX: Institutional Orders and Social Controls, II, Section 1: Religious Institutions.

ern capitalism. These types include pariah, political, booty, and colonial capitalism.[32]

I. *Pariah capitalism* is the capitalism of despised marginal traders who are originally strangers among host nations which allow them to fulfill economically welcome but morally impugned functions. Weber called such despised trading groups "pariahs" when they were socially ostracized: excluded from intermarriage and dinner table fellowship with members of the politically dominant group. And he used the term "pariah capitalism" in order to emphasize the marginal position which they typically occupy. Christian traders in the midst of Mohammedan Turks, Chinese merchants in Southeast Asia, the Parsee traders of India, and the Greek middlemen in Africa are cases in point, as well as, of course, occidental Jewry in the Middle Ages. Such pariah capitalists are often commercial capitalists, accumulating profits by the control of major trade routes for luxury commodities, such as spices, precious metals, and silks.

II. Under certain conditions even pariah capitalists may be welcome servants of political or ecclesiastical rulers. As market experts, they know how to raise credits for political and military enterprises. When any capitalist, pariah or not, undertakes services of this kind, we may speak of *political capitalism*.

Political capitalism tends to flower in states of chronic warfare or revolution. Many of the Jews, as well as Gentiles, of the European Middle Ages were protected by courts and participated in such capitalism. Thus the famous brothers Rothschild established themselves in Frankfort on the Main, as well as London, Paris, and Vienna. They helped finance the Napoleonic wars, on all sides of the battle lines, thus minimizing possible losses of the family as a financial community.

Political capitalism has assumed a number of different forms. Political rulers for example, in a fiscal capitalism, have often "farmed out" tax collection to private entrepreneurs. Such entrepreneurial gatherers of taxes existed in the late Roman empire, in which they enriched themselves by exploiting the provinces economically and using their private fortunes as stepping stones in political careers in Rome. Thus did Caesar squeeze Gaul. A similar stratum of "tax farmers" became significantly unpopular in prerevolutionary France under the absolutism of the *ancien régime*.

[32] Cf. *General Economic Theory*, *op. cit.*, and Max Weber, *op. cit.*

Rulers have frequently farmed out the royal mint itself to private enterprisers. The house of Mitsui, for example, floated the first government currency after the reformation in Japan. The house of Fuggers enjoyed minting rights as well as mining privileges. Such opportunities as tax gathering and money-issuing are direct state functions, which is why Weber called this type of capitalism fiscal capitalism—the term fiscal referring to the state as an economic agent.

Another kind of political capitalism involves the organization of armed forces by private entrepreneurs. The *condottiere* emerges when disciplined units of mercenary footmen prove superior to the individualistic, undisciplined feudal knight-in-armor. The Italian *condottieri* (Sforza), as well as the north Alpine organizer of mercenary troops (Frundsberg and Wallenstein), are best known. The later standing armies of absolutist European rulers were financed by a slowly emerging technique of regular tax collection, by political loans and subsidies from the outside (e.g., British subsidies to Frederick II of Prussia during the Seven Years War).

In contrast to the devaluation of pariah capitalists, fiscal capitalists have enjoyed great esteem, which, in part, has been due to their participation in royal functions and hence their borrowing of status. Jacob Fugger of Augsburg, who financed the election of an emperor was, and felt like, a kingmaker.

III. During the modern expansion of markets, overseas traders typically met tribal or other political communities which denied them access to harbor and trading opportunities. In such situations, the trader, in the absence of maritime and international law, used to go well armed, and if necessary open the door to trade at the point of a gun. Where persuasion to trade is implemented by the actual use or the threat of violence, one may speak of *booty capitalism*. The term is appropriate: under conditions of forced transactions one can hardly speak of an exchange of commodities by peaceful bargaining. The exchange is, in fact, a polite façade for direct appropriation by violence. Slaves have been one of the most favored commodities appropriated in this fashion.

IV. It has been an old tradition of occidental merchants to establish trading posts and stable places abroad. Thus, the Hanseatic League maintained trading posts on the Volga as well as on the Thames. Trading companies have engaged in overseas trade, and in due course acquired favorable sites, called "factories." Thus the

British East India Company established its factories in India. From such a "trading" post, resident stewards expanded their operations, and in due course, acquired considerable territorial domains. Increased holdings brought in their train increased tensions and dangers, political, military and economic. Accordingly, a military establishment had to secure the colony. Westerners residing in the trading posts and becoming acquainted with the problems of the surrounding territories naturally discovered occasions and opportunities for further expansion by entering the politics of the particular region and exploiting them for their own advantage. In short, booty capitalist adventures have led to *colonial capitalism*.

Colonial capitalism has typically established "the plantation system," which thrives on an intensive cultivation of tropical and garden produce such as tea, cotton, tobacco, sugar, and in the age of the automobile, rubber. It is a further characteristic of the plantation that it utilizes slave or forced labor. The most significant areas of such plantation systems have been in the North African grain belt, in the Portuguese, French, Dutch, and British domains in India, and in the Southern states before the Civil War.

Modern capitalist entrepreneurs have struggled against all the odds of jurisdictional handicaps, the closure policies of guilds and politically privileged monopolists, and the mercantilist police state. Their slogan, "laissez-faire," was directed against the feudal vestiges of guild policies, as well as against politically privileged monopolists. The autonomy of the pacified market appeared to them as the ideal field of operations, and the establishment of such a market as a fulfillment of freedom. The free market was thus the economic precondition and result of the free enterprise; this market became *world wide* and based in gold, and free migration of people knit together the system as a whole.

Nineteenth-century capitalism approximated the goal of an economic order knit together by markets. To be sure, vestiges of previous economic orders existed, especially in the rural economies of continental Europe, and a good many artisan establishments survived. But the dynamics of the economic order did not rest upon these vestiges; it was controlled by market-oriented free entrepreneurs. These agents enrolled a labor force in their expanding capitalist enterprises, which gradually came to permeate all branches of production and distribution. The right of the owner freely to dispose of exchangeable goods came to include such previously immobile items as land, and the initiative of the enterpriser fed upon continuously expanding business opportunities.

Legally guaranteed monopolies in trade, handicraft, and industry were broken down. Legislation which confined itself to the formal rules of the game replaced municipal statutes and guild rules that restricted those who could play the game. Free mobility became a recognized right of the citizen. Everyone could leave his place of birth and move where he pleased; emigration and immigration were legally facilitated through the free handing out of passports and the relatively free admission of newcomers to all localities. All national currencies had fairly stable relations to gold, and international trade in capital and commodities flourished.

States minimized direct political intervention in the economic order. For the implied assumption that ran through the laissez-faire system was that the automatic steering of the whole process of expansion would work out in the interest of all economic agents. A harmony of interests between the individual profiting in the process of expansion and the public weal was taken for granted by the advocates of the system. At the dawn of the system, it was possible for theoreticians like Adam Smith—the fountainhead of the theory of economic liberalism—to think in terms of further increasing the relatively equal distribution of private property. This was the central meaning of equality of opportunity: that every man of initiative and talent could enter the competitive race on equal terms with his competitors. Since at the start of the race, men were assumed to be more or less equally endowed, the different degrees of their success could be ascribed to their personal merit and initiative.

Such business depressions as occurred were declared to be temporary aberrations of particular branches of industries; such depressions in due course would be compensated for by a proportionate expansion of more profitable fields. Public opinion was optimistic to the point of enthusiasm, and the turbulent social unrest of the Chartist and similar movements was soon forgotten. Critics like Ruskin, Marx, and Saint-Simon remained outside the main drift. The severe human and social costs of this capitalism were overlooked in the scramble to get rich quick. In such virgin economic areas as the U.S.A., the unrestricted right of the private property owner often allowed for short-sighted exploitation of natural resources, profitable to the individual but costly to the nation at large and to later generations.

Under modern capitalism, private enterprises are (1) passed on as property to heirs and heiresses and (2) yield to these owners "unearned income" beyond the entrepreneurial salaries paid to managers and company directors, the interest due to investors and creditors, and the funds set aside for replacement and renewal of plant. Such properties are not the work-properties which Adam Smith had in mind when he thought of "private enterprise." The theorems of classical economics in fact have now become "ideologies" by means of which politically interested spokesmen apply the small-shop thinking of laissez-faire days to the giant enterprises of absentee owners in an age of monopoly capitalism.

The policies of the leading United States corporations today determine the economic fate of most other economic units in the United States, of many little businesses and family farmers, who are all dependent upon the price policies of the corporations that produce oil, farm machinery, electrical current, and artificial fertilizer.[33] The employment opportunities of employees—of wage workers and of the white collar people also—depend upon the strategic decisions of corporate managements. The structure of these corporations is bureaucratic, and the bureaucracy of an oil or a steel trust may be more powerful than that of many political states. Their decisions concerning investment and price policies pertain to far-flung production establishments, located in many countries and so having international ramifications.

Under such conditions, the meaning of "private" as applied to the leading American corporations means merely that their policymakers are not publicly accountable for their decisions—so long as they "stay within the law," which is often loosely defined and perhaps necessarily vague about the latest business practices.

In the big business establishment, all items of production, raw materials, labor, interest charges, and so on, are carefully calculated as "costs" and all income for goods sold is balanced against costs. The goal of production is to maximize the total assets, which means

[33] For a good introduction to this subject, see Caroline F. Ware and Gardiner C. Means, *The Modern Economy in Action* (New York: Harcourt, Brace, 1936); and David Lynch, *The Concentration of Economic Power* (New York: Columbia Univ. Press, 1946).

the long-run profitability of the corporation. This does not mean that the entrepreneur or the manager is necessarily motivated by "the profit motive." For he may take the profitablility of his operation for granted, and be motivated by the enjoyment of economic power, realizing the extent to which smaller, less strategically placed enterprises have to accommodate themselves to his price-policy lead or technological and organizational advances. He may enjoy the opportunity of providing jobs to so many employees, that is, the dependence of thousands of families on his skillful operation of the business. He may enjoy his freedom to brave government orders and find himself, as did Sewell Avery of Montgomery Ward during World War II, gently carried from his office in the arms of soldiers. The handling of colossal amounts of goods, the boom and din of machinery, the impressive figures of output, may all feed into a joyful sense of power, of the sheer momentum of the operation. Couched in moral terms, the powerful man of business may see the total enterprise as a going concern "demanding him," and so feel himself to be "indispensable." And in all these worries and gratifications, the "profit motive" may be but a by-product, even though, to be sure, analytically speaking, profitability is the indispensable prerequisite for continuous operation of the big business unit.

The principle of *technological* efficiency involves the solving of given technical tasks by the most efficient means available. The *economic* principle involves the attaining of optimum profits for a given outlay. These two principles are fused in the capitalist enterprise, and so capitalism has often been termed the embodiment of "rationality." Many observers, however, have doubted the "rationality" of the capitalist system as they have considered its operations and results over long periods:

They have noted (1) the wastefulness of its operations, as dramatically revealed during depressions; (2) the systematic unemployment of millions of men, as in post-World War II Europe, (3) the costs of wars and of colonies for raw material monopolies; (4) the costs of economic nationalism and protectionism; (5) the periodic breakdowns which displace in an unplanned and unconcerned way the careers of men, condemning some to permanent "unemployment" at the age of forty-five unless they change their vocations and "write off" their educational investments; (6) the distributions of both property and income, without rational linkage to merit or function; (7) the fairy-tale-like differences in consumption; (8) the expropriation of large masses of fixed income earners through inflationary processes benefiting the propertied; (9) the bombardment of low-income groups with a never-ending stream of advertised goods beyond their purchasing power; and so, the inculcation of wishes not to be satisfied; (10) the assertion of free consumers' choice to low-income groups who "have no choice." Even Max Weber, who of course accepted capitalism as "economic rationalism" incarnate, liked to cite Robert Wagner's phrase characterizing capitalism as "this masterless slavery."

The economic order is obviously related to other institutional orders. It is "costly" to build a church or to recruit an army. Whatever ends may be pursued, economic means limit or facilitate their attainment. When the state nationalizes or socializes the relevant means of production—the big land holdings, factories and facilities of distribution—and manages these establishments just as military property is now managed in the United States, then economic and political orders are fused. Even where there is private property, this process goes on, as during wartime, for the planning and technology required by twentieth-century warfare increasingly penetrates the economy—even during times of nominal peace. There are raw material allocations and a planned distribution of scarce labor; there are priorities and price controls and the rationing of consumers' goods; and there is possibly a control of private profits as well as major production for state-defined needs. At such times the production secrets of individual enterprises may be publicized and communicated to less efficient units in the economy in order to increase total output in the shortest possible time.[34]

Wartime planning under private capitalism, in short, is a considerable departure from "business as usual." It is when "all-out production" is the order of the day that the irrationalities of "business as usual," with its unused capacities and idle men, become most embarrassingly obvious. Rather than a promise of a policy, "full employment" becomes a fact. When men then consider such mobilization of production for the sake of more efficient destruction, when millions of men are taken out of production for years,

[34] Key books include: Alfred Vagts, *The History of Militarism* (New York: Norton, 1937); *Makers of Modern Strategy*, Edward M. Earle and others, eds. (Princeton: Princeton Univ. Press, 1943); and Speier, *op. cit.*, pp. 223-323.

and then millions of man-hours are spent for years for destruction, the irrational factors seem to loom larger. At any rate, since the 1890's, the periodic armament races of industrial societies have reduced Spencer's assumption of the peaceful nature of industrial societies to the bad joke of a "Little England" liberal.

6. The Military Order

The military order comprises the legitimate and institutionalized practice of violence. In modern industrial societies this order is of course a department of the state, but the practice of violence has come to be of such outstanding significance that it is convenient to single out the military order for separate analysis.

Arnold Toynbee has brilliantly outlined the sequence of pre-industrial warfare in terms of footmen and horsemen, either of which may be lightly or heavily armed. Accordingly, one may speak of (a) light footmen or (b) of light horsemen, and of (c) heavily equipped footsoldiers or (d) of heavily armed horsemen. Tribal horse nomads (the Huns), for example, represent light horsemen whose disciplined and swift attacks struck terror to the hearts of the men in Christendom; since that time, the term, "horde" has appeared in the vocabulary of all Western languages.

Toynbee sees in various civilizations a "David and Goliath pattern" of warfare: the small, quick maneuvering kind of man beats the massively armored giant. Toynbee's own materials, however, seem to us to show that in due course, heavy armor is more likely to be beaten by heavier armor—and heavier discipline. The Spartan phalanx won for a while; then an Athenian swarm of David's peltasts beat the phalanx, and then an improved phalanx, out of Thebes, with a formation in depth came to the fore. Later, everything went down before the Roman legionnaire, who as a versatile fighting man combined in his person a co-ordination of all known military skills and weapons—the light infantry man or the heavily armored hoplite, with throwing spear, sword, and huge shield. He was able to combine—and to use as occasion demanded—the maneuverability of the individual skirmisher with the driving force of the drilled formation.

Yet the legionnaire fell before the light horseman with bow and arrow and the heavily armed horseman with lance and shield. And this armored lancer, according to Toynbee, "kept the saddle for the next twelve hundred years . . . before he too, resting too long on his oars and so becoming an armor-plated travesty of his own beginnings, was decisively beaten by a David on horseback—a light horse archer of Nomad type and agility from the 13th century steppes." [35]

The alteration between the undisciplined hero—jousting as a chivalrous knight—and the disciplined formation of footmen may be repeatedly observed in military history. In ancient Greece the Homeric heroes were displaced by the hoplite army; in medieval Europe the feudal hero was displaced by armies of disciplined mercenaries; in ancient China the charioteers of the feudal age gave way to the army of footsoldiers; [36] in Great Britain the undisciplined fighting of the feudal lords proved technically inferior to the disciplined cavalry attack of Cromwell's ironsides. [37]

Before the rise of nation-states, warfare in agrarian societies was the privilege of princes. But since the American and French revolutions, the state has made warfare the concern of the nation as a whole. Mercenary armies, which were originally offered on a competitive basis to princes and to city states, became attached to the state as standing armies of mercenaries and impressed soldiers. Such armies, however, were costly, and the individual soldier, particularly after defeats, was not necessarily loyal to the respective prince or state. Men at war accordingly minimized open battles in favor of exhausting the adversary economically, threatening and shadowboxing without readily risking all-out battle. This military technique has been called the "strategy of attrition" a strategy pursued during World Wars I and II by naval powers who blockaded the central and Axis powers, blacklisted enemy-controlled firms in neutral countries, and purchased commodities in order to deny the enemy access to goods important for war.

Napoleon, however, revived and developed to new heights another type of strategy, the "strategy of annihilation." Its precondition is a patriotic army which today is recruited by universal drafts. The aim of the leader in annihilation warfare is to administer crushing defeats to the enemy's armies, to occupy his economically important areas and his capital city, and then, after unconditional

---

[35] *A Study of History* (London, 1951), Vol. IV, pp. 431 ff.

[36] See Max Weber, *The Religion of China*, H. H. Gerth, tr. (Glencoe, Illinois: Free Press, 1951), pp. 24 ff.

[37] See Sir Charles Firth, *Cromwell's Army* (London: Methuen, 1902).

surrender, to impose the victor's will. As a type of military strategy, annihilation has developed along with the political form of the state and with the industrialization of the nation. All twentieth-century warfare has been concluded by "unconditional surrender."

The mobilization of the modern nation's resources for war has reached a total state—in scope, intensity, and efficiency. The age at which soldiers are recruited has been lowered to eighteen years and raised to sixty or sixty-five; women have been drafted for military or production service; the difference between combatants and noncombatants has been abolished through blockade policies and the *tabula rasa* policy of the atomic bomb. Civilians behind the lines of invading armies are expected to wage guerrilla warfare and to practice sabotage. The co-ordination of all institutional orders involved in modern war leads to totalitarian measures of planning. All large-scale organizations in all institutional orders are co-ordinated to further the supreme end of victory. Art and science, religion and education are committed to the cause. The media of mass communications help to concentrate fears and aggressions, maximizing their intensity and directing them against the enemy as the "total threat." Accordingly, economic, psychological, political, and military warfare are so many special aspects of total war.

This co-ordination of a nation for war leads to unease and tension. For example, the lowering of the draft age, which is largely technologically determined, comes into conflict with the legal definition of adult status and the political definition of voting age. The Soviet Union and the states within her orbit have adjusted to this conflict by lowering the legal definition of adult status to eighteen years in Eastern Germany, to twelve years in the Soviet Union. The privileged status of youth before the courts has been abolished. In Russia a teen-ager in court is punished like an adult, rather than like a "juvenile delinquent." In the United States, such problems are still controversial.

Another tension results from the equal employability and compensation of men and women in military and other war work, and from the transferability of the worker to the army and of the soldier to the factory. The cartoonist Bill Mauldin caricatured such tensions expertly during the late war. As long as differences in income and in risk accompany such transfers, psychic compensations have to fill the gap. The invention and manipulation of such compensations require special policies and efforts, as well as large-scale measures of psychological warfare, by which leaders seek to control tension levels and insecurity feelings.

An increasing array of attitude, trait, and aptitude tests are used to "screen" masses of recruits in order to assign men to their most suitable roles. Moreover, psychological warfare now involves the study of suitable propaganda addressed to partners of the hostile coalition having diverse cultures and value preferences, which is thus intended to divide them, to maximize whatever tension state exists between them, to foment disloyalty to leaders and causes, to promote states of apathy and indifference, and finally, to produce "crises of conscience" which will weaken the will to fight or even induce a "change of sides."

The Russians were quite successful in such policies during the late war against Hitler, winning over and organizing captured "free German officers," and using them in their anti-Nazi propaganda. The Nazis, on the other hand, organized an army of Ukrainians under General Wlassow, who had deserted the Red army; although no Nazi, he made common cause with them for reasons of his own. During the same war, the United States and her allies were able to persuade Mussolini's ace diplomat, Dino Grandi, to abandon Mussolini and his regime, as well as the sinking Nazi ship, and to come over to the side of Victor Emmanuel and his following. With this, the Italian war was to some extent transformed into a civil war, as well as a war of liberation from the occupying Nazi army. Similarly, France was divided, the "Free French" under General de Gaulle, being cut loose from the Pétain-Laval regime, attacking the Pétain administration of Syria and Dakar.

The distrust characteristic of modern coalition partners is obvious when we remember the clause in President Roosevelt's destroyer deal with Great Britain which obliged his Majesty never to surrender the royal navy to Nazi Germany. The swiftness of events, the changes of sides by leaders who thus write off decades of verbalized sentiments and loyalties, the value cleavages by virtue of which Churchill had to order the sinking of the French navy "with a heavy heart," the transformation of Stalin's image from "Uncle Joe" to a scheming enigma—all such policies and strategies and images demand a subtlety of presentation to mass society and a short memory during the numerous changes in line.

In our times, speed is indispensable to success in total war, but of late, the mass training of hatred and friendship runs up against an ever-greater propaganda neurosis, and has had to overcome an increasing psychic inertia.

In present-day warfare, machines seem more important than men, who, in fact, often seem appendages to machines, rather than the manipulators of machines as fighting tools. In the United States air force during World War II, differences in the interacting personalities of the ten crew members of a bomber were irrelevant to their efficiency. Their tight-knit roles, based on the requirements of the plane, and their co-ordination to one another, shape individual men into uniform role takers. A rigid, straightforward patriotic feeling, and the ambition to be a proved hero are no longer, in the view of military personnel experts, unquestionable assets, at least not for all fighting men. Among bomber crews in the Eighth Air Force, such feelings and ambitions operated to repress anxieties, and so endangered performance as well as expensive equipment and training. Accordingly, such feelings were, as a policy, carefully discouraged in favor of a more candid admission of anxieties. Among parachutists, however, the reverse held: strong superegos, and so heroic postures, were encouraged.

7. Characteristics of Six Types of Armies

In order briefly to reveal the range of phenomena in the military order, we shall now discuss six quite different types of armies, in each case setting forth the following social and psychological characteristics: their legitimations and motivations for fighting, their social recruitment and their financing or provisioning, the technological implements they typically employed and the form of organization usually followed, and their typical strategy and tactical maneuvers. We believe that these are among the key typological features required for the sociological understanding of any army.

I. The tribal formations of Teutonic warriors and of a variety of nomads legitimated their wars for land and booty, or their migratory expansions due to population pressure, in traditional and charismatic ways. They are free men—although among their ranks are also adopted prisoners of war—self-equipped with club and sword, lance and bow, as well as, in the case of the Vikings and Homeric Greeks, ships. Their strategy is the raid, or the quick invasion, and their tactics include encirclement by swarms of lightly armed camel or horse bowmen, and the wedge formation of Teutonic warriors.

II. Patrimonial armies of the Eastern Roman Empire are recruited from among slaves and justified traditionally. They are organized in rational formations of legions or cohorts, and are equipped and provided for by their master or prince. Their officers are motivated by loyalty to the traditional head, and their ranks are often compelled by harsh discipline. Shoulder to shoulder they stand in a disciplined bloc—with lance, sword, and siege machinery, as well as road and bridge building apparatus. Their objective is to annihilate the enemy by frontal attack and envelopment, by a variety of rationally elaborated tactics.

III. The feudal knight of the Occident is a professional warrior, self-equipped from his fief; his violence is legitimated by personal charism and Christian blessings. He is motivated by personal honor, his oath of allegiance, and a sense of heroic adventure. He is also motivated by his interest in conquering fiefs which thus add to the domain and glory of Christian Knighthood. Since his tactic is to joust as an individual in the open fields, the organization for battle is a loose federation of individual fighting men. On horse, carrying lance, sword, and shield, and armored by metal and leather, his tactics include the individual duel and the taking of prisoners for ransom.

IV. Oliver Cromwell's army, recruited from the Puritan gentry, is legitimated by a religious cause. In part it is self-equipped, like the feudal knights, and in part, like modern national armies, provisioned by parliament. The men of this army are motivated by a discipline based on an absolute belief in their religious cause. They are organized in numerically defined units, in disciplined formations with stratified ranks of officers. They are a cavalry which, with pistol and saber, practice the tactics of the lineal frontal assault as well as the assault in depth for the strategical objective of annihilation.

V. The *condottiere* organizes soldiers of fortune, held by contractional obligations with a city-state or a prince or any other private or public body. The fulfillment of these contracts serves as his legitimation. As a private military enterpriser, he recruits mercenaries in a great variety of ways, including the shanghaiing of vagabonds. He is both self-equipped and provided for by his employer. The mercenary army is rationally disciplined and motivated by adventurous quests for profits and booty, including women; ranks of such armies are held together by coercion and expectation of wages and the general hatred of the population for these "strangers in the land" and disdain of the upper classes exploiting them. His implements vary with technological level, from pike and sword, musket and cannon, to frigate and aircraft. His tactics accordingly vary, as does the organization of the army, but his strategy tends to be that of attrition, especially the cutting off of the enemy from his base of operations and the financial exhaustion of the enemy.

VI. The violence of the modern national army is legitimated by the symbols and sentiments of the nation and its cause; the men of this army are disciplined for obedience to a hierarchy of staff and line officers. Discipline rests upon acceptance of the nation's cause and is guaranteed by sanctions—including loss of status and career chances and, in the last analysis, capital punishment. Although voluntary enlistments are permitted or encouraged, the mode of recruitment is compulsory service for all citizens judged fit. The national army is organized as a national bureaucracy, equipped by the state or by the lend-lease of other friendly states. Historically, equipment has ranged from rifle and cannon to the machines of modern industrial war. Tactics include every type from "Indian war" with rifle and grenade in small quick attack, to trench warfare of position and maneuver and break-through, as well as saturation bombardment from above. The strategical objective is to wear down, and in the end, to obliterate the enemy, occupy his territory and impose the victor's will. Since major wars are global, the power blocs of nations aim at division and redivision of the world, and in the last analysis at world domination.

Institutional Orders
and Social Controls, II

1. Religious Institutions

By "religious order," as we have already noted, we refer to all those institutions in which men organize the collective worship of God or gods at regular occasions and at fixed places. In religious conduct men use supernatural means—prayer and sacrifice, for example—in an effort to attain supernatural ends. In various ways religion has to do with salvation from suffering or, as in many Oriental religions, with mysticism—a fusion of the person with the All-One.[1]

Magic, which is often associated with religion, involves the use of supernatural means in an effort to control natural phenomena. The ends of magic are thus naturalistic—for example, long life, or good health, or many offspring, or victory in the hunt or in war, or control of the weather. But the means or techniques of magic are supernatural. Magic is used for occasions at hand: the chief is sick and so the medicine man is called in. Magic is not usually practiced at fixed establishments, but wherever it seems needed.

Today the great world religions (Hinduism, Buddhism, Judaism, Christianity, Islamism, Confucianism, and Taoism) have super-

---

[1] For systematic classifications of religious phenomena, see J. Wach, *Sociology of Religion* (Chicago: Univ. of Chicago Press, 1944). William Howells' *The Heathens* (New York: Doubleday, 1948) is a good account. See also E. Durkheim, *The Elementary Forms of the Religious Life* (Glencoe, Illinois: Free Press, 1947), and Max Weber, *From Max Weber: Essays in Sociology*, H. H. Gerth and C. Wright Mills, trs. and eds. (New York: Oxford, 1946), Part III.

seded and largely transformed magical practices and beliefs. Accordingly, in our necessarily brief discussion we shall emphasize the world religions.

The scriptural prophets of Judaism, from the ninth century B.C., were the first "men of conscience" about whom we have literary documents and so historical knowledge. They stand out, in the course of history, as the first men ready to obey God rather than other men. They were active prophets, who considered themselves instruments of God and, as divinely compelled men, volunteered to bring forth their prophetic oracles and exhortations, in the form of a divinely inspired mission, to their people and to their kings.[2]

It was characteristic of them to withdraw from society into solitary states of brooding ecstasy or stolid trance, and then to "return" to the market place, to the Temple of Jerusalem. There they agitated as religiously motivated demagogues for true Judaist conduct in daily life, for religiously inspired political isolationism in the face of Egyptian and Assyrian aggression. Max Weber has called such men "emissary" prophets.

In the canonical books of the Old Testament, Amos represents the first, Zechariah the last "prophet," the prophet who prophesied against all prophesying. Since then in Judaism only "false messiahs" and "false prophets" have made their appearance. For a time a temple priesthood was restored to power in Jerusalem; but under the Roman Emperor Hadrian, this second temple was destroyed, and since then the Diaspora existence has been decisive for the course of Judaism as a world religion. The rabbi—the religious teacher—became the decisive leader of this religion. The establishment of the state of Israel marks a new epoch for Judaism.

Both Christianity and Islamism were developed out of Judaism's legacy. The decisive event in the development of Christianity from a Jewish sect into a world religion was Paul's success over Peter, in defining "liberty in Christ" as the renunciation of the ritualistic commandments of Judaism. For this eliminated from Christianity the self-segregating features of Judaism. In the orbit of the Roman Caesars, Christianity was successfully propagated—in competition with Judaism, with innumerable ancient cults, with local and func-

[2] Cf. Max Weber, *Ancient Judaism*, H. H. Gerth and D. Martindale, trs. (Glencoe, Illinois: Free Press, 1952).

tional deities of the Greek Olympia, with the Egyptian cult of Isis and Osiris, and especially Mithras, as well as with the impersonal godhead of Plato, Aristotle and the Roman Stoics. The following major factors were decisive in Christianity's victory: [3]

I. Like the Old Testament prophets, the Christian apostles made it their rule to live for religion rather than to make their living off religion.

II. The ethical code of the ten commandments—of course also taught by the Pharisees and the synagogue—was readily taught to children and to uneducated masses as the divine imperative of an invisible, though personal and majestic, God.

III. And quite apart from its simplicity, the Christian message proved attractive to the people of later antiquity. Jewish messianism was mixed with the Greek and Oriental mythology of a dying and resurrected God; its family model upheld the image of a loving God who was the just and merciful Father of His faithful children; and its majestic conception of an omniscient, omnipotent, and omnipresent figure held out eternal salvation of the immortal soul in a blissful beyond to the faithful—that is to the obedient—believer, and eternal damnation in hell to the nonbeliever.

IV. The dropping of Judaist ritualistic prescriptions of diet, the Sabbath, and circumcision—the self-segregating features, as we have said—made joining the Christians much easier for the pagans.

V. Finally, during the centuries of persecution, when public agitation by preachers and prophetic figures was impossible, the Christians managed to transform each administrative hearing, and each circus show of the death of Christian martyrs, into an impressive public demonstration of faith in a world without hope. The processional burial which followed was a highly visible testimony of the inner-directed man of conscience who would obey God rather than man, who would reject this world and not shy away from suffering, who would in fact seek suffering in imitation of Christ and for the status of sainthood, in order to gain eternal salvation in the hereafter.

Since then, with the emergence of a Roman and a Byzantine oriented priesthood, Christendom has been divided into an Eastern

[3] See Karl Holl, "Early Christian Propaganda," H. H. Gerth, tr., which will shortly be published by Beacon Press, Boston. See also Edward Gibbon's famous chapters on the rise of Christianity in *The Decline and Fall of the Roman Empire* (Modern Library Edition in 3 vols.).

and Western Church. And since Martin Luther (1483-1546), Ulrich Zwingli (1484-1531), and John Calvin (1509-1564), Western Christianity has been differentiated into the Roman Catholic Church, the Calvinist and Lutheran Churches, as well as numerous Protestant sects.

The religious monopoly of the Catholic Church was, in part, broken because of Gutenberg's invention of printing by movable types, about 1450. For this soon made possible thousands of editions and copies of the Bible. An intelligentsia, which was opposed to the pope but found patrons in the princes, emerged. The crisis within the church led to reform movements of poor friars and cardinals, of students and other migrant propagandists. Two urban strata arose which followed their own courses—smaller middle-class entrepreneurs, who developed toward inner-worldly asceticism,[4] and smaller artisans, who tended to mysticism and the perfection of contemplation. In Central Europe all during the fourteenth century, the peasantry was in revolt. The journeymen were in revolt against the closing of the guilds, and they as well as the poor in the guilds were against usury and political capitalism, and thus took sides with the peasantry. German princes protected the heterodox movements, which thus allowed them to emancipate themselves from the Holy Roman Empire, under the Hapsburgs and the pope.

Today in America there are Mennonites and Catholics, Quakers and Baptists, Old Order Amish and Methodists; the United States, in fact, exceeds all other countries in the number of denominations it embraces, there being between two and three hundred.[5] Since the advance of the Red army into Central Europe, Protestantism has been reduced to a minority status on the continent; Catholicism, although suffering grievous losses in Eastern and Southeastern Europe, prevails from Hesse to Spain.

It has been characteristic of Western religion that religious leaders—saints and founders of monk orders, reformers, plebeian prophets, and evangelizing artisans—repeatedly democratize and reactivate Christianity. Tendencies toward an aristocratic intellectualism of the cultured have been repeatedly submerged; accordingly, by numerous compromises and concessions, Christianity

[4] See below, pp. 360-63.
[5] Cf. R. H. Abrams, ed., "Organized Religion in the United States," *The Annals of the American Academy of Political and Social Science*, March 1948.

has permeated the daily life of the masses in quite diverse societies. This is one meaning of the "emissary prophets" of Christianity, who as active men seek to transform the world.

In this perspective, Protestantism, by renouncing the religious aristocracy of the priesthood, and of religious orders, has eliminated the split between professionals and laity. Christian asceticism was developed behind monastic walls for especially organized elites; it was democratized by the code of "inner-worldly asceticism," which was especially effective in Puritan Calvinist denominations and countries.

Max Weber, in *The Protestant Ethic and the Spirit of Capitalism*,[6] ascribed world historical consequences to this turn of events. Inaugurating one of the great intellectual debates of the social sciences, he asserted that modern industrial capitalism could not have emerged without the "inner-worldly asceticism" which contributed to the personality formation of the entrepreneurial middle classes. In these strata, systematic vocational work was religiously hallowed; success in one's work was religiously interpreted as indicative of one's place among those predestined by the hidden God's inscrutable resolve. Hence, religiously motivated fears for one's salvation were mobilized for the conscientious self-discipline of the vocational man. This man sets out to "master" this world, which at the same time he rejects, in order to help produce the kingdom to come. He does not withdraw from the world into contemplation, nor build a specialized monastic world withdrawn from the larger world; on the contrary, he stays in this world yet is not of it; he actively tackles the world by work in order to realize his ethically inspired quest for mastery. Whether in his workshop, in the market, or on the battlefield, he aspires to be a crusader for the kingdom to come; and wherever he finds them, he fights the devil and all evil.

Weber's explanatory scheme for the emergence of capitalism among the rational bourgeoisie may be summarized in more detail as follows:

The religious doctrines of Luther, and especially of Calvin, defined anew the Christian's relation to his everyday work. In the English and in the German languages—and in them only since

[6] See also R. H. Tawney, *Religion and the Rise of Capitalism* (New York: Harcourt, Brace, 1948).

Protestant Bible translations—the terms, "calling" or *Beruf*, refer both to one's occupation and to one's religious destiny. According to Calvin's doctrine of predestination each man was to be saved or condemned by an inscrutable judgment of the stern Lord. This doctrine released in the pious believer great anxieties lest he be among the condemned, and these anxieties could not be relieved by withdrawal from the world into monastery life or into extraordinary religious conduct, like the medieval saint's. For these avenues were blocked by the theory that God had placed man in the world of his creation, coupled with the doctrine that the Lord had chosen or condemned all men. Therefore pious works, like donations to churches, extra prayers and pilgrimages, became senseless and frivolous attempts to interfere with God's inscrutable will. There was indeed only one way to gain signs of one's state of grace as a portent of one's being elect; namely, the methodical adherence to a God-pleasing code of conduct in whatever position the pious found himself.

This code of conduct, as historically developed by puritan sects, Weber called "inner-worldly" or "this-worldly asceticism"—an abnegation of the enjoyment of worldly pleasures in the midst of the world. The puritan thus undertook to live a quasi-monastic life without becoming a monk, to carry forth the norms of this-worldly asceticism, and so to "conquer the world" rather than to withdraw. To follow through this program required the methodical and systematic observation of self and an ever-renewed self-discipline. The minimization of impulses and deviations from the religious code served the pious puritan as an indication of his selected status in the eyes of God. The religious code, however, by denying indulgence in joyful revelry and dancing, in sexual gratifications, and even in sleeping (the ideal of the long hard day), left the puritan the concentration on work as his major ascetic technique. The pious man must always renew his efforts, because no final guarantee or security is held out to him. In the face of possible condemnation, any exertions and tribulations in this valley of tears weigh but lightly. Accordingly, guilt spurs his intensified work: the vocational man is now the man who pleases God.

The religious ethic of the puritan makes it impossible for him to invest the fruits of his work in ostentatious consumption, like horses and carriages, mansions and feudal estates; on the other hand, he believes that he who does not work shall not eat. Therefore, Catholic alms to beggars, vagrants, and the like are denied. For puritan philanthropic enterprises organize uniformed orphans and vagrants, beggars and the aged in institutions set up for the purpose. There is only one way in which the puritan may use his private accumulations of wealth: to invest and reinvest them in productive enterprises. For this allows for the extension of salvation opportunities to so many more beggars. The puritan businessman thus saves their souls by using them as his labor supply, and they, the labor supply, acquire a new work discipline by becoming the employer's brethren. For salvation's sake, they forego many popular and colorful days, festivities, mysteries, and plays which were holidays from work for the medieval Catholic worker. Thus the puritan becomes the restless worker making sure of his state of predestination, and, as a particularly saintly man, earning the respect of his fellow believers the more he expands his establishment.

Weber's analysis reveals the impact of a creed upon the formation of a type of character. Religiously motivated insecurity and its religiously designated escape place premiums upon specific psychic attitudes and traits like thrift, hard work, control of "idle words," humility, continuous self-control, purposiveness. This character structure, in turn, becomes economically relevant in that it guarantees competitive advantage over traditionalist and less frugal economic agents.

The necessity of the puritan to maintain himself in the eyes of his sectarian brothers allows for the emergence of the new morality of everyday business. The puritan does not higgle in the market, and contracts are sacred. Hence the puritan is a safe credit risk, and has the highest credit rating in the business community. This, in turn, fructifies his business advance, and the puritan sect thus becomes a selective, and at the same time a breeding agency, for that personality type best fitted to develop and propagate industrial capitalism as a system.

Religious ideas became psychologically relevant to character structure; they place a premium on specific traits, and these traits become incentives for a new style of economic conduct. As religious organizations, the sects are fit to stabilize such personality types into an organized elite. Their conduct and religiosity can be propagated, and hence expanded. The long-run result of these changes, namely all that goes with modern capitalism's success, was neither intended nor foreseen by its puritan pioneers.

Religious developments seem to occur by revivals and by secularizations, which alternate with each other. Accordingly, we speak of the "great revival" of Protestantism in England during the late eighteenth century, when the Methodist movement sprang up and put an end to the "merrie old England" of the Restoration period. Catholicism has also had its revivals, the most prominent being the renewal of religious ardor during the Jesuit-led "counter-reformation," which recovered Southern and Southeastern Europe from Protestantism, leaving only scattered islands of Calvinist and Lutheran Protestanism in Hungary and Romania, which were eliminated by the advance of the Red army during World War II.

Catholic and Protestant revival movements occurred at the end of the Napoleonic epoch. Romantic intellectuals were converted to Catholicism under Metternich; and nowadays we witness the successful endeavors of Catholics to win over such intellectuals as Jacques Maritain, the late Heywood Broun, the ex-editor of the Daily Worker, Budenz, as well as influential upper-class persons such as Clare Boothe Luce and Henry Ford II.

The role of the convert merits special attention for his ardor may be especially intense. He may be motivated more by his resentment against what he leaves behind than by positive and loving identification with what he has come to embrace. Tertullian is the often quoted case of such "resentful" Christianity. This concept of "resentment," as developed by Nietzsche,[7] asserts, in fact, that all Christianity is nothing but the uprising of the slaves in morality, which means that since direct aggression is denied to the slave, he must "repress" his aggression and thereby sublimate it into a wish for delayed aggression, or revenge. This desire for revenge, in turn, becomes conscious and is then repressed, but it is repressed from a new vantage point, from a presumably higher value positon resulting from a "transvaluation of values." Not the strong, the high, or the mighty are accepted as highly valuable types of men, but the lowly, the suffering, the meek, who "shall inherit the earth." It is the uncomely and the despised of this world who are the beloved of God.

According to this theory, the righteous can condescendingly

---

[7] For an excellent account of Nietzsche's thought, see Walter A. Kaufmann, *Nietzsche* (Princeton: Princeton Univ. Press, 1950), especially Chapters 7, 8 and 10.

anticipate the dire fate of the godless and unrighteous—a fate which God is preparing for them on "doomsday" or on "The Day of Judgment," of which the Christians sing. Nietzsche, in thus construing neighborliness and Christian love as a "compensation" for denied aggression, takes up Hobbes's assumption that human nature is "originally" evil and aggressive, and that profession of love is a compensatory derivation of hatred and frustrated aggression.

One may, to be sure, readily discern features of resentment, as well as resentful men, in the Jewish as well as the Christian tradition. But to "explain" these religions, in all their complexities, in terms of "resentment" requires that we reduce their specific value preferences and their ethos to a naturalistic bias concerning the nature of love. Max Scheler has convincingly juxtaposed the conception of Christian love with that of Greek antiquity's "eros." The Greek philosophers conceived of love in terms of scarcity consciousness: Men should allocate their scarce love to those men and to those values that "merit" love; hence they should want to prefer the "higher" value or the higher type of man to the "lower." The Christian idea of a loving God, in contrast, is predicated on the assumption that love is "infinite." The loving God and the loving Christian are not thought to be striving, in a competitive context, towards something higher and higher but rather from the outset as standing high and holding out infinite love and mercy to the creature who is in his failings and in his weakness lowly. It is a conception foreshadowed by Isaiah's hope for a new covenant with a merciful God, who will consider "not the circumcision of the foreskin but the circumcision of the heart." It is foreshadowed also in Isaiah's idea of the Servant of Yahweh. "Love" in Christianity is thus conceived, not as a naturalistically limited impulse, but as a spiritual and psychic act of unlimited capacity.

William James, in a quite different context,[8] gives expression to this idea of loving empathy as being a prerequisite of discernment rather than a compensation for a frustrated "will to power." "Every Jack," he wrote, "sees in his own particular Jill charms and perfection to the enchantment of which we stolid on-lookers are stone-cold. And which has the superior view of the absolute truth, he or we? Which has the more vital insight into the nature of Jill's existence, as a fact? Is he in excess, being in this matter a

[8] See F. O. Matthiessen, *The James Family* (New York: Knopf, 1947), p. 404 ff.

maniac? or are we in defect, being victims of a pathological anaes-
thesia as regards Jill's magical importance? Surely the latter; surely
to Jack are the profounder truths revealed; surely poor Jill's pal-
pitating little life-throbs *are* among the wonders of creation, *are*
worthy of this sympathetic interest; and it is to our shame that
the rest of us cannot feel like Jack. For Jack realizes Jill concretely, and we do not. He struggles toward union with her inner
life, divining her feelings, anticipating her desires, understanding
her limits as manfully as he can, and yet inadequately too; for he is
also afflicted with some blindness, even here. Whilst we, dead clods
that we are, do not even seek these things, but are contented that
the portion of eternal fact named Jill should be for us as if it were
not. Jill, who knows her inner life, knows that Jack's way of taking
it—so importantly—is the true and serious way; and she responds
to the truth in him by taking him truly and seriously too. May the
ancient blindness never warp its clouds about either of them
again."

The relevance of the religious order to other institutional orders
depends upon the organizational principles of the religion involved, and in particular, upon whether or not the religion is
compulsory or voluntary. American democratic society, for example, with its innumerable voluntary organizations, is greatly
indebted to Puritanism and to the multiplicity of denominations
and sects. At the opposite extreme, state and church are led by one
man who combines the roles of supreme priest and emperor. This
is Caesar-Papism, as exemplified by the Japanese Mikado, the Confucian Emperor of ancient China, the Roman Emperors after
Augustus, the Russian Tsars after Peter the Great, or the German
Lutheran princes.

The oldest, and in the West, the largest, ecclesiastical structure
—the Roman Catholic Church—is headed by the Pope who is unani-
mously elected by a college of seventy cardinals. The Pope
legitimizes his claim to Catholicity, that is, to universal authority,
by the dogma of the apostolic succession from Peter, the first Bishop
of Rome. The authoritarian structure of this priestly organization,
however, has accommodated itself to constitutional democracy. If
the state should attack the church, the church is likely to enter the
political order more explicitly than it has in the United States by
lending its support to the organization of a special Catholic Party,

as is to be found in Germany, Italy, Belgium, and other European countries. If the state, in its public schools and universities, should not allow religious instruction, the church is likely to organize a parochial school system of its own up through the university level, as in the United States where 15 per cent of the school population is enrolled in such Catholic schools. Celibate monks and nuns can compete effectively with more expensive secular teachers. Where the legal order permits the free accumulation of property, the church can add to its corporate wealth.

In those large cities in which the Catholic Church controls the majority vote, the official "separation of state and church" is, in a way, bypassed on the municipal level. Direct and indirect subsidies can be allocated under diverse headings. In the United States, Catholicism was originally a religion of plebeian immigrants—of Irish, German, Italian, and Polish descent. During recent decades, however, Catholics have added propertied and educated elites to their ranks, who can and who do exert significant influence in foreign and domestic political decisions. The combination of the Democratic Party, the Catholic clergy, and the trade unions under the presidency of Franklin Roosevelt is a well-known political coalition.[9] In the face of attacks, the Catholic Church of course claims democratic rights and liberties for itself, but where the church is established and represents the great majority of the people it is unlikely to grant Protestant minorities the right to proselytize. The strife and tension in Italy, in Spain, and in Colombia are recent cases in point. In France, the Catholic Church has twice been disestablished—during the French Revolution, and in 1904-05 under the Millerand coalition of socialists and bourgeois liberals. Under Pétain, the church was re-established, a measure that has been honored by postwar governments.

Where religious authorities take over the administration of the state, we may speak of a "theocracy." World famed examples include the theocracies of ancient Jerusalem under Ezra and Nehemiah and later under the Pharisees; Calvin's rule at Geneva; the rule of the Puritan divines in colonial New England; and the Jesuit state in Paraguay in the seventeenth and eighteenth centuries.

[9] For a knowledgeable account of such matters, see Samuel Lubell, *The Future of American Politics* (New York: Harper, 1952); and Paul Blanshard, *American Freedom and Catholic Power* (Boston: Beacon Press, 1949).

It is characteristic of Western Christianity that at various times it has been in tension with political authorities and economic powers, with military, scientific, philosophical, and artistic movements. Christianity has held revolutionary as well as conservative positions—at different times and in different contexts. Accordingly, generalizations of the political orientations of Christianity are bound to overlook or to bypass pertinent aspects and ramifications of its varied adaptations to Western social structures. As Hegel has observed:

"The Christian religion has sometimes been reproved, sometimes praised, for its consistency with the most varied manners, characters, and institutions. It was cradled in the corruption of the Roman state; it became dominant when that empire was in the throes of its decline, and we cannot see how Christianity could have stayed its downfall. On the contrary, Rome's fall extended the scope of Christianity's domain, and it appears in the same epoch as the religion of the barbarians, who were totally ignorant and savage but completely free, and also of the Greeks and Romans, who by this time were overcivilized, servile, and plunged in a cesspool of vice. It was the religion of the Italian states in the finest period of their licentious freedom in the Middle Ages; of the grave and free Swiss republics; of the more or less moderate monarchies of modern Europe; alike of the most heavily oppressed serfs and their overlords: both attended one church. Headed by the Cross, the Spaniards murdered whole generations in America; over the conquest of India the English sang Christian thanksgivings. Christianity was the mother of the finest blossoms of the plastic arts; it gave rise to the tall edifice of the sciences. Yet in its honor all fine art was banned, and the development of the sciences was reckoned an impiety. In all climates the tree of the Cross has grown, taken root, and fructified. Every joy in life has been linked with this faith, while the most miserable gloom has found in it its nourishment and its justification." [9A]

2. Characteristics of World Religions

We may grasp the main features of a religion if we know the following facts: its attitude toward the status quo, its representa-

[9A] Georg Wilhelm Friedrich Hegel, *Early Theological Writings*, T. M. Knox, tr. (Chicago: Univ. of Chicago Press, 1948), pp. 168 ff.

tive class or leadership; the sources of its religious authority; its type of religious assembly and organization, the chief end of life it holds out, its views of the superhuman and of life after death, its sexual code, its magical features, if any, and its attitude towards politics, work, and education. In the following paragraphs we characterize each of the great world religions in these terms.[10]

I. Confucianism accepts the present order as good, for the emperor who reigns is the Son of Heaven. It is the religion of cultured erudites who find their source of religious authority in the writings of· Confucius and the Confucian tradition. It involves ancestral and political festivals, and understands the major end of life to be the preservation of the social order. A multitude of spirits populates its world, although Heaven is rather impersonally imagined. Confucianism is not concerned with the salvation of immortal souls. It scorns women, although it stresses the perpetuation of the family. It officially disowns the magical beliefs and practices of vulgar Taoism, which are widespread among the masses. It upholds filial piety as a cardinal virtue, which ties it to ancestor worship. Discouraging independent thinking, it glorifies rote learning and feats of memory among its scholarly leaders. Man's work, according to this creed, is and should be under the control of the tradition-minded family, or when it is office work, under the control of the Confucian hierarchy headed by the emperor as the Son of Heaven.

II. Hinduism, both classical and popular, looks upon its world of castes as eternal and unchangeable, for there is no beginning and no end of the immortal soul of man. Accordingly, it upholds and at the same time makes more tolerable the caste system. Classical Hinduism is represented by the Brahmins—an hereditary, intellectual aristocracy; popular Hinduism, by the gurus (i.e. mendicant monks) and by holy men of quite different caste origin. For its classical form, the Brahmins interpret ancient writings and tradition; for its popular form, the gurus interpret tradition and folklore. Both forms involve pilgrimages to holy places. The Brahmin identifies himself with the cosmic spirit—that is the chief religious

[10] See E. J. Jurji, ed., *The Great Religions of the Modern World* (Princeton: Princeton Univ. Press, 1946); H. L. Friess and H. W. Schneider, *Religion in Various Cultures* (New York: Holt, 1932), as well as the works of Max Weber cited elsewhere in this volume.

end of his life; the masses seek to improve their status in their next rebirth. For these masses, there is a vast pantheon of nature and functional gods; for the Brahmin, a more or less impersonal cosmic spirit. But both, as Hindus, believe in the transmigration of souls, the next incarnation according to the karman doctrine being determined by one's adherence to one's "dharma": the ritualistically sanctioned code of one's hereditary caste. The Brahmin scorns women, for they interfere with contemplation; among the masses cults of various sorts prevail. Among both, magical features are in evidence, although much more so among the popular than the classical forms of Hinduism. Education is limited to the aristocratic class, with an emphasis upon classic writings in Sanskrit. Work is completely controlled by the hereditary and endogamous caste system, and all innovations are discouraged.

III. Buddhism regards the present world as evil and unchangeable. The Buddhist monks—the representative class of this religion —interpret ancient writings and tradition, and religious assemblage is limited to monasteries and to certain festivals. The chief end of life is conceived to be the escape from suffering, that is, escape from the wheel of life with its rebirths for more of the same. There is a continual rebirth through desire, but if one escapes from desire there is the eternal rest of nirvana. Celibacy and the avoidance of all desire is sought by means of complex spiritual exercises and the achievement of extraordinary psychosomatic states. There is no image of the superhuman in classic Buddhism, although spiritism is rampant in popular forms of the religion. Magic is forbidden in the former, but abounds in the latter. Accordingly, education is limited to the monasteries and to those trained there. As routine work would distract from the holy path, it is despised by the mendicant monks.

IV. Judaism views the present order with resolute hope for the future. Its religious cohesion rests upon faith in being chosen by Yahweh for a covenant fellowship with him as a party to the contract. Its representative religious leaders are Levites and Torah teachers, charismatic prophets and hereditary temple priests. Of special significance has been the demilitarized, pacifist, peasant, shepherd, and plebeian strata of cities. Since the destruction of the temple and its priesthood, the law and the prophets are its holy books; its sources of religious authority and its religious assemblage is the synagogue. Life is a waiting, a tarrying, for a new and better social order; in ancient Judaism there is no idea of personal survival after death. There are relatively few magical features in Judaism and its monotheistic God is personal and ethical. Aside from some cult prescriptions of chastity, there is no asceticism; priests, prophets, and rabbis marry—and the family is sanctified. Education consists of general instruction in the Torah and in history. The orthodox Jew views work rationally and practically, although since the exile, work has been hampered in various degrees by ritualistic separation.

V. Originally Mohammedism was a prophetic creed of a crusading order of warriors; now Islamic society largely accepts the present order as fate. The individual interprets the Koran; there are private devotions as well as pilgrimages and mass meetings. The chief end of life is to realize the will of Allah, who is a personal and monotheistic God. Originally there was a conception of a warrior's paradise, with houris and carousing. Nowadays there is a crudely conceived heaven and hell, and magical practices and beliefs are much in evidence. Women are isolated, popular education neglected, and the attitude towards work is indifferent.

VI. Christianity, in both its Roman Catholic and Puritan form, conceives of man as in the present world but not really *of* it, as forming a super-social fellowship. Catholicism is inclined to support each of the varieties of status quo in its vast domains; Puritanism, to stand in defiance of the world and attempt to remake it. The representative Catholic leaders are saints, celibate priests, monks, and nuns; of Puritan sects, the "middle classes." The sources of religious authority for Catholics are the Bible as interpreted by religious, priestly guidance, and *ex cathedra* pronouncements of the pope. For Puritans the Bible, as interpreted by the individual who is qualified for sect membership by his "inner light," is the source of authority. Catholics have a heaven, a hell, and a purgatory; Puritans—in fact, all Protestants—have only a heaven and a hell. Both, however, entertain images of individual salvation, although the Catholics' is in a future heaven, the Puritans' in a kingdom to come. The Catholic assemblage is the mass; the Puritan, common worship. Both are Trinitarian in their images of the godhead, although the Catholics also revere the saints and the Virgin Mary. Magic is much in evidence in Catholicism—the sacrament being thought to work by virtue of the ritual. Puritanism has fought and eliminated all magic as devilish. Sacraments, for example, the Lord's Supper, is considered a festival in memory of Christ's last supper; Catholic priests are professionally trained; other Catholic education varies in level according to competitive or monopolistic situation, and is determined by the interests of religious conformity. Like Judaism, Puritanism lays great stress on and pays zealous attention to mass education of the laity, and has encouraged exploratory thinking in science and technology, and education for businessmen. In Catholicism there is celibacy for the holy, marriage, though considered a sacrament, being a concession to human frailty and belonging to "the natural order." In Puritanism, the same ethical demands hold for clergy and laity, marriage involving a love of sobriety. Work, for the Benedictine monks especially, represents the burdensome legacy of man's fall. The religious zeal of Puritanism, as we have noted in detail above, is channeled into work of this world.

3. The Kinship Order

The kinship order—we have noted above—is composed of institutions which regulate and facilitate legitimate sexual intercourse, procreation, and the rearing of children as well as the transmission of private property.[11]

All social structures institutionalize sexual activities and thus regulate them, but often such activities are accompanied by illegitimate forms of relation that are more or less tolerated. When the kinship order is taxed beyond capacity, the load is shifted to men, women, or children not belonging to legitimate, domestic groups but offering erotic services to its members. Hetaerae, mistresses, concubines, prostitutes—male and female, sacred and profane—all play such supplementary roles. The idea that only women have honor (and hence can lose it) reflects thousands of years of male dominance. If the gigolo were revealed throughout world history

[11] See W. Goodsell, A History of Marriage and the Family (rev. ed.; New York: Macmillan, 1934); and A. W. Calhoun, A Social History of the American Family (New York: Barnes & Noble, 1945).

as is the female prostitute, then men too could lose their honor, and in this connection be equal with women. Illicit erotic relations are most likely to occur when economic conditions keep the biological adult from assuming the role of provider. The socially unplaced erotic overhead is thus transferred to erotic specialists, to the prostitute, or on higher-class levels, to the mistress.

When we emphasize the economic aspect of the kinship order, we speak of the "household"; when we stress the kinship aspect we speak of the "family." [12] In the remote past, and in many contemporary preliterate societies, the economic and the kinship orders are not differentiated. In fact, all "economy" was once "domestic economy."

Max Weber has noted that the kinship order is generally comprised of sexually enduring communities of father, mother, and children. Economic functions, although historically linked with those of kinship, can of course be analytically separated from them. Conjugal relations and parent-child relations are based on the kinship order, but purely sexual relations are highly unstable and problematic. In order to be enduring, they must be instituted, and they have most frequently been instituted with reference to economic conditions. Thus the father must provide for the mother; and, until the child is able to provide for himself, the mother must so provide. Relations between siblings are not necessarily important until they involve attachments to a common source of provisions. But even in societies where men are bound together communally in bachelor quarters for military and economic purposes, mother and children are likely to remain in common residence.

Marriage can only be defined with reference to larger organizations than the family; accordingly the kinship structure is usually a dependent order. Marriage, as a legitimate sexual relation, presupposes larger groups which sanction the relation, against the will

[12] On the relation of economic functions and types of families, see Max Weber, *The Theory of Social and Economic Organization*, Talcott Parsons and A. M. Henderson, trs. (New York: Oxford, 1948), pp. 341-57. See also the excellent articles by Alfred Meusel, "National Socialism and the Family," *The Sociological Review* (British), Vol. 28, 1936, pp. 166 ff. and 389 ff. "From an economic point of view the family is (1) an institution to transmit private property, (2) a system of productive relations directed by patriarchal authority" (page 167).

if necessary of one or both of the partners. These larger groups which thus sanction marriage—we may call them "frame groups"— may be sib or clan, or of political or economic, religious or status nature. Only those descendants who are borne as full members of such association involved may consider legitimate marriage. This is the sociological meaning of legitimate or illegitimate birth. There must be agreement by the frame groups and certain forms must be met. Marriage thus takes its arrangement and content from these associations, and not from the merely sexual relations of man and woman, or the rearing of children.

Sexual relations are economically important because they lead to the common concerns of a household. The household requires a degree of planned production; in fact, it does not typically exist in preagricultural societies. But the household is central in a society where there are sedentary agriculturalists of relatively low technological development. When agriculture is more advanced, domestic authority is placed under the jurisdiction of larger frame groups. As members of these groups, individuals gain more rights as family members, or even against domestic authority. For example, when larger associations lend rights to the mother of the house so as to separate her property from that of the husband, patriarchal power declines.

The household is the most widespread economic community, and at the same time is the bedrock of piety and authority, which, in turn, are the substructures of many sentiments involved in other institutional orders. For the cardinal sentiment of the domestic group under patriarchal authority is a strong sense of piety, which holds it together. Patrimonial duties for the women, and filial piety for children and servants complement the tradition-bound authority of the patriarchal head, who freely bestows his favors and chastisements upon his "dependents." In extreme cases—ancient China is the great example—this filial piety is elaborated into the belief in ancestral spirits, and a family temple implements the worship of ancestors. And almost everywhere the household unit stands for in-group solidarity, for common residence is essential to the domestic group in its pure type, and its locale is accordingly sentimentalized and the object of nostalgic and xenophobic attitudes.

On the basis of piety and common residence, there is in the household a communism of consumption of every day goods. In the economics of late medieval and Renaissance Italy, business ventures were engaged in by several households, which are thus prototypes of partnerships and joint liability.

For all their importance, we do not consider kinship institutions as more "natural" than any other institutions. The bond between mother and child may be "natural," yet, as we have seen, it may be up to the father to determine whose offspring shall be ascribed to his wife, whether her own or her maid's—witness the story of Leah and Rachel. Throughout antiquity, the infanticide of unwanted infants was accepted as "natural." The "legitimate child" is defined to be such by the rules and agents of the kinship orders, and so there is a gap between "biology and human nature" which institutionalizes the roles of father and mother.

In industrial and urban societies, kinship orders have tended towards the small, two generation family, consisting of parents and children. In such an institution, children do not have much contact with older people, and respect for old age is at a discount; even the patriarchal image of Santa Claus may assume the character of just another funny man.

Today in America more people are married than was previously the case, and they tend to marry earlier. Although monogamy is guaranteed by legal and religious sanctions, the Kinsey report [13] reveals that actual conduct deviates widely from professed norms and moral codes. Even if we make allowances for shortcomings in Kinsey's technique, and even if the figures are not perfect, the proportions of illicit relations are impressive; they fit too well with what is known from less formal data to be written off. The evidence shows that premarital chastity is not strictly enforced for women, and that men no longer place decisive weight upon it. The emancipation of women, and the dissemination of contraceptive information, has brought about her sexual freedom. For themselves, men have never honored the demand for premarital chastity; "sowing one's wild oats" has been tolerated as a "natural privilege" of man. The monogamous family, in the meantime, is psychologically upheld, positively by love, negatively by the "jealousy" of the lover against any threat by a third party to his or her exclusive rights to the erotical services of the partner. Accordingly, where jealousy is discounted or depreciated, "monogamous love" is indirectly threatened.

[13] Alfred C. Kinsey, Wardell B. Pomeroy and Clyde E. Martin, *Sexual Behavior in the Human Male* (Philadelphia and London: Saunders, 1948).

The combination of "love" and marriage is of course a specifically modern linkage. We know from Thomas's and Znaniecki's study of the *Polish Peasant in Europe and America*—and we may generalize the point for the Old World peasantry at large—that marriage is closely connected with the property and status considerations of the two families who are to be linked by marriage. The couples themselves are not euphorically infatuated with one another; on the contrary, they maintain a stylized respect in which they see one another as "members" of their respective families rather than as heroized individuals. In this, the peasant family is comparable to dynastic and noble houses. King Edward VIII was not permitted to be king and also to marry the "woman I love." He might of course have had her in a "lefthanded" marriage, or —possibly as a royal mistress—anything, but not for a queen. The case is interesting—as Kingsley Martin in *The Magic of Monarchy* has shown—for its revelations of the status sentiments of *arrivé* bourgeois society, which in its ascent has acquired an understanding of proper background and status as being more relevant for marriage than the "mere love" of movie fans and pulp magazine readers.

The combination of modern marriage with love is a contribution of the rising middle classes. Since the Italian opera and the eighteenth-century British novel, this linkage has been glorified and widely diffused. What, by the way, do we mean by "love"? Certainly more than mere "sex," for sexual activity and gratification is possible without "love." If sexual impulse is culturally stylized; if it is spiritualized, refined, or "sublimated," we may speak of "eroticism." Coquetry and flirtation are forms of erotic playfulness. To have an "affair," however, still falls short of "true love," in that it lacks the permanent commitments of the loving partners.

Just as we find types of marriages without "love," we also find true love relationships without marriage. Ever since the French Revolution, in fact, the institution of marriage has been criticized in the name of "true love," as over against the possibly mercenary motives leading to "marriage without love," or the marriage *à la mode,* or the "marriage of convenience." Anticapitalist movements, socialists and anarchists of all sorts, including Marx and Engels, have criticized marriage without love as "bad." Here is a recent voice: "There are illicit and extramarital relationships which are in reality more moral and more decent than those often found in marriage.

Love without marriage is in its essence far more moral than marriage without love." [14] Sometimes status inequalities may preclude
marriage, but not love; occasionally legal barriers—for instance barriers against the employment of both husband and wife in public
employment, or on the same teaching staff—may make marriage
"inexpedient" for the lovers.

We thus find types of sexual relations consisting of (1) marriage
combined with love, (2) love without marriage, (3) marriage without love, as well as (4) relations outside of marriage and devoid
of love—the transitory "purely sexual" partnership available in
houses of prostitution, which all over the world count soldiers
and sailors, traveling salesmen and itinerant artisans, as their fore-
most clientele.

The highest ideal of the modern marriage would seem to involve the following elements: (a) the permanent and exclusive
attachment of the partners to one another, "for better or for worse,
in sickness or in health," the attachment implemented by a sense
of moral responsibility for one another; (b) erotic elements present in the degree to which the partners "charm" one another; and
(c) sexual gratification. Where the puritan ideal of "sobriety" and
the ascetic factor remain strong, erotic elements are suppressed
as "idolatry," or as creature worship. Women must not "adorn
themselves," must not be proud of their "beauty," either in appearance or in gestural behavior; dancing, for example, is out. Vestiges
of puritan society survive in rural America, especially in small
sectarian communities of Mennonite groups, or the Old Order
Amish.

Role-differences between men and women, and their concomitant traits, may be ascribed to presumably "natural" differences of
sex: "Women are just naturally this or that"—"That's just the way
men are. . . ." Philosophers, from the time of Aristotle, have specu-
lated on "masculinity" and "femininity," in terms of man being
rational and discreet, women being "emotional" and given to "talka-
tiveness." The ideological legacies of patriarchalism and of male
dominance clearly extend into Sigmund Freud's psychology, which
makes "penis envy" the hub of "feminine character." [15]

[14] A. L. Wolbarst, *Generations of Adam* (New York: Stokes, 1930), p. 240.
[15] For an astute analysis of the various ideologies revealed in schools of
psychology, see Viola Klein, *The Feminine Character* (New York: International Univs. Press, 1949).

4. *The Educational Sphere*

In societies which allow or encourage special institutions for the transmission of skills and values to the young, we may speak of an educational "order." But the educational sphere, which comprises schools of all sorts, is rarely autonomous, which is why we call it a "sphere" rather than an "order." [16]

There are in the political order, party schools and national compulsory public schools; in the economic order, there are trade schools, for in-service training; in the religious order, sectarian schools, as well as official schools for the priesthood. The military order has its own military academies; and the kinship order has, for a long time, had as one of its aspects the training of the young. In fact, all institutions train people for skills and loyalties.

Nevertheless, we may make a distinction between apprenticeship—in which the novice enters a respective role as a novice to be trained as well as to work—and formal education which is a vicarious set of roles available outside the institutional sphere in which the student will eventually play them. The educational sphere is thus a world of models. When such a world occurs and is autonomously instituted, we have an educational order. Key sociological questions about education include the following: (1) Who gets educated? (2) By whom are they educated? (3) How are they educated? (4) For what roles are they educated? (5) When are they educated? (6) Where are they educated?

Education is a deliberate attempt to transmit skills and loyalties, as well as forms of inner cultivation and conventional deportment required by status group membership. All education aims at developing loyalty towards the educator at the same time, for he is a trustee of the group loyalties which he would impart. In a society dominated by salon ladies, girls go to finishing schools; public schools in England turn out gentlemen with an inner sense of bearing and dignity.

[16] See Thorstein Veblen, *The Higher Learning in America* (New York: Viking, 1918); I. L. Kandel, Essays in Comparative Education (New York: Teachers College, 1930); E. H. Reisner, *Nationalism and Education Since 1789* (New York: Macmillan, 1922); and Walter M. Kotschnig, *Unemployment in the Learned Professions* (London: Oxford, 1937).

In a very general way, we may speak with Max Weber of three types of education: first, the attempt to call forth and to test allegedly inherent traits of the individual, to allow them to unfold, to be realized.[17] This is generally characteristic of charismatically sanctioned institutions and status groups. Second, by rote learning and moral exhortation, by drill and imposed habituation, the attempt to stereotype the individual into line with traditional routines, which is generally characteristic of traditionalist societies. Third, the attempt rationally to transmit to the individual certain traits, to train him for specific skills by challenging him to think and act independently—which is generally characteristic of educational spheres of rational bureaucratic organizations.

In the occidental Middle Ages, traditionalist educational institutions were attached to the religious order, to the upper-class household of the warrior noble, to the middle-class household, and to the workshop of the guild master. Nowadays, rationalist educational spheres are attached to political institutions, as in "public school systems," as well as to the religious order, as in parochial schools. Modern totalitarian regimes attach part of their educational spheres—charismatically oriented—by means of youth organizations, to the ruling party. There was thus the Hitler Youth, and there are the Communist youth organizations in the Soviet Union and other states of the Soviet bloc. Special educational spheres of varied sorts in different social structures may thus be attached to religious, military, economic, and other institutional orders.

Only under quite special conditions do professional educators emancipate themselves from the control of superordinate institutional orders. The situation of "private universities," like Harvard or Oxford, Yale or Cambridge; of independent artists' studios; of various types of contemporary progressive schools; of the Athenian philosophers' "circle of disciples"—these are rather the exception than the rule.

In the United States in the middle of the twentieth century, some 84 per cent of all schools are elementary, 6 per cent of them being "private"; 15 per cent are secondary schools, 4 per cent of them being private; only 1 per cent of all schools are colleges, universi-

[17] See *From Max Weber,* op. cit., p. 426.

ties, or professional schools, but 65 per cent of them are "private."[18]
It is characteristic of the United States that elementary education
rests in the hands of 853,967 "schoolma'ams" who do not always
make education their permanent careers, teaching in the interval
between the family of their descent and that of procreation.[19]

Because of the steady increase of educational requirements for
an increasing range of specialized occupations, the opportunities
to climb the ladder of occupational success becomes more and
more dependent upon education. During the last half century the
educational level of the American people has risen accordingly;
enrollment figures indicate that in 1900 some 94,883 adolescents
graduated from high schools, but by 1940 their number had increased to 1,221,475.[20] This impressive quest for higher education
is not due to any sudden outburst of intellectual enthusiasm but
may largely be attributed to the function of education as a "social
elevator" in an epoch of scarcity-consciousness and social fence-
building. Degrees have become indispensable for entrance into
preferred occupations. Yet, at the same time, many people have
come to realize that education alone is not enough for "success."
The bitter phrase—"it's not what you know but whom you know"
—is indicative. The traditional Jeffersonian optimism about education as *the* answer has given way to an increasing tendency to
view educational policies in connection with social stratification,
and to assess educational goals statistically in terms of their function for later adult life.

Since the great depression, there has been an awareness of social
rigidities and institutional strains in the United States. This awareness has been reflected in a vogue of inquiries into the function of
the school in a democratic society, and the worthwhileness of education as an investment of long years for hopes of social ascent.
Yet the gulf between the educated and the uneducated in the
United States is not felt so deeply as it is in Europe, or, in fact,
is not felt to be a gulf at all. To American eyes, a smooth broad
ascent leads from elementary to higher education. And, on the
whole, the smooth gradation of institutions of higher learning—
from the best to the not-so-good; from lower grades to higher—

[18] Computed from *The World Almanac*, 1951, p. 580.
[19] Cf. Frances Donovan, *The Schoolma'am* (New York: Stokes, 1938).
[20] Table 154, *Statistical Abstract of the United States*, 1947, Washington, D. C.

and the readiness of American educators to teach new subjects as well as popular hobbies and fads, have made for a successful linkage of higher education and the population at large.

The demand of the state and of corporations for trained civil servants and qualified experts of all sorts has been decisive for the modern development of universities. The displacement of patronage and spoils systems by the "merit system," and the decline of administration by amateurs, however high-minded and notable, has been one result of this. Lorenz von Stein correctly called the modern university "a school for bureaucrats." Germany is a neat case in point.[21]

During the late eighteenth century, German princes "reformed" the universities, using Göttingen as the model. The universities of Bonn and Berlin were founded during the Napoleonic era, which also witnessed the establishment of engineering colleges in Germany. With industrialization and the expansion of administrative functions of all sorts, universities were shaped to answer the needs of a more complex and swiftly urbanized society. At the same time, they became social elevators for the middle classes. Of course, wage workers and small-holding peasants were sidetracked from that educational ladder that led to the university, being given instead vocational training, which was combined with apprenticeship systems, first in quasi-guilds of craftsmen, and later in big industries.

Under the Weimar Republic—in fact through 1935—a sociologically-minded census was taken of university students. This census provides unique data on the social composition of the student body in the twenty-five state universities of a major industrial nation. In the years between 1928 and 1935, about one-third of the students came from upper-class homes; about 60 per cent from a middle-class background; and only between 4 and 8 per cent from lower-class families. Over half of the students were the sons of officials, army officers, or professional men. The universities thus served as a means for the hereditary appropriation of bureaucratic positions. Despite broad discussions of university reform in post-

[21] For details on school enrollments in Germany, see *Deutsche Hochschulstatistik* and *Die Deutschen Hochschulen, Eine Uebersicht ueber ihren Besuch* (Berlin, 1936); cf. also Hans H. Gerth, "Germany on the Eve of Occupation," *Problems of the Postwar World,* T. C. McCormick, ed. (New York: McGraw-Hill, 1945), pp. 422 ff.

World War II Germany, as far as the question "who shall study" is concerned, nothing essential has been changed in Western Germany. The enrollment of the University of Münster, in Westphalia in 1947, conformed almost to the decimal point to the old picture.

In Eastern Germany under Russian rule there has been a speed-up of education developments, in accordance with the model of the Soviet Union itself. The over-all slogan is "cadre training," which in sociological translation means the displacement of all elites by loyal communist vanguards.

Eastern Germany is typical of all totalitarian regimes. Family influence is weakened by removing young children from their homes and placing them in publicly sponsored kindergartens. The number of kindergarten schools, teachers, and students has greatly increased since 1946.[22] This development provides young women with semiprofessional opportunities; communist aspirants from lower classes can readily be found and properly indoctrinated in the new loyalties. The kindergarten development also permits the increasing employment of housewives in industry.

Whereas the wealthy formerly sent their children to private schools, now private schools have been abolished. Whereas middle- and upper-class children once were separated from lower-class children after four years of elementary education, they are now separated only after eight years of public school education. A minority of fee-paying students used to attend high school from the time they were ten until they were eighteen years of age; they then passed a stiff examination which was a prerequisite for university attendance. Under Soviet occupation, most children now leave school at the age of fourteen, and those who wish to be apprenticed as "skilled workers" have to attend a vocational school once a week.

By August 1949, the top administrator of Eastern Zone schools stated that of the 65,000 teachers 80 per cent were "new teachers." [23]

[22] On schools in Eastern Germany, see Annemarie Jacobs, "Der Kindergarten als Vorstufe der Einheitsschule," *Die Deutsche demokratische Schule im Aufbau* (Berlin, 1949), p. 7. Der Fünfjahrplan zur Entwicklung der Volkswirtschaft der DDR (1951-1955), *Informationsdienst* (Berlin, n.d.).

[23] These facts and figures are taken from various East German publications, cited by Erich Hoffman, *Cadre Training in East Germany* (unpublished MA thesis, University of Wisconsin, 1952).

All teachers must be organized in various communist organizations, and naturally party membership, though not compulsory, suggests itself to the ambitious young teachers. The universities offer compulsory training courses for teachers in Marxism-Leninism, and at all schools have been formed communist teachers' groups which are affiliated with the Communist Youth. All educational institutions, in fact, are a sphere of party-controlled institutions.

All university students in Eastern Germany receive a monthly salary, which is graded by class background and political activity in favor of the active communistic, working-class student. Working-class sons made up 40 per cent of the student body by 1949. The total student body has been considerably expanded, and although standards of instruction and learning have been considerably lowered, a new plebeian intelligentsia is emerging which fills the ranks and the offices of the completely remodeled bureaucracies. The impressive mass euphoria of the two and one half million youths who in May 1951 were concentrated in Berlin to march behind Stalin posters may in large part be ascribed to the opportunities open to working-class youth under such policies. Thus may the educational sphere be linked with dominant political and economic institutions.

5. Types of Social Control

In the institutional orders and spheres of various societies we observe certain uniformities of social conduct which represent conformities with expected patterns, and may thus be said to be "socially controlled." The major types and bases of such social controls may also be classified according to their subjective meanings to the individual actors involved, and according to the types of sanctions, if any, employed against people who deviate from them.[24]

I. A custom, or a folkway, is a pattern of conduct which rests upon long familiarity. If people do not follow such rules no exter-

[24] The essentials of the definitions given below are abstracted and paraphrased from various contexts of Max Weber. Cf. also, Karl Mannheim, *Man and Society in an Age of Reconstruction* (New York: Harcourt, Brace, 1940), pp. 311-66.

nal sanctions will be called into play, although they may be inconvenienced. People may not even be conscious of these customs; if they are, they may merely feel that it is more comfortable to conform than not to do so. Thus, although conformity is not "demanded" by anybody, there is a general expectation that people will do the usual things, and this in itself makes for the stability of the custom.

The routine metropolitan day involves the interlocking of many activities; it is customary to adapt to this routine. The times for meals, the lunch hour for example, are of consequence for the rush-hour traffic, and for peaks of demand on restaurants and newspaper stands. The stray latecomer may be inconvenienced: this or that item on the menu "is out." Other restaurants, in turn, advertise "meals served at all hours" for the irregular patron. Economically determined routines of urban mass life make for an adjustment of the program structures of the mass media to the peak availability of specific mass publics and audiences. The statistically calculated coverage of leisure-time hours by mass media of communication and other machinery of amusement—radio's soap opera for housewives weekday afternoons, Metropolitan Opera Saturday afternoons, NBC symphony concerts Sunday afternoons —contributes to rigidly disciplined, routinized, and therefore predictable patterns of customary mass behavior.

In continental Europe the sharper differences in the ways of life of diverse classes and status groups—folkways of village peasants as against urban factory workers, of academicians as against bohemian artists and intellectuals, of salesladies and other white-collar groups as against civil servants and their wives, of rural nobles and ladies of leisure as against artisans and craftsmen—these status differences make for greater diversity of routinized schedules. The parallel habituations of millions who adjust and accommodate to the customary ways of doing things result in regularities of behavior which have caused thoughtful men such as Lord Bryce to posit inertia as one of the fundamental traits of man. Social and personality change stands out in such a perspective as the exception demanding explanation. Both the tradition-bound folkways of agrarian societies and the interlocking matrix of time-clocked metropolitan ways of life, in work and in leisure, seem to result in equally predictable stability of what man takes for granted as the usual thing, as the realm of the customary.

II. Fashion is a usage which rests on appreciation of new
appearance values as indicative of status claims in a dynamic and
stratified society. Fashions are *new* enough to be discernibly different from "last year's model," yet *old* enough so as not to affront
conventions of propriety.

Both fashion and conventions, which we shall presently consider, usually rest upon claims of prestige; when internalized
they are obeyed because of expectations as to what is "proper,"
or what is "smart," which means what is accepted in the style of life
of given status groups.

III. In the case of the customary you may "take it or leave it"—
part your hair on the right or the left side, eat your soup with or
without salt—but this is not true of "conventions" or, as William
Graham Sumner termed them, "the mores." Conventions are more
exacting than customs, for they rest upon the expectation that
deviation from them will result in a general reaction of disapproval. Conventions are generally recognized as binding, or at least
definitely expected, and are protected against violation by sanctions of disapproval, including informal boycott and ostracism.
Convention is the "respectable thing to do" at the right time and
the right place, as against the things that "one just doesn't do."

The "enforcement agency" for conventions is not a specialized
staff, but rather community opinion at large, or at least the opinions of one's status circle. The expectations of general disapproval,
if one breaks with convention, may be internalized, and then
form part of the generalized other, which thus operates as a further psychological motive for conventional conformity. The motive
for adherence to convention, as to fashion, thus involves one's
status or prestige, for the violation of deeply internalized conventions may lead to loss of self-esteem or self-respect.

Different ways of life are shot through with conventions which
all sorts of groups, communities, and institutions consider as binding for their members. Body hygiene in America is subject to conventional standards of cleanliness and propriety—we use tooth-
brushes, mouth wash, and handkerchiefs, and we control body
odor by use of soap and perfume. The enjoyment of meals is a
purely biological process only in extreme situations; usually, we
eat just as much with our eyes and ears as with our mouths. Hence,
table manners and codes of propriety and esthetics serve to facili-

tate our appetites and our ways of "setting the table," of using our knife, fork, and spoon in the proper ways, of taking in the proper amount of the proper food at the proper tempo. We learn to suppress vulgar noises by chewing with our lips closed.

There are standards of sociability, controlling, for example, the preferable, permissible, and tabooed subjects for light or serious conversations and requiring us to be sensitive to the personal tempo of our partner's responsiveness of thought and feeling. The demand to be "tactful" forms part of the conventional code of "polite" behavior. Most of these conventions have been elaborated by occidental court nobilities. The very words used for courteous deportment—"curtsy" and "courtship," for example—remind us of their social-historical origin: to behave as people do at court. Where such conventions become rigid and complex we speak of "codes of etiquette." In formal contexts, such as diplomatic functions, or state dinners in high society, there may be a specialist— the chief of protocol—who devotes his professional skill to questions of etiquette, determining who should be invited to what functions, who might take offense at being "overlooked," who can be left out without harm, who shall sit where, and so on.

The best sellers of Mrs. Emily Post and Miss Lillian Eichler during the last thirty years indicate the spread of certain conventions of high society, prevailing about 1900, to the growing middle classes.[25]

Forms of intimacy are conventionally stylized to guarantee what we demand as our "right to privacy" even from our marriage partner or lover. To be sure, in the euphoric phase of courtship we seek to minimize all social distance, taking offense and feeling hurt at every distancing response of the intimate other.

The "conventional lie" serves the purpose of securing "distance" from the other. "Tell him I am not at home" hurts less than the candid "I don't wish to see him." "Young man, you are a genius and I am afraid this job does not give the proper opportunity to your talents" hurts less than "You are fired," although the occupational results are of course the same.

---

[25] Lillian Eichler's *The Book of Etiquette* sold over a million copies between 1921 and 1945, Emily Post's *Etiquette* from 1922 to 1945 sold more than two-thirds of a million copies. Cf. Arthur M. Schlesinger, *Learning How to Behave* (New York: Macmillan, 1946); and Edmund Wilson, *Classics and Commercials* (New York: Farrar, Straus, 1950), pp. 372-82.

IV. Law, as a type of social control, is distinguished by two features: First, as a pattern of conduct it is upheld by the fact that deviation will probably be met by sanctions aimed at compelling conformity or by punishment. Second, these sanctions are applied by a staff of agents who are especially empowered to carry out this function. It is clear that in this rather broad sense, "law" may exist in any institutional order; in modern societies, however, the legal order of the state is the most inclusive in jurisdiction.

The state, as the most powerful organization of contemporary social structures, regulates through its legal apparatus the power that may be wielded by and in other institutions. Thus a husband may use force against his children or against his wife only to the extent that administrative agents and courts permit it. In some parts of the United States, divorces are granted for slight cases of "mental cruelty"; in other nations, the husband or the wife just has "to take it." A schoolteacher's use of the rod may be outlawed or at least restricted by agents of the state. The laws of the state mediate between the politically determined distribution of power and the economic order, for the legal apparatus defines dispositions over goods and services and other "assets" by the "owners" of goods and the employers of men. It is one of the main functions of law to guarantee, define, and endorse rights over "property"— public, joint, and private.

Laws differ from conventions in that they are enforced by a staff. In the case of deviation from conventions anyone may express disapproval, anyone may apply the sanction and thus publicly represent the generalized other. Institutional patterns per se, as we have seen, are guaranteed by an authoritative other, the head of the institution. Law, as one type of institutional control, involves a specialized staff. Or, in other terms, orientation to conventions, as Émile Durkheim and Max Weber have pointed out, is guaranteed by socially diffuse sanctions, whereas orientation to legal codes is guaranteed by organized sanctions. In the case of convention, any member of a given group or institution may volunteer to "punish" a breach of conventional proprieties, of standards of hygiene, of beauty, or truthfulness. In the case of law, it is the agents or agencies of law enforcement that may take action. As Justice Holmes said, "The prophecies of what the courts will do in fact, and nothing more pretentious, are what I mean by the law." [25A]

Even in Biblical days, we hear of the elders and judges sitting "at the gates," that is, holding court on the town squares behind the city gates. One of the great legacies of ancient Rome are the "Roman Digests" which inform the "canonical law" of the Roman Catholic Church, as well as Anglo-Saxon law, and which stand back of modern legal codes. Among these modern codes, the Code Napoléon has found the widest diffusion and the greatest authority because of its lucidity and simplicity. On the European continent legal education became a university subject at an early time. In the Anglo-Saxon tradition, the bar, essentially a guild of the

[25A] Oliver Wendell Holmes, *Collected Legal Papers* (New York: Harcourt, Brace, 1921), p. 167. Especially pertinent for the social scientist are the essays of Roscoe Pound, "Interests of Personality," 28 *Harv. L. Rev.*, pp. 343, 445 (1915); "A Survey of Social Interests," 57 *Harv. L. Rev.*, p. 1 (1943); "A Survey of Public Interests," 58 *Harv. L. Rev.*, p. 909 (1945); "The Lay Tradition as to the Lawyer," *Mich. L. Rev.*, Vol. XII, No. 8 (June 1914); "The Causes of Popular Dissatisfaction with the Administration of Justice," *Transactions of the American Bar Association* (1906); "Common Law and Legislation," *Harv. L. Rev.*, Vol. XXI, p. 383 (1908). For his survey of the "Sociology of Law" see *Twentieth Century Sociology*, ed. by Georges Gurvitch and Wilbert E. Moore (New York: Philosophical Library, 1945), pp. 297-341. *Social Control Through Law* (New Haven: Yale Univ. Press, 1942) presents a summary statement of the "Dean of American Jurisprudence." Simpson and others in their three-volume *Cases and Readings on Law and Society* (St. Paul, Minn.: West, 1948-49) have attempted to do what has been so much talked about—correlate law with the social sciences. Of special value to the social scientist are the essays of K. Llewellyn. See "Law and the Social Sciences—Especially Sociology," *Harv. L. Rev.*, Vol. 62, p. 1286 (1949).

The best one-volume history of American legal institutions in the perspective of social history seems to us to be Willard Hurst's *The Growth of American Law* (Boston: Little, Brown, 1950). A translation by Max Rheinstein of Max Weber's monumental *Sociology of Law* is due to be published soon by the Harvard University Press.

Given the instability of the American family and the wide interest of social scientists in family and personality problems, we may draw attention to the recent symposium of the *Conference on Divorce*, February 29, 1952, The Law School of the University of Chicago Conference Series, No. 9. Cf. especially the brilliant paper of Max Rheinstein, "Our Dual Law of Divorce: The Law in Action versus the Law of the Books," pp. 39-47. The linkage between the psychopathology of behavior disorders and the law is well presented in Manfred S. Guttmacher and Henry Weihofen's *Psychiatry and the Law* (New York: Norton, 1952).

legal profession, has for centuries retained the transmission of skills and knowledge in the form of legal apprenticeship. University training has moved in the direction of textbook systematization; apprenticeship has retained close contact with legal practice.

Conventions and laws may be quite intricately related, but, briefly, here are four broad, possible combinations: (1) A convention may be guaranteed by law, as in the case with most ordinances enforcing proprieties of dress in public. (2) Both the legal staff and the public may co-operate in suppressing "crimes" against person and property. (3) A convention may rule out a legal conduct pattern. In Tsarist Russia, for example, it was a widespread popular convention to protect revolutionary intellectuals against the police, that is, "denunciation" in accordance with the law was conventionally tabooed. It was considered "dishonorable" to denounce a revolutionary. Hence, the political fugitive from the law could "vanish among the people." (4) A legal code may conflict with a convention, i.e., the lawmaker may seek to "break up" a conventional code of conduct. Thus the Volstead Act was an attempt to "outlaw" drink. Conventional behavior proved stronger, to the point where the law was repealed. In Europe, laws against dueling have by and large proved effective—although army officers, nobles, and some student fraternities, in Germany for instance, take a chance and surreptitiously transgress the law.

If there is general moral indignation about someone's breaking with an institutional pattern, we may say that conventions buttress institutional controls. Institutional roles, however, may or may not be thus upheld by conventions. What is essential to the institution is that the roles it organizes are upheld by the power of the head over institutional members.

Legal sanctions may be differently applied to persons of different social standing. Where justice involves the "bail" and legal counsel is costly, for example, lower-income groups are automatically at a disadvantage. The motives for conformity to law range from calculations and fear of possible sanctions to an absolute belief in the justice or other ethical qualities of the law. The convicted offender may feel deeply guilty, or he may feel himself to be the innocent victim of a "miscarriage of justice." Either extreme of attitude may of course deviate widely from what the facts warrant. Some people may take into account what courts are likely to enforce as a rationally calculated cost factor; others may view the law in all its majesty with simple awe.

Vigilantes, who "take the law into their own hands," or the hooded men of the Ku Klux Klan, who practice "lynch justice," usurp the public prerogative of applying violent and coercive sanctions. Where public authorities do not care to repress the denial of justice to the underprivileged, we encounter situations where conventional violence is honored by men who do not trust the law to "take its course."

Responsibility for a breach of law or convention may be ascribed informally, or by widely different trial procedures with varying rules of evidence, to the individual actor or to one of his community, family, sex group, age class, school class, status group, army unit, mass organization, or nation. Accordingly, we speak of personal or of joint responsibility, of individual or of collective guilt. In one African tribe, the Ila, all of the male population "may be held responsible for any disparagement by the women of the group." [26] The rules of conduct are thus enforced by a sexual group. Moreover, the sanctions are not directed against the individual directly "responsible" for the breach but must be borne by the entire male population. Still another case is found in the patterns of the old Japanese Kumi, in which some five family heads were jointly responsible for public work and tax quotas. If any one of these five ran away from the village, the other four had to make up his work. Similar conditions of joint liability existed in the Mir, the village commune of Tsarist Russia, as well as in ancient China.

Max Weber has distinguished three main types of legal administrations and staffs, which parallel his types of political authority and his types of education: charismatic, traditionalist, and rationally bureaucratic.

A. The law of the charismatic leader is the law of the leader's will. The justice of charismatic leaders is always "emergency justice"; it is by definition personal and arbitrary—if one wishes, it is "justice without law." It does not follow precedents, but estab-

[26] W. I. Thomas, *Primitive Behavior* (New York: McGraw-Hill, 1937), p. 78.

lishes them from case to case, and its legitimation is the followers' faith in the presumed extraordinary qualities of the leader.

This is the sort of justice meted out by successful revolutionaries such as Robespierre and the Directoire, who did not feel bound to traditional codes, time-honored rules, or precedents when dealing with "enemies of the state." More recently, there was Hitler's usurpation of judicial prerogatives when, in June 1934, he arrested Röhm, the leader of the Storm Troops, at night in his home. Röhm and other Storm Troop leaders were "court martialed" by the Leader's bodyguard after ten-minute hearings. Other men, such as Generals Bredow and Schleicher, were murdered by Elite Guards in their homes, without form and in plain daylight.

The justice of Ibn-Saud, King of Saudi-Arabia, is similar.[27] Ibn-Saud takes his seat on the sun-lit steps of his palace, hears a case, for instance, against a man who stole a saddle, convicts him and promptly has one of his Negro slaves cut off the man's hand with a sword and dip the arm in a bucket of hot oil.

B. Traditionalist justice has been called "cadi justice," for in this legal system, the judges consider the case, as does the Mohammedan cadi, with precise regard to the person. Cadi justice differs from charismatic justice in that it usually follows religiously sanctioned norms and time-honored precedents. There are no rational rules of proof and evidence, and ordeals and duels may be considered magically significant tests of guilt or innocence. This realm of traditional norms, in the absence of rational definitions of terms and rules of evidence, is supplemented by a realm of personal arbitrariness in which judicious wisdom and psychological astuteness enter the procedure and the verdict. King Solomon's justice readily comes to mind, as does that of Chinese judges of old and the Biblical "Elders at the Gate." Both charismatic and traditionalist justice bespeak the rule of men, not the rule of law.[27A]

C. The rule of law, in a rational, bureaucratic manner, is a late and specifically Western attainment, built on the legacy of Rome. There a prestigeful group of legal practitioners—the jurisconsuls—

[27] Cf. H. C. Armstrong, *Ibn Sa'ūd, King of Saudi Arabia* (Penguin Edition, 1938).

[27A] Said Elihu Root in his Presidential Address to the American Bar Association in Chicago, in 1916: "The vast and continually increasing mass of reported decisions which afford authorities on almost every side of almost every question admonish us that by the mere following of precedent we should soon emerged, who offered professional advice to their clients. Roman law demanded that the complainant file his charge in legal terms. Court procedure allowed the court to judge the case only in terms of the original charge, regardless of what facts might be disclosed during the court hearings. This necessitated legal aid. Moreover, under the Caesars, the bureaucratization of public authorities, and the development of administrative and other laws of great subtlety, made it necessary for the politically ambitious man to study law as well as forensic rhetoric. This allowed jurisconsuls to establish free schools of law and rhetoric. A practical bent of mind combined with a ritualist traditionalism, reminiscent of peasant background, made the Romans eager to state whatever new problems faced them in terms of old norms by construing them with the necessary interpretive twist. The hairsplitting finesse of legal definitions, the logically unambiguous distinctions, and the deductions made are all appraised by experts as unique and unsurpassed in legal history.

V. *"Rational Uniformity"* involves the orientation of persons to similar, ulterior expectations; it is an action by which men strive to exploit opportunities in their own self interest. Rational uniformities are only expediently oriented to norms, duties, or to felt obligations. Their stability as patterns of conduct rests on the deviator's running the risk of damaging his own interests. Although rational uniformities of conduct may be a feature of any institutional order, the economic actions of agents in a free market, who by their interpersonal calculation and bargaining determine the price of commodities, are outstanding cases of rational patterns of conduct.

VI. *Ethical rules* are standards of conduct, or conventions, to which men attribute intrinsic value. By virtue of this attribution, they treat these patterns as valid norms governing their decisions and conduct. Such rules may have profound influence upon human action, even in the complete absence of external sanctions. If they are really effective, abstractly formulated ethical rules become part

have no system of law at all, but *the rule of the Turkish cadi who is expected to do in each case what seems to him to be right;* and then the door would be thrown wide open for *the rule of men rather than the rule of law,* and for the exercise of personal injustice as well as personal justice. We are approaching a point where we shall run into confusion unless we adopt the simple and natural course of avoiding confusion by classification." [Our italics.]

of the conventional patterns, being supported by the danger of disapproval and the loss of prestige. They may even become part of law, and accordingly be enforced by special staffs.

VII. *Institutional controls* are of course most important for our conception of social structure. They are patterns upheld by the heads of institutions or by their agents. The roles played by members of a household for example, are guaranteed by parental authority; employees are subject to the control of owners and managers; soldiers are subject to the authority of the commanding officer; parishioners stand under the jurisdiction of church authorities. Whatever ends the organized and interacting partners may pursue, and whatever means of "authority" or "leadership" exist, sanctions against infractions of the "rules of the game" are expected by those who to any extent deviate. Institutional controls are thus upheld by the expectation and the fact that deviation will probably result in the head of the institution or his authorized agents taking action of some kind against the person who deviates.

In terms of internal sanctions, institutions mean that the generalized other which operates in the persons involved is likely to include the head of the institution as a particular other. The king of a political order or the father of a patriarchal kinship order are particular others—the most significant others of persons who are psychologically members of the institution. The kinds of external sanction which this head will take against offenders have a wide range—disapproval, expulsion, or death.

The types of social controls which we have defined and illustrated often seem to cluster around or be limited by the institutional framework. They specify and formalize institutional control —as with law, which is of course a specific formalization of institutional control in general; or they diffuse and generalize institutional regulation—as with convention, which involves reactions to more than specific institutional heads. Institutional orders form, as it were, typical limits in accordance with which other social controls normally tend to operate.

6. *Orientation to Social Controls*

Whether a code is sanctioned by staff action, as in law, or by diffuse agents, as in ethical rule or convention, it may have a wide range of personal and social orientations. Wherever there are norms and codes, ideals and aspirations, the social psychologist has learned to expect "trespasses" and failings, and in the case of religious commandments, "sins." We have accordingly to distinguish between behavior and attitudes with regard to norms: broadly speaking, four such orientations to conventional, moral, or legal codes may be located by means of this simple chart:

ATTITUDE TOWARD THE IDEAL OR NORM

		+	−
CONDUCT WITH REFERENCE	+	I	II
TO THE NORM OR IDEAL	−	III	IV

I. There is the type of man who cherishes or affirms a given norm and in his behavior abides by his conviction. If he is given to judge others, we may call him an ethical rigorist, with reference to moral issues; a saintly man, with reference to Christian demands; or a militant liberal, with reference to the American creed.[28]

Such persons have successfully internalized the "codified" value —whether it is a religious imperative, a standard of hygiene, a conception of the beautiful, the true, or the good. Socially, such internalization leads to standards of "good taste" and "decorum," of *savoir-faire* and "decency"; psychologically, it leads to the actor's ascribing traits such as "politeness," "tactfulness," or "uprightness" to others and to himself. Internally, the person of type I subscribes to the respective values, verbally affirming them; externally, in his conduct, he abides by these standards.

In matters of food, appropriate thresholds of disgust secure the person against dropping below his dietary standards. So the pious, orthodox Jew will not consume pork, will not enjoy the "blood" in rare roast beef. He will be as "disgusted" as was the sober Roman with drunkards, for the Roman identified drunkenness with "barbarism," just as the Hindu Brahman identifies "beef eaters" with Barbarians. Religious and ritualistic taboos, as well as hygienic standards and simple childhood habituation to what is "usual," contribute to the establishment of such thresholds of disgust. Men like to eat what they are used to eating.

[28] Robert K. Merton has applied this scheme to ethnic and racial tolerance in his essay printed in *Discrimination and National Welfare* (New York: Institute for Religious Studies, 1948).

Most peoples or groups sentimentalize certain food habits and are even proud of them, and this is all the more so if they conceive of these habits as badges of group distinction. The Britisher enjoys being a "beef eater"; the Frenchmen conceive of the "Paris cuisine" as a contribution to world civilization; the Spartan enjoyed his "blacksoup," which disgusted the Athenian ambassadors; to the Scotch-Irish, Woodrow Wilson attributed the whisky bottle, just as the stereotyped German is assigned his "stein of beer," the Indian his "peace pipe," and the modern American his "cocktail." "National beverages" and food preferences, and differences between, for example, the tea-sipping salon society and the plebeian "beer garden" folks come to mind, not to mention the "potato-eating Irish" of the nineteenth century. Such standards and preferences, with their accompanying images of "disgust," often serve then to implement group hatreds. Thus the French consider the Boche sauerkraut eaters; the Germans consider the Russians drunkards; and Erasmus considered the British "dirty."

II. There is also the spurious conformist or opportunist. Outwardly he conforms to the code, inwardly he does not subscribe to it. He conforms externally for reasons of expediency, or because he deems it "cheaper" to do so. He "goes to church" in a kind of Sunday obsequiousness although he does not believe in the creed. Sören Kierkegaard thought that with the exception of himself all Christians in his time were spurious Christians. The motivation of this type of person is thus an attitude of expedient opportunism and a fear of sanctions, not a love of the respective value.

Since the values involved in the code are not internalized in moral contexts we may speak of this type as the pretender. Thus there is the sham patient, the malingering soldier, the disguised royalty, and many other masters of pretense, respectable and unrespectable. No matter how outwardly correct his conduct, the pretender's lack of conviction and integrity, the "mask-like" nature of his role enactment is often discernible, in the "give away," the slip, the inconsistency—no matter whether the actor "deceives himself" *and* others, or whether he is self-conscious about what he is doing. Moral philosophers from Pascal to Nietzsche have contributed to the discernment of such phenomena.

III. The person who subscribes verbally to a code but deviates from it in conduct represents a third type. Here is the hypocrite whose verbal cant is the tribute vice pays to virtue. When such a person acts in good faith we speak, in modern terms, of "rationalization" whereby the actor substitutes a socially acceptable vocabulary of motives for his socially unacceptable motives. The pejorative connotation of the term "cant" implies the demand and expectation that the verbalizer of "cant" potentially could and actually should realize his double standard, the incongruity between his words and his deeds. Such disparities often emerge when the horizon of the actor's awareness is restricted, and he does not face up to the implications and ramifications of his conduct. Thus, free enterprisers during a depression may discharge workers, denying them job opportunities. But regardless of whether the workers by habituation then become lazy, or whether they are only too eager to work, the entrepreneur may readily blame their unemployment on their laziness. Or a similar situation may occur when the social structure does not offer to dependent workers adequate incentives, when the experience of generations has taught them that additional efforts remain fruitless. And it may, in fact, be so: effort not paying off because it remains without compensation, because geographical factors offer no opportunities to improve one's lot, or because an oppressive tax system deprives the subject of the fruit of his labor. The ruling class, at this point, may be only too eager to vilify the slave, peasant, or worker, who thus has no other means of retaliation than skillfully withholding his efforts.

Such a vocabulary of motives—of laziness and general no-good—lends to the status superior the secondary advantage of implementing his superiority of property and power by a sense of moral superiority; it enables him to "rationalize" social differences into "moral" differences, with all the moral benefits accruing to himself. Even the suffering patience of the downtrodden is held against him as "lack of agility" and "stupidity," as "lack of initiative" and as "docility." Thus do status snobbery and human pride often feed on the misery of the others.

Criticism of upper classes and of the codes and motives they impose also finds its point of attack. The professed values are played off against those who profess them, as the intellectuals, acting as the conscience of their time and society, contrast professed values with actual conduct, and thus "debunk" and "unmask" the hypocrite, the "Tartufe," the "Elmer Gantry."

IV. This type represents the consistent deviationist, the nonconformist of word and deed. Here we find the rebel and the revolutionary who openly renounce the dominant norm and break it in their behavior. We also find the criminal, who differs from the revolutionary in that he has no counternorms. Naturally "criminals" might also belong in Type III, being persons who acknowledge the law in words and often wish others to abide by the code, whereas they do not feel bound by it: tax delinquents may, for example, readily be found in this category. It is the difference between the role of the "citizen" and that of the "bourgeois," in Marx's sense, that we have in mind here. One wishes to be considered a respectable citizen—but such respectability must not cost too much. Abuses of all sorts—from corruption in high office to food adulteration and other evasions of government regulations—are due to the fact that profit interests get the better of civic highmindedness. Whereas the heroic *citoyen* of France criticizes the corruption of kings and nobles and establishes his own rules after the revolutionary overthrow of the *ancien régime,* once he is in the saddle and has developed into a plutocrat, his "republican virtues" may crumble and disintegrate in the face of "tempting" or "unique opportunities." On a large scale we also see repeated the cycle of many monastic orders, whose members work hard for the glory of God, then becoming rich, succumb to the temptations that seem to go with wealth. But, then, looking around them, they find another and new movement, and begin the same cycle. Municipal administrations also have their cycles of "reform" under the slogan "throw the rascals out"; then comes the relaxation of civic endeavor and the return to "taking it easy."

In Type IV, we also find principled opponents of the code, who may be complete cynics, skeptics in the face of the respective value. These opponents may even publicly uphold emergent countervalues and thus be revolutionaries or precursors of revolutions to come. In this case, such a person would be inspired by a rival value to promote the establishment of "countermores," which are usually linked to an actual or imagined "reference group" whose members may supposedly or actually sustain him. Whether he actually is their "representative" or merely wishes to be, he may think on "their behalf" or "in their interests."

Intellectuals and their activities deserve special attention in this connection, for they often play important roles during periods of transition from one social structure to another. They criticize as already "dead" what actually exists, and they do so in the name of the as yet unrealized, and perhaps even unrealizable, "utopian" standards. Thus, during the decline of the Hebrew kingdoms, solitary prophets arose who, in their religiously motivated dema-goguery, developed grandiose eschatological expectations and visions of divine punishments to come on the Day of Yahweh, after which a pious "remnant" would be saved and its hidden glory brought to light. Such Biblical eschatologies, combined with the rational utopian construction of a "good society" for which Plato provided the model in his "Republic" and "The Laws," were fused in the postmedieval utopianism of Renaissance political thinkers—such as Thomas More and Campanella—and in the work of the Enlightenment philosophers of the dawn of democratic con-stitutionalism, as well as in the socialist critiques of capitalist so-ciety, from Saint-Simon and Robert Owen to Marx and the Marx-ists.

The problems of subjective and objective orientation to norms and codes become more complex when moral and legal codes conflict. Sociologically speaking, as we have seen, such conflict means that a staff-enforced code deviates from a group-cherished convention which is guaranteed by diffuse or unorganized sanc-tions. Such situations may occur where the lawmakers and their staffs seek to break up certain special mores of particular groups.

This simple fourfold scheme may be useful for any situation containing norms; applied to marriage in Western societies, for example, we would have under I the loyal, monogamous married couple; under II persons who conform to the conventional regula-tion of acceptable marriage partners although they do not "believe in them"; the white girl who shrinks back from accepting the marriage proposal of her Negro lover, or vice versa. Under III we have the adulterous husband who "believes in monogamy," or the adulterous Christian minister. And under IV there is the con-firmed Mormon of old, or Goethe who in his drama "Stella" re-solved an erotic triangle by a "happy ending" in bigamy. Goethe, who married for the first and for the last time at the age of fifty-seven, practiced the "freedom" he believed in, and in his novel, *Elective Affinities,* appraised monogamous marriage as a story of tragic resignation.

In this as well as in the preceding chapter we have discussed the range of institutions in each of the institutional orders which comprise a social structure and some of the types of people which may best be understood in terms of these institutions.

In discussing the *political* order, we have paid particular attention to various kinds of power—especially as power is organized in the state and associated with the various sentiments of "nationalism." And we have devoted attention to the major types of states of the twentieth century: democracy and dictatorship. In regard to the *economic* order, we have studied the development of capitalism, especially in terms of rationality, and described in brief its major types and the kinds of roles men play in each of them. We have tried in a brief account of the *military* order to relate some of the historical practices of violence to types of military men, and we have paid special attention to the sociological and psychological characteristics of six contrasting types of armies. In discussing the *religious* order, we have pointed out selected aspects of the six world religions, especially the type of generalized other they inculcate in their adherents, and their typical relations to the other institutions existing in the social structures of which they have been components. With respect to the *kinship* order, we have discussed various types of families and the type of generalized other they tend to form, as well as how the kinship order has been historically related to the economic order in the "household," and hence to role differences between men and women. We have also indicated some of the intricate ways in which marriage and love may be related. The *educational* sphere refers to those aspects of any institution which transmit skills and values. Every institutional order may to a greater or a lesser degree have an educational sphere, the types of skills transmitted in each case being relevant to the ends of the respective order. We have suggested that educational institutions are rarely autonomous, and illustrated the services educational institutions may perform for the state by reference to the case of modern Germany.

In conjunction with these institutional orders, we have discussed certain major types of social controls and norms which guide the enactment of roles by persons. These controls include custom, fashion, convention, ethical values, and the several types of law. In connection with such controls, we have pointed out that persons may react—objectively and subjectively—to such controls in a variety of ways, and that to understand these, as well as the motivations involved, we must observe both public conduct and private attitude.

Persons accept or reject various roles—and leaders make known their expectations—by means of symbols. Moreover, whether or not persons accept the demands made upon them is in part dependent upon their positions in the prevailing system of stratification. Accordingly, before we consider how institutional orders are variously combined into total social structures, which we shall do in Chapter XII, we must elaborate the conception of symbol spheres, in Chapter X, and we must relate our scheme of institutional orders to systems of stratification, in Chapter XI.

C H A P T E R

X

Symbol Spheres

LANGUAGE is central to the concerns of social psychology because it has to do with the functioning of institutions as well as with the socialization of the individual. By considering the social and the personal functions of language we can relate intimate details about the person and the psychic structure to broader conceptions of institutional organization. To understand how any given person strives, feels, and thinks we have to pay attention to the symbols he has internalized; but to understand these symbols we have to grasp the way in which they co-ordinate institutional actions.[1] For symbols mediate entire institutional arrangements as well as the conduct and roles of persons.

In the psychic structure, language articulates and patterns the objects and noises which we see and hear; we come to know many of our feelings and wishes in terms of specific vocabularies. By singling out targets for action, language helps turn impulses into defined purposes, inchoate sensations into perceptions, vague feelings into known emotions.

In the person, symbols lend motives to conduct, and signal the expectations of others. Symbols provide the person with a frame of reference for his experience, and this frame of reference is not only "social" in general, it may be definitely related to the operations of specific institutions.

If we examine the content and functions of communication within institutions, or within the various institutional orders of a social structure, we notice that certain symbols tend to recur more frequently than others in given contexts. This universe of discourse—the vocabularies, pronunciations, emblems, formulas,

[1] See Chapter IV: The Person, and Chapter V: The Sociology of Motivation.

and types of conversation which are typical of an institutional order—make up "the symbol sphere" of this order.

Such symbols may be acoustic—as in music or in speech—or they may be visual—as in written and printed imagery and signs. The distinctions and symbols of a symbol sphere of a given institutional order are related to the preoccupations and practices of persons in that order. For since language helps us to co-ordinate social activities, it reflects the objects with which persons of the order deal and the conduct patterns with which they do so.

Thus the myths of religion, the incantations of magic, the technical jargon of an occupation, the high-brow pronunciations and slang of status groups, the tête-à-tête of lovers, and the table-talk of families—all these represent modes of speech which reflect different institutional contexts. We become more aware of this when we examine foreign languages. Arabic, for example, "contains about 6,000 names for 'camel,'" or derived from camel—for breeding-camels and running-camels and for female camels in all the various stages of pregnancy.[2] The practices and objects involved in a society of camel breeders are reflected in the content and distinctions which make up the symbol sphere of their society. The Teutonic languages have terms for horse, steed, mare, stallion, all of which to the Greek were simply *hippos*.

Religious institutions develop their own rhetoric and liturgy—the hymn, the prayer, the sermon, the benediction. Similarly in the political and economic orders we find genres of talk and of writing—the sales talk, low- and high-pressure; the election speech, stump or fireside. And, of course, the bulk of our modern fiction is a symbolic elaboration of love and kinship relations. Not all societies, of course, develop identical symbols for the same pursuit; the increasingly precise notation, and hence the symbolic recording, of musical sound patterns is peculiar to occidental civilization. In like manner, not all institutions of the same order have identical symbols. Puritanism, for example, suppressed instrumental music as well as opera and the dance. Catholicism, however, has made rich use of all the arts, with the exception of dancing, as symbolic means of religious worship.

Certain emblems and modes of language not only recur in

[2] See W. I. Thomas, *Primitive Behavior* (New York: McGraw-Hill, 1937), p. 68.

given social contexts but seem to be more important to the maintenance of certain institutions, to their chains of authority and to the authoritative distribution of their roles. The contexts in which these symbols appear may seem to be "staged"; they are dramatic, solemn, weird. They carry more "weight." These symbols may be repeated every day by everyone; or they may be used only on extraordinary occasions and by specifically authorized persons. As we have seen, the symbols which thus justify a social structure or an institutional order are called symbols of "legitimation," or "master symbols," or "symbols of justification."

By lending meaning to the enactment of given roles, these master symbols sanction the person in re-acting the roles. When internalized they form unquestioned categories which channel and delimit new experiences; they promote and constrain activities. When public justifications are privately internalized, they make up the stuff of self-justification, operating as reasons and motives leading persons into roles and sanctioning their enactment of them. Indeed, no self-justification is likely to be entirely private; unless it is accepted by others it does not secure the private self in feeling that all is well. If, for example, "individualistic" institutions are publicly justified, then reference to self-interest may be acceptable as justification for individual conduct. Personal reasons are thus related to public legitimations.

While the symbols typically found in any order comprise the symbol sphere of that order, those symbols that justify the institutional arrangement of the order are its master symbols. To the social scientist such master symbols are of special interest in that they allow us to understand the cohesion of role configurations, their permanence and change, and their function in the intrapsychic life of persons.

The more refined symbol elaborations of the philosopher, theologian, publicity director, scientist, or artist may not be so immediately important for the understanding of a period and society as are the doctrines which do not seem to be "doctrines" at all, but rather *facts*. In the experience of men enacting the roles of their time, they seem "inevitable categories of the human mind. Men do not look on them merely as correct opinion, for they have become so much a part of the mind, and lie so far back, that they are never really conscious of them at all. They do not see them, but other things *through* them. It is these abstract ideas at the center, the things which they take for granted that characterize a period." [3]

Those in authority within institutions and social structures attempt to justify their rule by linking it, as if it were a necessary consequence, with moral symbols, sacred emblems, or legal formulae which are widely believed and deeply internalized. These central conceptions may refer to a god or gods, the "votes of the majority," the "will of the people," the "aristocracy of talents or wealth," to the "divine right of kings," or to the allegedly extraordinary endowment of the person of the ruler himself.

Various thinkers have used different terms to refer to this phenomenon: Mosca's "political formula" or "great superstitions," [4] Locke's "principle of sovereignty," [5] Sorel's "ruling myth," [6] Thurman Arnold's "folklore," [7] Weber's "legitimations," [8] Durkheim's "collective representations," [9] Marx's "dominant ideas," [10] Rousseau's "general will," [11] Lasswell's "symbols of authority," or "symbols of justification," [12] Mannheim's "ideology," [13] Herbert Spencer's "public sentiments" [14]—all testify the central place of master symbols in social analysis.

[3] T. E. Hulme, *Speculations* (London: Routledge, 1936), p. 50.

[4] G. Mosca, *The Ruling Class*, H. D. Kahn, tr. (New York: McGraw-Hill, 1939), pp. 70-71.

[5] John Locke, *Two Treatises Concerning Government* (London, 1924).

[6] Georges Sorel, *Reflections on Violence*, T. E. Hulme, tr. (New York: Viking, 1914).

[7] Thurman W. Arnold, *The Folklore of Capitalism* (New Haven: Yale Univ. Press, 1937).

[8] Max Weber, *The Theory of Social and Economic Organization*, Talcott Parsons and A. M. Henderson, trs. (New York: Oxford, 1948), Chapters I and III.

[9] Émile Durkheim, *The Elementary Forms of the Religious Life* (New York: Macmillan, 1915).

[10] K. Marx and F. Engels, *The German Ideology* (New York: International Publications, 1939).

[11] Jean-Jacques Rousseau, *The Social Contract* (New York: Hafner, 1947).

[12] H. D. Lasswell, *World Politics and Personal Insecurity* (New York: McGraw-Hill, 1935), and *Politics: Who Gets What, When, How.* (New York: McGraw-Hill, 1936). See also Kenneth Burke, *Attitudes Towards History* (New York: New Republic, 1937), Vol. II, pp. 232 ff.

[13] Karl Mannheim, *Ideology and Utopia*, Louis Wirth and Edward Shils, trs. (New York: Harcourt, Brace, 1936).

[14] Herbert Spencer, *Principles of Sociology* (London, 1882-1896), Vol. II, Book 1, pp. 319 ff.

1. Symbol Spheres in Six Contexts

In modern social structures, it is sometimes difficult to classify the prevailing symbols according to the institutional orders which they justify or according to the roles to which they lend meaning. The modern expansion of mass communications has made for a wide and rapid diffusion of symbols and vocabularies, which may arise in local areas for special purposes. Nevertheless, if the interrelations of the different orders, in terms of their symbol spheres, are to be grasped, one must attempt to sort them out.

Since the roles of an institutional order involve specific modes of conduct and the social integration of these modes, it is only natural that special vocabularies should arise. These vocabularies are shorthand ways of referring to common tasks; they integrate the behaviors which go on within the order more readily and precisely than could symbols from general discourse. Thus, in addition to master symbols (which justify and sanction the authority of institutions and lend meaning and motivation to the enactment of roles), symbol spheres also contain many generally less important specifications and implications that are, in fact, specialized ways of talk and writing.

In discussing some symbols which "belong to" the various orders we are able to illustrate some of the general points we have made about symbol spheres.

I. The vocabulary is a major element in the style of life which sets off different status groups. It is one of the first things we notice about a person. In terms of his speech, his choice of words and pronunciation, we place a person in the hierarchy of the status sphere. The words that may with propriety be used on given occasions are circumscribed by status conventions, which may be maintained esthetically in terms of "good" and "bad" taste, or magically, in terms of "foul" language, or religiously by taboos being placed upon certain modes of speech, for example, cursing. Conformity to the status conventions of the symbol sphere is upheld by the formal and informal educations of status group members.

Such vocabularies change, and may even be subject to fads and fashions. No matter how much formal education persons are exposed to, they may never be able to learn the innuendoes of a situation and respond to it with the proper symbols unless they have imbibed it, so to speak, with their mother's milk. For there are differences in enunciation and in the scope of vocabulary which depend upon the variety of contacts and travel and dinner companions over long periods of time. The conventionalization of language by an upper-status group is usually conservative. It slows up the drift of linguistic change, as does education, which makes persons sensitive to "good form" and "usage." Changes in language therefore, tend to drift upward; the "uncontrolled speech of the folk" today provides advance information about proper usage tomorrow.[15]

Where stratification is rigid, the vocabularies of the various strata may not diffuse very readily. Social position is thus "closed" to others by the development of an "exclusive" conventional language. Then, by listening to conversations one can identify the speaker's status level (in Confucian China, highly educated people could do so by the calligraphy of the writer). In Java, five vocabularies may be used in connection with the status stratification, and in old Siam, as well as in seventeenth- and eighteenth-century Europe, the court-centered nobility spoke French rather than the national language or the regional dialect of commoners, just as the old Russian court spoke French and, before 1914, English. In Polynesia, among the Tonga, a similar situation prevails, there being three vocabularies. Prince Hohenlohe, German chancellor around 1900, wrote to his wife only in French; German for him was public language, French was the private language. Frederick II of Prussia, a contemporary of Kant, considered German a boorish and vulgar idiom, which the king need not master.

A speaker may "emphasize the superiority of the person addressed by using the vocabulary above that of his rank, or his inferiority by using that of the rank just lower."[16] In England, "gentleman," a term designating a status type, has tended to spread and include certain abstract character traits rather than all well-born persons who need not engage in routine work for livelihood. Yet status groups tend to close up their ranks by means of language. The use of medieval Latin thus excluded the uneducated, just as

[15] See Edward Sapir, *Language* (New York: Harcourt, Brace, 1921), p. 167. This point may require modification under mass communication conditions.
[16] W. I. Thomas, *op. cit.*, p. 83.

the use of foreign languages by upper-status groups excludes lower classes and status groups.

Germans in Goethe's time referred only to noble-born girls as *fräulein;* today for Germans it is a common form of address for unmarried young women; for many American soldiers it means sexually available women. In the United States such terms as "sir," or even "Mr." reflect status stratification. In classic China, with its ancestor worship, there was no word to designate "one who is old" in a socially neutral, chronological way. The Chinese words carried overtones of deference so that in this language it was difficult to raise the ethical question of whether one should or should not treat old men with respect.[17]

The prestige of national languages may be implemented by the prestige of works of art integrating language and music. Thus Italians and Germans have profited from the diffusion of Italian and German operas sung in the original language, especially Verdi and Wagner, and the lied, from Mozart to Mahler. Together with the works, star performers also have migrated: the Italian tenor and the "Wagnerian soprano."

II. In the *economic order,* the jobs that men do together give rise to specialized trade jargons. Changes in the technology connected with the job give rise to new terms connected with novel tools and their use (kilowatt, X-ray, video, static). Such terms may spread to persons and to strata that are not connected with the new technology. Most craftsmen and engineering groups develop specialized workshop vocabularies which may be quite seperate from the terminology they are formally taught. Where speed is at a premium, as in a news agency, "shop languages" tend to develop which aim at a skeleton language that, for economic reasons, drastically reduces the number of syllables, using only those that are indispensable for comprehension. In part, the prose style of *Time* magazine represents an overt cultivation and publicizing of such normally shop-restricted language, thus giving readers the illusion that they are "on the inside." This is a comforting feeling at a time when, due to the concentration and secrecy of key decisions, so many people feel "on the outside" and have learned to

[17] Cf. I. A. Richards, *Mencius on the Mind* (New York: Harcourt, Brace, 1932).

distrust the news organs to the extent of a "propaganda neurosis."

A good deal of American "common sense," for example, deals with the necessity of a man's "earning a living," and the "practical" is generally identified with the "pecuniary" or the profitable. The pecuniary may also inform moral vocabularies: he is a sterling character, worth his weight in gold. Some tombstones, in fact, inform us that a deceased child was "worth a million dollars."

In the United States many master symbols of the social structure are derived from and primarily legitimate the economic order. "Free Enterprise" and "Private Property" are practically unquestionable symbols, even when they are not very skillfully used. The autonomy and power of the laissez-faire economic order, as guaranteed by formal law, has thus been a major factor in shaping all U.S. symbol spheres.

For over a hundred years, lawyers and politicians, journalists and academicians have taught, argued, and presented economic issues in terms of the "competitive model" of laissez-faire capitalism essentially derived from Adam Smith. The disturbing facts of an economic life now dominated by giant corporations has led to a popular view of them as deviant institutions, as "monopolies," and the word has about it a ring of righteous indignation against monopolistic "abuses" of power.

One of the characteristic legacies of puritan America is the moral conception of property as stewardship. In early days, in the face of the "roving Indian," this concept sanctioned the American seizure of hunting ground and the placing of it under the God-willed plow. In the face of presumably "improvident" and propertyless masses it has made philanthropy obligatory, at least from the deathbed of the millionaire. Symbols of stewardship and some accompanying practices have thus blended with other legitimations of the dominant economic order.

III. Families may develop special terms understood only by its members. Such terms or phrases may originate from some experience which the family feels to be unique and wishes to recall by symbols that carry its overtone or mood. Or, a baby's mispronunciation may be considered so cute that it is thought worthy of being preserved.

Everyone knows that lovers develop little phrases so intimate and subtle that only they could ever understand them. Some words, like cute and nice, are specifically feminine. Others seem to arise from the conduct of women in handling babies: dydee for diaper, booties, goodies, teeny-weeny. Others refer to objects connected with the tabooed sphere of sex: "unmentionables," or "lingerie" for underwear.

An extreme instance of the segregation of language by sexual groups is provided by the island Caribs who have "two distinct vocabularies, one used by men and by women when speaking to men, the other used by women when speaking to each other, and by men when repeating, in *oratio obligua*, some saying of women. . . ." [18] The institutions of exogamy and of exclusively male war councils appear to underlie such sexual divisions of vocabulary.

Words referring to "young girls" are likely to take on moral connotations: "In French, one word after another that has meant a young girl has dropped out of polite usage because words signifying this sweet creature too easily take on the meaning of what some of the weaker of the sweet creatures may become. Thus *Bachele, mescine, touse, garce* and even *fille* have in succession been demoted." In English one has similar trouble with words like "mistress, lover, and even woman." [19] The sociological analysis of such shifts in meaning reveals the interdependence of words, conduct, and conventions within given institutions.

In Western civilization the "sanctity of the home" is a legitimation of the privacy maintained at the family abode. The political order in the United States guarantees this feature of the monogamous family, the fourth amendment to the Constitution holding that "The right of the people to be secure in their persons, houses, papers, and effects, against unreasonable searches and seizures, shall not be violated . . ." Although the practical expediencies of local authorities have modified the interpretation of this amendment it still stands as part of the formal sphere of political symbols which guarantee privacy.

Reporters intent on making headlines with "the human interest story" caused the Lindberghs to leave the country. Wire tapping and the secret installation of equipment for overhearing and over-

[18] Cf. the passage from *The Mystic Rose*. Reprinted by W. I. Thomas in his *Source Book for Social Origins* (Boston: Badger, 1909), p. 521.

[19] Cf. Isaac Goldberg, *The Wonder of Words* (New York: Appleton-Century, 1938), p. 269.

seeing what goes on in the home of suspects under police surveillance often seem to make the legal rights to privacy quite tenuous. Some private citizens disdain the verbal invasion of their neighbor's legitimate privacy by dismissing it as "gossip."

The German equivalent of "gossip" is *Klatsch,* and it is perhaps no less characteristic that one speaks of "Klatschbase"—a gossipy woman—but not of a man. Hence one may wonder whether they were not men who were in the lead in depreciating "gossip" in the name of a "broader horizon" of public concerns in the light of which women's housebound talk appeared "trivial." It is no less characteristic that philosophers, like Aristotle and Bacon would preferably ascribe "garrulity" to women.

At any rate, the demand for conventional protection of privacy emerged along with the greater individuation of families and the sharper definition of "private" and "public" segments of the personality. When the workshop and the home of the guildmaster were still under the same roof, when the master's wife was an important authority also in the workshop, such segmentalization of "private" and "public" life could not emerge. It was the differentiation of workshop and home, office and home, of private fortune and business capital, of "bourgeois" and "citizen," which allowed for the drawing of a line between "private" and "public" life.

For democratically elected leaders of the community the line between public and private is differently drawn than for persons having lower "representative value" to the community. The public claims the right to know more about the leader's life than merely the official aspect. Thus baby pictures of the President as well as photographs of his home and hobbies are publicized to satisfy "human interest." The moral conduct of teachers, ministers, civil servants outside the class room, church, or office has a bearing on their positions of public trust, yet this is not true for a salesman.

Another feature of the symbol sphere of kinship orders that is associated with the political order is "the oath." Western civilization generally has been guaranteed by religious and secular state symbols, rather than by blood. Fealty, loyalty, and the magical sanctions involved in the taking of oaths have centered around these two orders, whose symbol spheres have been used to guarantee the roles and contractual relations of other orders, including that of kinship. Thus the marriage oath—a vow of constant and exclusive love—is taken in terms of the state and on the Bible.

IV. The symbols of the *political order* may be visual or auditory, like the flag or the national anthem, or they may be sentimentalized places like "the Capital," or written documents as in the constitutional states of modern democracies. In discussing political symbols, our chief concern is with those which sanction political authority.

The party politician will, in one way or the other, use the master symbols of the political order, and will also develop special rhetorics: both the content and the delivery of his speech will become stereotyped around those modes that are felt to be effectively persuasive appeals. He names events and personalities in the stereotypes of his viewpoint: "radical" or "progressive," "regimentation" or "regulation," "dole" or "home relief," "alien" or "foreign," the "New Deal" or the "Raw Deal."

The symbols which legitimate a political order may be so deeply embedded in mass media and popular mentality that countersymbols are avoided—even if they stand for programs or policies which people actually want. Thus a majority of certain groups may be in favor of specific policies for which "socialism" stands, but reject the "socialist party" or socialist terminology. Stereotypes of the symbol sphere, and not issues, may thus determine political orientation and conduct.[20]

V. The symbol spheres of the *military order* and of the political order are blended in the modern national state. This symbolic integration follows the integration of the institutions making up the two orders. The state monopolizes the instruments of violence and permits only those who are authorized to wear the uniform of the army, navy, or police to have access to them, and then only when "under orders." The uniform is a symbol of this authorized access and use.

In modern armies special premiums are placed upon such character traits as courage and bravery, and the risk involved is not compensated in money to the same degree as it would be if

[20] On the use of stereotypes in political conduct, see the experimental study of G. W. Hartmann, "The Contradiction Between the Feeling-Tone of Political Party Names and Public Responses to Their Platforms," *Journal of Social Psychology*, 1936, 7, pp. 336-57; S. S. Sargent, "Emotional Stereotypes in The Chicago Tribune," *Sociometry* II, (1939), pp. 69 ff.; Thurman W. Arnold, *op. cit.;* and *The Symbols of Government* (New Haven: Yale Univ. Press, 1935).

anyone ran the same risk in a civilian job. Therefore, special weight and a heavy emotional aura are characteristic of the symbol sphere of the military order. Medals and other tokens of honor become important as psychic compensations and incentives which enable and inspire men to risk their lives in the fighting role of the soldier or sailor.

In addition to these honorific accentuations of the traits needed for the soldier, most armies tend to develop specialized vocabularies which reflect the feelings, situation, and needs of the soldiery. The organizational complexities of large-scale armies and navies bring about special "command languages" which officer candidates have to learn. It takes skill to write out unambiguous "orders" with the utmost economy of words and yet perfectly lucid simplicity. The speed of transmission and the choice of proper "channels" of staff and line officers who have to transmit the supreme command with the appropriately classified "military secrecy" have helped to influence and foster such developments in the technology of means of communication, codes, ciphers, deciphering. These developments in turn have been transferred to other institutionalized orders. "Radio," as developed during World War I, is only one, though a most telling, example. Since the age of railroading and the telegraph, modern business needs and modern military requirements have often coincided.

An army is made up of diverse population elements; it contains men who are performing new roles, segregated from ordinary social routines; accordingly these men develop specialized viewpoints and modes of protest. In the bureaucratically disciplined army, there is repression of spontaneous impulses and individual differences. That is why there is so much cursing and griping in armies. Since the sexes are segregated, a major restraint upon profanity is removed. Cursing in an army is a safety valve of men in situations where obedience is stereotyped. The extent to which such blowing off of steam is necessary will vary with the levels of the personnel. The sergeant in all armies, for example, has traditionally been a man of violent language. That is because he does not formulate very many of the orders which he gives, yet he must enforce them directly upon those who execute them.

VI. In the *religious order* the symbol sphere is very important, since the contents with which religion deals and the sanctions it employs are "psychic." The basic symbol which legitimates the authority of any of the salvation religions is some image of God, or of gods. All roles within the religious order—of prophet and of priest or of believers—are justified in terms of some such symbol. Theology is the doctrinal elaboration of the concepts of deity to which the religion is bound. Religious symbols and the image of God are manipulated and argued over, or silently accepted, by those in pursuit of salvation. The modern sermon, which has been considerably shortened, is still delivered with such tonal quality and gesture as to make the sound of the voice identifiable as a minister's, even without reference to content.

The extent to which religious symbols may be internalized and linked to the psychic structure may be indicated by the following: ". . . the very name of Jesus was of so sweet a taste in her mouth [the mouth of the Venerable Sister Serafia] that on uttering it she frequently swooned away and was therefore obliged to deprive herself of this joy in the presence of others till she was given sufficient robustness of spirit to repress these external movements." [21]

Language produces "action at a distance": from a distance it "wakens hope or fear . . . excites the dangerous or useful action. From this comes the belief in the fruitfulness of invocations, of incantations, of all that is action by speech: thus came into being magico-religious techniques. . . ." [22]

The symbols of magic, if verbal, may not be in the grammar of ordinary language, and may not refer to ordinary objects of the tangible everyday world,[23] yet in the feelings and consciousness of the believer they refer to extraordinary realities and weird powers. The symbols which are thus used may be verbal—as in the casting of a spell, like abracadabra or sesame; or they may be manual acts—like the handling and eating of the dead brave man's heart in order to garner bravery for oneself; or they may be both —as when the verbal incantation is accompanied by the ceremonial

[21] See Norman Douglas, *Siren Land*, quoted by Isaac Goldberg, *op. cit.*, p. 121. Cf. also J. Wach, *Sociology of Religion* (Chicago: Univ. of Chicago Press, 1944).

[22] Célestin Bouglé, *The Evolution of Values*, H. Sellars, tr. (New York: Holt, 1926), p. 154.

[23] See B. Malinowski, *Coral Gardens and Their Magic* (New York: American Book, 1935), Vol. II, pp. 213-14.

rite. Such wishful analogies may occur in the symbol spheres of almost any order, although historically they have been most closely associated with religious orders.

2. Monopoly and Competition of Symbols

The degree to which master symbols are publicly unquestioned —and the depth to which they are internalized in persons—varies from one institutional order or social structure to another. Two contrasting situations may be constructed.

I. Where master symbols are not questioned or even invoked by anyone except those authorized to do so, such key terms monopolize the symbol sphere and, other things being equal, are likely to be deeply internalized. Then they are so implicit in the prevailing speech, feeling, and thought that they require no explicit justification. Indeed, they do not require systematic articulation, much less promotion. This deep internalization is characteristic of traditional societies with relatively homogeneous institutional composition. The chances for master symbols to remain unquestioned, and hence internalized, are also increased by the extent that the communication channels are monopolized by persons who secure and justify authority by means of particular symbols.

When such conditions prevail there is not much need for taboos against challenging the master symbols, for no one is likely to do so. The symbols are part of the person's life, that is, so tied in with his roles that he identifies himself with them as he learns his roles. Giving meaning to his motives for role-enactments, they may be linked in turn to his psychic structure, so that his very impulses are mobilized to sustain the symbols and the roles which they guarantee. They are the "existential" categories of which the prevailing philosophers speak. If referred to at all, they are preceded by "of courses" and they make up the higher "common sense" of a period and order. It is difficult to examine them critically; as alternative symbols, much less symbols of protest, do not exist. There are no ideas available to compete with the master symbols and a unity of style characterizes the symbol sphere of the whole social structure and the reflective activities of its more articulate members. "Happy indeed," Harold Lasswell once remarked, "is that nation that has no thought of itself; or happy at least are the few who procure the principal benefits of universal acquiescence." [24]

II. If the master symbols are questioned and articulated by some persons, but not by others, "countersymbols" may arise. These countersymbols may not justify any actual institutional arrangements, but in time those who hold them may project them as part of an ideal community of the imagination. Then they may strive to realize this community in actuality. With such competition, the master symbols will be cognitively elaborated and thus reinforced. It is in controversies that symbol systems are tightened up. Theology—the expert elaboration of the creed which legitimates a religious order—emerges in response to controversies over, or attacks upon, its symbols. The political treatise may serve a similar function. The modern conservative thinking of Edmund Burke, De Maistre, and Justus Möser crystallized only in answer to the criticism of traditionalism by the philosophers of the "Enlightenment."

The rise of competing symbols of protest and their interplay with symbols of justification may take the following schematized form: (A) There is doubt of the correctness of interpretation and management of the master symbols. (B) This leads to a more deepgoing doubt, of the master symbols themselves, although this debunking may not yet be in the name of any set of articulated countersymbols. (C) The originally implicit master symbols will, to meet this attack, be explicitly reshaped by apologists. Thus, what was simply "traditionalist" becomes "conservatism": the self-reflection of traditionalism. And what was a simple piety becomes an elaborated theological orthodoxy: a weapon against heterodoxy.

The critical themes of the opponent will in part be countered directly and in part they will be "fruitfully misunderstood" and thus taken over into the master perspective. Each major concept will be answered by a counterconcept, each theme by a countertheme. Thus, the "spirit of the times" and the "awakening of the people" was countered by the conservative romantic theme of the "folk spirit" and the "slow and silent forces" of folk tradition. Blind spots—that is, unanswered themes—are of course highly

[24] *Politics* (New York: McGraw-Hill, 1936), p. 30.

symptomatic of bias.[25] Thus, Max Weber—author of the major critique of Karl Marx—was not interested in the problem of the business cycle as crucial for capitalist dynamics, for it did not fit his conception of capitalism as the apex of "rationality." (D) All these developments, in turn, may tend to make what was merely a protesting heterodoxy into an explicit rival creed.

If the rival creed cannot be liquidated and is itself not strong enough to establish another monopoly in the symbol sphere, a "duopoly" may arise. This is a situation of accommodation to a tolerant though competitive co-existence. Both of the churches or parties may unite against any newcomer and the newcomer may make the most of this chance by playing off the first "two big ones" against each other. The third camp may have more chance to use the technique of general ridicule or cynical deprecation ("The Laughing Third").

In a territorially expanding society complete control of new groups may be impossible because they have ample opportunity to escape in a physical sense. The history of religious tolerance in America, up to the Mormons, illustrates this tolerance by emigration.

In the course of time, former conflicts recede and are forgotten. Then new mergers become possible: differences which make no difference in practice will in time be forgotten as differences in theory. The interpretation of theological fine points is neutralized —for the sake of institutional weight and the advantages of bigness. This is the more likely to occur in the face of a common foe: United States Protestant sects, which once competed with one another, may put up a common front in the face of an expanding Catholicism. The Southern and Northern Methodists officially came together two generations after the slavery issue had been settled. Thus out of competition there occurs a move toward concentration.

One or several of the competitors increasingly wins out, and the smaller units, eager to avail themselves of the prestige of the big winner, will jump on the band wagon. Symbol cartels will thus be formed. In such situations there will be a lowering of standards for the sake of more effective and "open" propaganda. Another general mode of concentration occurs by the alliance of a few big units

[25] Cf. Karl Mannheim, *op. cit.*

for the more effective suppression of a number of small fry who are thus gobbled up.

On the other hand, a practically insignificant unit may make a virtue of necessity. Its very lack of appeal may motivate its adherents to consider their alienation and their withdrawn ways of life and thought as superior. Rigid exclusiveness for the sake of maintaining standards of purity and orthodoxy are frequently observed among sectarians. With the expansion of adherents, leaders may become more "broadminded," and viewpoints with previously sharp profiles may become more diffuse and blurred.

Three factors are important in giving rise to competition among symbols of legitimacy: (A) a diversity of institutional composition, (B) a rapid turnover, or dynamic, of institutions, and (C) a relatively easy access of persons holding differing opinions to the channels of communication. This latter condition may come about by the rise of new media and techniques of symbol diffusion. Thus Luther was able to capitalize on the invention of movable type carried by itinerant printers and to outcompete the hand-copying monk. Such conditions increase the chances that no one set of symbols will monopolize and unify the orders which make up the total society. They lead to the onset of the dialectic of competing creeds which we have outlined above.

Institutional diversity and conflict may exist (A) among the institutions which make up a single institutional order, as when two religions compete for adherents, or when two revolutionary parties agitate in and over the political order. The master symbols which compete will then be different symbols yet of the same order. The diversity and conflict may, however, (B) be between different orders within a social structure, as when religious institutions conflict with those of the political order. Then state and church, secular and religious parties, compete for loyalties, and specialists, as in totalitarian dictatorships, may seek to debunk, prevent, hollow out, or otherwise take over for their own ends those religious symbols that conflict with undivided allegiance to the charismatic symbols of the dictator's claim. Finally (C) the disharmony may be between two different social structures, as when nations compete within each of their respective confines and/or across a third country for the adherence to their respective symbols of national loyalty.

When the roles men enact change more rapidly than the legiti-mating symbols which lend meaning to them, individuals may be-come alienated from the symbols and even abandon them for some competing set. During revolutions role structures may be broken up and made meaningless to practice. Men wake up, the morning after, believing firmly in master symbols they had not thought of during the time of terror and panic. Then self-elected elites may say, with Yeats: "The best lack all conviction, while the worst are full of passionate intensity." [26]

If, through competition, the master symbols are made articulate, symbols venerated as absolutely true by some may by others be treated or even believed in as "mere opinions." It is in such a situation, when beliefs are less absolutely held, that tolerance may emerge. Tolerance and compromise as features of a symbol sphere are found where former contrasts of either-or have become less compulsive, and indeed, no longer vital to the persons involved.

When one set of religious institutions forms the only "religion" available, and the religious order is dominant in the social struc-ture, then its symbols will not be questioned: absolute adherence to them is the only road to salvation.

But in a social structure where the religious order is not domi-nant, and where the symbols of religious institutions are diverse and contradictory, the tolerant belief arises that one set of symbols may be as true or as wise as another, or at any rate that other per-sons who hold differing symbols, or even none at all, may not be entirely damned. Religious agencies such as "Bible Institutes" may argue about whether Buddhism is worse or better than Christianity, or a Lessing (in his "Nathan the Wise") may expound tolerance and the equal worth of the three rings, Christian, Mohammedan, Hebrew. Many may feel that all the diversities are equally worth while, and few will ostracize those who adhere to differing sym-bols. Symbol experts fulfilling official roles in religious institutions —teachers of theology, for example—may try to solve the problems of the variegated symbol sphere by talking from such an abstract level as to find that, after all, they are "basically," or in the last analysis, the same.

And similar processes work in the political order. Wilsonian

[26] W. B. Yeats, "The Second Coming," *The Collected Poems of W. B. Yeats* (2nd ed.; New York: Macmillan, 1950), p. 185.

idealism of World War I could not be effectively renovated during World War II, nor could it be revived in connection with the United Nations. The disillusionment in the wake of World War I, and the many crises between the two wars prevented it. Political tracts advocating "faith for living" are usually more indicative of the will to believe than of the actual faith.

If symbols are held as absolute, their adherents may be intolerant of beliefs different from their own. Absolute belief justifies and motivates the actions of the propagandist who would convert others and thus spread his faith. On the other hand, the decline of "crusading" democracy and the growth of a conscious propaganda of democracy in the late thirties in America may mean that the symbols of this kind of political order are not felt to be held with sufficient surety in the face of the threat of war with dictatorial political systems.

The tolerance and compromise allowed or available in given symbol spheres vary according to the estimation and condition of the orders in which the symbols are anchored. In a typical American town, tolerance of economic and labor-business differences has "increased markedly in recent decades," whereas tolerance of "deviant" religious creeds and practices has diminished." [27] If men don't really care about the issues at stake in a given order, they are likely to be tolerant in that order. Thus by examining what men are intolerant about one finds out what really matters to them. In contrast, when men believe that only their enemies have the power to be successful bigots, they see the value of tolerance. Two religions, each claiming to monopolize the only toll bridge to salvation, will tolerate each other if they are persuaded that they cannot destroy each other.

Tolerance in the symbol sphere must of course be distinguished from toleration of deviant and threatening practices. Symbol differences may be tolerated only by those who do not expect them to be translated into threatening practices. This means that those who are thought to be less powerful ("ridiculous" and "harmless") may be the more readily tolerated. "Parlor Socialism" for gentlemen may be permitted, even though labor unions for workers are frowned upon or forbidden. A skillful ruler acting for the status

[27] See Robert S. and Helen M. Lynd, *Middletown in Transition* (New York: Harcourt, Brace, 1937).

quo may absorb new threats by the cynical opportunism of kindly tolerance and adroit compromise. In conversation the politely nodding head of tolerance may hide timid ignorance and that genial hypocrisy which is the death of thought. The decisive question of tolerance is always: *tolerance in whose favor?*

A strong ruler unafraid of some "tangential" challenge may "tolerate" it and thereby "take the wind out of its sails." All modern constitutional regimes have "tolerated" more and more voters to come to the polls—to the extent to which stronger party organizations could effectively control such voting. The strategy of British Empire politics may also be recalled, as well as the history of compulsory education and the expansion of newspaper circulation. The original sponsors of "equal rights for women"—socialists and progressive suffragettes of bourgeois background—found that many housewives, following patriotic and religious appeals with prompt attention, vote more conservatively than do their husbands. In this case, "tolerance" was an adjustment of authority which buttressed the dominating structure rather than challenged it.

Tolerance may, however, work in favor of the intolerant; the Weimar Republic and Nazism is a recent example. Hitler and his movement were ridiculed as "playing the soldier," and were able to profit by this minimization of their stature. Being tolerated they could bide their time and wait for their opportunity, which was provided by depression. The "playing soldiers" were thus held intact and ready to capitalize on the decisive shift in votes. The question of tolerance, therefore, becomes a question of what sort of organization is built up under its protection. In England and other countries there has been an intolerant outlawing of "private uniforms" and political haberdashery.

Relative strength and the espousal of tolerance as a value may be briefly systematized in this way:

I. A strong party can afford to be tolerant of deviation or even of opposition—at least up to a point. This characterizes a ruling stratum of multiple elites without over-all bureaucratic organization. Or, as Madame de Staël once remarked, "If a nation is to have the courage to laugh at itself, it must be conscious of its superior strength." [28] II. A strong party can also afford to suppress all opposition and criticism by organizing ruling elites and functions and

[28] Cf. *De L'Allemagne,* critical edition prepared by Comtesse Leon de Prange (Paris: Hachette, to be published).

all authoritative positions into a central machine; for example, the totalitarian party. III. A weak party may plead for tolerance, which means the freedom to continue in its own ways of conduct and thought. Thus, during their struggle for power, totalitarian parties will most jealously plead for "the democratic liberties" which, once in power, they promptly suppress. IV. A weak party may be intolerant of internal deviation, enforcing strict discipline upon the in-group members, and imposing upon them a pattern of "organized thought" in order to increase their cohesion and striking power.

In summary, symbol spheres may be monopolized by one set of legitimating symbols which are so deeply internalized they do not need to be defended. If they are questioned, persons become articulate about them and jump to their defense as absolutes. The existence of such symbol spheres is conditioned by institutional harmony within and between various orders, by a slow rate of institutional change and by a monopoly of the channels of communication and persuasion. When the reverse of these three conditions exists, the chances for countersymbols of legitimacy to emerge are increased. When there is competition among symbols, some of them may be debunked, and various persons may hold them merely as "opinions," whereas others may be completely alienated from them; indeed, whole populations may become alienated from one set of symbols and shift allegiance to other symbols which make more sense in terms of actual or expected practices. In certain competitive situations, tolerance and compromise may emerge as general features of the symbol sphere. Thus the legitimacy of public competition in ideas has been part of the creed of parliamentary democracy of the modern constitutional state. Totalitarian parties and states have typically claimed "the freedom to propagandize" in the name of "democracy" in order to overthrow this system.

3. Communication

Out of the total range of symbols socially available, each person picks up certain symbols which he passes on to others. Each person who faces the total volume of symbols transmits a selected number and a selectively arranged portion of the total. Generally, we speak of manipulation or management of symbols when this channeling and rearranging of selected symbols is done consciously and in an organized way. Competition among symbols referring to given objects or legitimating different institutional roles may lead to the purposive manipulation or management of the spheres of symbols by symbol experts.

In a stratified society is it possible to debunk or to build up a given stratum by selecting the symbols which are used to represent it. To devaluate a religious, political, or ethnic group, one selects the lowest representative of the group—of the Jewish community, e.g.—and generalizes him as "*the* Jew." To build up a group or stratum one focuses upon the "best" representative, selecting those traits that are most approved of by those to whom one would build up the group, and generalizes him as "*the* Jew." Such images are known as stereotypes. They are symbols built out of a selection of alleged traits yet represented as the whole truth. Stereotypes which debunk or build up a group may not be set forth in their totality at any one time. A newspaper, for instance, may use the symbol "Negro" every time a Negro commits a petty crime, but avoid mentioning "Negro" when a Negro performs some meritorious act. The stereotype of "Negro" is thus built from an accumulation of incidents with which the symbol is associated.

When a small-town youngster goes to a big city and does well, the town's newspaper may carry the story: Podunk boy makes good. But if he gets lost in the anonymity of the city and wanders into crime, the local newspaper may not play the fact up. By selecting from the totality of world, national, and local affairs, the story of the local youngster who grew up to make $50,000 a year, the glory of his success is reflected on the symbol, Podunk. His success is shared; ascribed in part to the community. His failures are ignored, or ascribed to him alone. The stereotyped image of Podunk is built up by the accumulation of such stories and by the omission of other types of fact. At the same time, a generally optimistic tone of individual success is maintained in the sphere of symbols.

We may distinguish several ways in which conduct is positively or negatively stereotyped, and ascribed to the individual alone or to groups to which he belongs by virtue of actual or past membership:

I. Meritorious conduct may be strictly ascribed to the individual, as in the case of Homer's build-up of Achilles, or as in the modern cult of genius. In legend, the family of descent is often entirely eradicated by means of an ascription of divine origin, or by "foundling" sagas. II. Liabilities of conduct may be ascribed strictly to the individual, as in contemporary democratic court proceedings. III. Meritorious conduct may be ascribed to the individual as a representative of a group whose members are eager to share in the prestige accretion of their outstanding members. This occurs in the construction of self-images by groups and collectivities, as when Americans see themselves as in the "land of the free and the brave," or nineteenth-century Germans saw themselves as a "nation of poets and thinkers." IV. Conduct liabilities may be typically ascribed by dominant groups to the individual as a representative of despised lower or hostile out-groups. In the Soviet Union and its orbit, "bourgeois" descent—for the failure— is never an "accident," just as in Nazi Germany "Jewish descent" was the reference point for alleged criminal dispositions, despite all statistical evidence to the contrary.

In the selecting and editing of symbols referring to nations, all these processes may be observed. Nations compete for prestige with other nations in terms of symbols and events which are associated by symbol manipulations, with stereotyped images of the whole. To an inhabitant of nineteenth-century India, "the British" may be an irate man with battleships, troops, and whipping canes; a beef-eating barbarian who consumes alcohol on so supreme a religious occasion as The Lord's Supper. But in the edited sphere of symbols, "British" may appear to Englishmen as a rotund gentleman surrounded by "tricky natives," or a nation of small shopkeepers trying honestly to get along in the world. During wartime, "Uncle Sam" gets a fierce compelling look in his cartooned eyes as he points his finger at *you*. The superegos of some members of the public may be stimulated by such compulsive figures. The guilt feelings thus engendered may increase the participation of fortune, time, and life in the war effort.

A nation becomes "one and indivisible" through a continual process of communalization. This communalization is directed by those strata that successfully address their political expectations to the rest of the population in the name of the "nation." To the extent to which this process is successful, "a nation one and indivisible" exists. The most effective symbols implementing the process are those of common historical fate, of common triumphs of the past: national history bespeaking of grandeur; a national mission; assurance of the nation's worth for mankind. The emphases, as between the past or the future, may shift. When the "American dream" is no longer stressed, or does not seem unilinear and unambiguous, the press may demand greater emphasis on instruction in the nation's history as beneficent to civic morale and patriotism. History teaching is, of course, subject to selective emphases and stylizations stemming from patriotic loyalties rather than scientific detachment.[29] Much of the national historiography of the nineteenth century falls under the same heading: Germany had her Treitschke, Great Britain her Seeley. The American Mahan, as the philosopher and historian of "seapower," could hardly have emerged on Prussian soil, and neither could a Delbrück, the German historian of warfare, arise in a great maritime power. "History," it is often said, is concerned with the past that is "dead," but as an ongoing enterprise it is of vital concern to the living in an age of nations with rival claims to disputed areas, new boundaries, and opportunities seized and justified in terms of "historical rights."

In a world where primary experience has been replaced by secondary communications—the printed page, the radio, and the picture screen—the chances for those in control of these media to select, associate, manipulate, and diffuse symbols are increased. In the twentieth century, a unified symbol sphere, one monopolized by certain master symbols, is more likely to be the result of a monopoly of the channels of communications, and of a forceful tabooing of countersymbols, than the result of any harmonious institutional basis. It is more likely to be imposed than to grow. But the symbols which are thus made masterful are not likely to be so deeply and unquestioningly internalized as those arising as adequate and meaningful expressions of a harmony of institutionalized roles. Where there are deep antagonisms in the institutional structure, men seeking to transform power into authority may grasp all the more compulsively for the channels of mass communication, but their monopolization of these media does not necessarily mean that the symbols they diffuse will be master symbols.

[29] See B. Pierce, *Civic Attitudes in American School Textbooks* (Chicago: Univ. of Chicago Press, 1930).

4. The Autonomy of Symbol Spheres

In the scholar's study or the agitator's den the symbols which legitimate various kinds of political systems may be rearranged, debunked, or elaborated. But such logical manipulations of master symbols by intellectuals do not of themselves change the legitimating symbols to which the great bulk of persons are attached. For changes in the *legitimating* symbols to be realized, masses of people must shift their allegiances.

Hulme, from whom we have quoted above, believed that the master symbols are "the source of all the other more material characteristics of a period"; not "men" but "ideas" make history. This is an unfortunate manner of statement; as a matter of fact, it is magic. Unless symbols are tied to the roles enacted in institutional orders, unless they lend meaning and even sacredness to these roles, they will not even be master symbols. They will merely be little marks on paper or breath going over vocal cords. Symbols can "make a difference" only if they answer to some feature of the character structure and the roles of individuals, and these character structures and roles are shaped in large part by institutional arrangements. To the extent that the symbol sphere is truly autonomous, it does not count in the dynamics of the institutional structure. An autonomous dynamics of the symbols sphere implies the detachment of persons from it, and detachment is a step towards alienation. To say that there is no symbol *order*, but rather a symbol *sphere*, or symbol spheres, is to deny this "idealistic" theory of history and society. And only if one set of symbols were successfully imposed upon virtually all of a population could we speak strictly of "common values."

If the character of the master symbols sets the character of a social structure, then a monopolization of the communication of symbols would enable the monopolizers to create new institutions by diffusing certain kinds of would-be master symbols. And we know that this is not the case. Propagation of symbols is effective only so long as they have some meaningful relevance to the roles, institutions, and feelings which characterize a people. Symbols cannot create these roles. It is in terms of their relevance or lack of relevance to persons and institutions that the free competition of autonomously developed symbols will be decided. Only in this sense may we speak of the autonomy of symbol spheres in certain kinds of social structure. "Governments" do not necessarily, as Emerson put it, "have their origin in the moral identity of men." This is to confuse the legitimations of government with its causes. Just as often, or even more so, the moral identities of men have their origins in governmental institutions which successfully impose their symbol spheres.

One hundred years ago the matter was fruitfully discussed in terms of the assumptions typically made by many of those who believe that the dynamics of the symbol sphere is self-determining and that it may dominate history: [30] (A) The symbols which justify some authority are separated from the actual persons or strata that exercise this authority. (B) The "ideas" are then thought to rule, not the strata or the persons using the ideas. (C) In order to lend continuity to the sequence of these symbols, they are presented as connected in some "mystical" way with one another. The symbols are thus seen as having an autonomous "self-determination." (D) To make more plausible the odd notion that symbols are "self-determining," they are "personalized" or given "self-consciousness." They may then be conceived as the concepts of history or as a sequence of "philosophers" whose thinking determine institutional dynamics.

Symbols which are often written about as "values" are historically and sociologically irrelevant unless they are anchored in conduct. They become relevant when they justify institutions, and/or motivate persons to create or at least to enact roles. There is undoubtedly an interplay of justifying symbols, institutional authority, and role-enacting persons. At times we should not hesitate to assign causal weight to master symbols—but not as a, much less *the,* theory of social unity. There are ways of constructing unity that are more flexibly geared to a lower level of generality, closer to empirically observable materials.[31]

It seems to us the better procedure to build up to such symbolic unity or "common values" as a social structure may display by examining the symbol spheres of each of its institutional orders, rather than to *begin* by attempting first to grasp "common sym-

---

[30] Cf. K. Marx and F. Engels, *op. cit.,* pp. 42 ff.
[31] As we shall see below, Chapter XII: The Unity of Social Structures.

bols" and then in their light to "explain" the society's composition and unity.

There is of course a symbolic aspect to social integration. If all, or nearly all, members of an institutional order internalize the order's legitimations, accept and adhere to these symbols, we may speak of "common values," or in other terms, master symbols of legitimations. Such legitimations do involve an evaluative aspect; as the terms in which obedience is claimed, master symbols are used as yardsticks for the evaluation of the conduct of institutions and actors. Such symbols ramify throughout the institutional order so as to "define the situations" of various roles. Social structures, which are thus integrated through universal adherence and acceptance of such central symbols, are naturally extreme and "pure" types.

At the other end of the typological scale, we find societies in which a dominant institution controls the total social structure and superimposes its values and legitimations by violence and the threat of violence. This need by no means involve a breakdown of the social structure; all institutions and roles for technical reasons simply involve the effective conditioning of persons by formal discipline so that unless they accept the institutional demands for discipline the majority of the actors do not have any chance to earn a living. A skilled compositor employed by a reactionary newspaper, for example, may for the sake of making a living and holding his job conform to the demands of employer discipline. In his heart, and outside the shop, he may be a radical agitator. Many German socialists allowed themselves to become perfectly disciplined soldiers under the Kaiser's flag—despite the fact that their subjective values were those of revolutionary Marxism. It is a long way from symbols to conduct and back again, and not all integration is based on symbols.

The emphasis on such disparities does not of course mean a denial of "the force of rational consistencies." Just as discrepancies between words and deeds are often characteristic, so also is the striving for consistency. The question whether or not discrepancy or consistency is socially effective and predominant can be decided *a priori* neither on the basis of "human nature" nor on the "principles of sociology"; it must be decided in terms of socially and historically situated responses. We might well construe a pure type in terms of perfectly disciplined social structure in which all dominated men, for a variety of reasons, cannot afford to quit their institutionally prescribed roles, but who nevertheless share none of the dominator's values, and thus in no way believe in the legitimacy of the order. Such a social structure would be run like a ship manned by galley slaves; due to the disciplined movement of the oars, the individual is reduced to a cog in a machine, and the violence of the whipmaster may only rarely be needed. The galley slaves need not even be aware of the ship's direction under their propulsion, although any turn of the bow might evoke the wrath of the master who sees ahead and steers the boat.

Between these two polar types—of a "common value system" and of a superimposed discipline incapable of being broken by the institutionalized members of the structure—there are numerous forms of social integration. For example, it takes a long time for a social structure to be totally revolutionized. Most occidental societies have been able to incorporate many divergent value orientations, as long as the legitimacy of the political order could be successfully imposed. The origin of such a dominant order has been quite various, ranging from forceful imposition to the instituting of an order by a covenant of its beneficiaries. In the former, the submission of the subjects to the superimposed order may be a result of accommodation, compromise, or renunciation of their own values; in the latter, joint agreement precedes the order.

Such unity, involving various degrees and mixtures of legitimation and coercion, may be found in any order, not only in the political and economic. A father may impose a specific order over all family members by threatening to withhold inheritance or his necessary consent to a minor's wishes, or by the use of such force as the political order may allow him. But, in any case, "common values," as a unified symbol sphere, are not necessary in order to secure integration and unity.

Fruitful questions about symbol spheres are usually quite specific: What kind of conduct or institution does this or that symbol motivate and guarantee? In what orders are given symbols to be found and what is their precise function therein? Symbols may influence conduct if they are relevant to the roles men enact; roles, in turn, are components of institutions. And the dynamics of institutions, and of their component roles, determine the content, range, and character of spheres of symbols more than the symbols determine institutional history.

A person may incorporate, believe in, and use a symbol which motivates a role which he does not enact, or legitimate an institution to which he does not belong. It is not necessary to be a priest in order to repeat the formula about the doctrinal infallibility of the pope. Yet this formula is important primarily in the college of cardinals, where it insures against open dissent and unwanted discussion. Wage workers in modern capitalist states may repeat the formulae of laissez-faire, although these symbols may be against the economists' imputation of the workers' rational interest, that is, his interests as "adequate" to his economic and political position within the whole system were he to act "rationally" as an "economic man." Such "mislocated" adherences are increased by modern techniques of mass communication which are, on the one hand, monopolized in favor of some one type of institution, system, or authority, and on the other, used to satisfy irrational fantasies and distract from both art and reality.

The institutional patterns of different orders are not equally or evenly implemented by means of symbols. The dominant symbols of a whole social structure will tend to be in the symbol sphere of its dominant institutional order. These symbols will legitimate the symbols and practices of other orders as well as those of its own. If the economic order is the weightiest one within a social structure, the legitimating symbols of the whole structure will likely be related to the economic order.

Specific interests of different institutions are defined in terms of specialized symbols appropriate to their respective contexts. There are, however, symbols which with but slight modifications may hold for various institutions serving quite different ends. By our definition, all institutions contain a distribution of authority. The head of the household, the principal of the school, and the army officer have "authority" over the household, the school, and the army unit. The symbols implementing this distribution of authority may be the same in all these institutional contexts: the "democratic" process may be stressed in which the head claims no more than the position of the first among equals, or an authoritarian discipline may pervade the relations of institutional leader and subordinates. The father may be the stern family despot to his children, as the officer may be to his soldiers and the teacher to his pupils. In the latter case "orders are orders," and there is to be "no back talk," only harsh silence.

The parallelism of such symbols in different institutional orders may result from the fact that one institutional context is acknowledged as the model for others. By identification of teacher with military officer, or of officer with father—by studious imitation of the higher prestige bearer's conduct—the diffusion of types of authority and their concomitant symbols is effected. Which institutional order sets the model for others and to what extent depends upon special historical and social situations. At any rate, our analysis, to be complete, must proceed as a search for such "transmission belts of authority."

The rich symbols of medieval Europe were anchored as a sphere of the religious order, and the institutional structure of that society was in part dominated by religious institutions and in part by decentralized hierarchies of knights bound by oaths to their feudal superiors and their Christian emperor. Out of the religious order and its symbols, the master images and preconceptions of a whole society were elaborated. Symbolic elaborations which were thought irreconcilable with those of the religious order were tabooed or repressed. This anchorage of the institutions and the master symbols of a society in the religious order has affected most philosophical work in Western societies, and may still be seen in the attempts of various symbol experts to "reconcile" the symbols of modern science and modern modes of living and dying with subtilized and attenuated symbols and images of the Christian religion. An order thus seeks to extend its symbols and publicize them as applicable to all conduct. In their competition with other agencies for the use of increased leisure time, modern religious institutions have striven to publicize and adapt their symbols to changing circumstances. Books have been written to show how Jesus was after all a businessman in mentality and outlook, thus attempting to adapt religious symbols to those of the dominant economic order. On the other hand, an order may seek to hide its sphere of symbols: a priesthood may hide its formulae and doctrines as too esoteric and holy to be broadcast, while at the same time developing an exoteric set of symbols for the laity.

We may note in passing that much of the symbolic materials of the twentieth century are created for the complex equipment of the communication industries, for radio, phonograph, television, and movies. The movie actress does not play before an audience, but before a small committee of visual and acoustic experts; the poet reads, and the musician plays not before an audience of appreciative laymen and journalists, but before committees of recording experts.

The distributed product, whether it is seen on the screen or heard from a disk, is a performance that has been carefully selected from a series of less flawless trials. The mass availability of such performances by star actors, orchestras under star conductors, and so on require the communication and amusement industries to establish and market their products as "brands," to command attention by the excellence of performance and reproduction standards. In fact, these items often gain ascendancy over the content or message of the work of art itself. Interest in mass marketing also promotes the selection of what is "safe"—the accepted and proved work. The established work of art—that is, the noncontemporary or the "classical"—stands in the center, and enjoyment of art is not enjoyment of the unheard of and hitherto unseen, of the experimental thrust and the eye opener, but of the acoustically stereotyped and soothing brand, in terms of which the recognition of the composer, opus number, and star performer become conversationally prestigeful, and accordingly train for regressive listening. The reduction of a Beethoven symphony or a Verdi opera to the acoustic dimension of a living room, the photographic "blow up" or enlargement of a pictorial detail, or the photographic reduction of life size to pocket-book size, immerse twentieth-century men in a great stream of mechanically reproduced visual and acoustic images which tend to treat the cultural legacy of the ages as raw material for industrial processing. The original work, torn from its context and aura, tends to be swept away by the flood of its varied reproductions. For this is the age of the mechanical reproduction of art.

In the face of all this, the contemporary artist unless he turns to "commercial art" (which is to say, the implementing of the advertising interests of business or the propaganda interest of political groups) is pushed to the sidelines. The more his work uncompromisingly expresses the agony of the sensitive individual, the more it is felt to be shocking, perverse, or intellectually mannerist. Business advertising, however, like totalitarian propaganda, flatters the escape-seeking, untutored masses by endorsing their regressive nostalgia under the slogan, "the customer is right."

Language is the major key to an understanding of many problems of both character and of social structure. We have seen, particularly in Chapter V, that it provides us with many clues to the motivations of the person. In the present chapter, we have seen that language—conceived as a sphere of symbols—is necessary to the operations of institutions. For the symbols used in institutions co-ordinate the roles that compose them, and justify the enactment of these roles by the members of the institution. Our discussion has thus involved the various ways in which such master symbols justify and sanction institutional authority and at the same time motivate personal conduct in the economic and kinship, the political and military and religious orders.

Stratification
and Institutional Orders

IN New York City some people taxi home at night from Madison Avenue offices to Sutton Place apartments; others leave a factory loft in Brooklyn and subway home to an East Harlem tenement. In Detroit there is Grosse Pointe, with environs, but there is also Hamtramck, without environs; and in a thousand small towns people live on either side of the railroad track. In Moscow, leading party members ride cautiously in black cars along well-policed avenues to well-policed suburbs; other people walk home from factories to huddle in cramped apartments. And in the shadow of swank Washington, D. C., apartment houses there are the dark alley dwellings.

In almost any community in every nation there is a high and a low, and in some societies, a big in-between.

If we go behind what we can thus casually observe and begin to examine in detail the twenty-four-hour cycle of behavior and experience, the twelve-month cycle, the life-long biographies of people in various cities and nations, we will soon need to classify the people and their behavior. Otherwise we cannot easily understand our observations. We might well decide to make our classification in terms of valued things and experiences; to find out just which people regularly expect to and do receive how many of the available values, and in each case, why. Such classifications are the basis of all work in stratification.

Whatever the value may be that most people seem to want, some people get more of it than others, and some do not share in it at all. The student of stratification is bent on understanding the ranking of people with respect to such values, and in finding out in what respects these ranks differ and why. Each rank or stratum in a society may be viewed as a stratum by virtue of the fact that all of its members have similar opportunities to get the things and experiences that are valued: things like cars, steady and high incomes, toys, or houses; experiences, like being given respect, being educated to certain levels, or being treated kindly. To belong to one stratum or another is to share with the other people in this stratum similar advantages.

If, again, we go behind these strata of people having similar life-chances, and begin to analyze each stratum and the reasons for its formation and persistence, sooner or later we will come upon at least four important keys to the whole phenomenon. We call these "dimensions of stratification." Each provides a way by which we can rank people in accordance with the specific opportunity each has to obtain a given value. And all together, these dimensions, if properly understood, enable us to account for the whole range of these different opportunities. These four dimensions are occupation, class, status, and power:

By an *occupation* we understand a set of activities pursued more or less regularly as a major source of income.

Class situation, in its simplest objective sense, has to do with the amount and source (property or work) of income as these affect the chances of people to obtain other available values.

Status involves the successful realization of claims to prestige; it refers to the distribution of deference in a society.

Power refers to the realization of one's will, even if this involves the resistance of others.[1]

Each of these four "keys" may be related to our conception of institutional orders and spheres, and in turn, to social structure. In fact, these dimensions of stratification may be understood as ways of focusing upon certain features of certain roles in quite various institutional orders.

[1] These definitions are loose formulations of Max Weber's terms. In the course of the present chapter we shall make them more elaborate and precise. See E. Shils and H. Goldhammer, "Types of Power and Status," *American Journal of Sociology*, September 1939, and C. Wright Mills, *White Collar: The American Middle Class* (New York: Oxford, 1951), especially Chapters 4, 13 and 15.

The conceptual relations of dimensions and orders are not, how-ever, neatly "systematic"; class and occupation are, of course, ways of referring to selected aspects of certain roles in the eco-nomic order. But each may be deeply and intricately involved in the other orders.

As a sphere (not an order), status may be based on, expressed in terms of, and cashed in or realized in any order, and each aspect of status may involve different institutional orders. Status is not necessarily anchored in any order; it is often the shadow of them all and always the shadow of one or the other. A man's status may be based primarily on his military occupation but he may express his status claims in the educational sphere, and cash in on these claims in the political order; thus a general, on his way to the Presidency becomes a college president. The top positions of various institutional orders and occupational hierarchies may in-creasingly be interchangeable—just as are the bottom, unskilled roles. When social structures are in fluid change, status has less of a chance to determine conduct; when society is, as it were, frozen, status may become a major determinant.

As with status, so with power: all roles that are instituted, no matter in which order, involve authoritative relations—the family no less than the political, military, economic, and religious orders. The power of a person thus depends on a great variety of possible roles, in any one or more of the available institutional orders and spheres.

The availability of the two schemes (institutional orders and social strata) invites us to elaborate the very intricate range of pos-sible relations that may exist among these dimensions of stratifica-tion, as well as between them and the institutional orders char-acterizing any concrete society.

1. Occupations

As a set of activities which provides a livelihood, occupations are economic roles, part of the economic order. Yet these economic roles may at the same time be part of any of the other orders. Any role in any order that is "paid for" may be an occupation. Occupa-tional roles may thus at once be oriented to a job market, providing goods or services, and yet serve by their enactment the functions of other than economic institutions. The civil servant as well as the political boss are "gainfully occupied." The professional general and the draftee fill occupations in the military order. The priest and the minister pursue occupational roles instituted in the religious order and paid for by religious devotees; and teaching is, of course, a job in the educational sphere. Even in the kinship order, the household servant, the private tutor, and the governess may be included in the domestic circle. The "unpaid family labor" of children and wives is an important borderline case, especially in many small businesses and on farms.

From the individual's standpoint, occupational activities refer to skills that are marketable. These skills range from arranging mathematical symbols for $1,000 a day to arranging dirt with a shovel for $1,000 a year.

From the standpoint of society, occupations as activities are functions: they result in certain end products—various goods and services—and are accordingly classified into *industrial* groups within the economic order.

As specific activities, occupations thus (1) entail various types and levels of skill with which roles are performed, and (2) their exercise fulfills certain functions within a system of functional specialization.

We speak of occupations only when (a) there is a division of labor in which distinct, functional roles have been developed—such as farmer, artisan, scribe, priest, warrior; (b) when a certain regularity exists—an enduring linkage between the person and what he does for a living, his "routine"; and (c) when what he does is intended to win for him a regular income.

If an urban patrician of Rennaissance times once in a while made a profitable deal, he was not necessarily a "merchant"; if a covetous man "wins" even large sums of money at cards, he is not necessarily a "professional gambler." A man who happens to save a drowning man for the sake of winning a "reward" does not thereby become a "lifeguard."

On the other hand, a gentleman who likes to spend his leisure working at masonry (like Churchill) is not thereby a "bricklayer," nor is he a professional artist because he regularly plays the piano, or paints pictures. A hobby is not an "occupation." This distinction between the two does not reflect the "seriousness" *v.* the "lightness" of the pursuit, for some men take their vocations "lightly" and their hobbies "seriously." Similarly, play—an activity enjoyed for its own sake—may be taken quite seriously. Some men, in fact, may feel a defeat in a game of chess more severely than defeat in their work.

In industrial nations today the most publicly obvious strata consist of members of similar occupations. However it has been and may now be in other societies, in contemporary United States occupations are the most ostensible and the most available "way into" an understanding of stratification as a whole. For most people spend the most alert hours of most of their days in occupational work. What kind of work they do not only monopolizes their wakeful hours of adult life but sets what they can afford to buy; most people who receive any direct income at all do so by virtue of some occupation.

As sources of income, occupations are thus connected with *class* position. Since occupations also normally carry an expected quota of prestige, on and off the job, they are relevant to *status* position. They also involve certain degrees of *power* over other people, directly in terms of the job, and indirectly in other social areas. Occupations are thus tied to class, status, and power as well as to skill and function; to understand the occupations composing any social stratum we must consider them in terms of each of these interrelated dimensions. And we must understand how they limit or even determine the noneconomic roles and activities open to their occupants.

The most decisive occupational shift in the twentieth century has been the decline of the independent entrepreneur (the "old middle class") and the rise of the salaried employee (the "new middle class"). During the last two American generations the old middle class has declined from 33 to 20 per cent of the total occupied, the new middle class has bounded from 6 to 25 per cent, while the wage workers have leveled off, in fact declining from 61 to 55 per cent. In the course of the following remarks we will pay brief attention by way of illustration to these three occupational levels in the United States.

2. Class Structure

Classes are anchored, by source and amount of wealth, to the property institutions and occupational roles of the economic order. But the laws of property are part of the political order of a society and the income from work may be, as we have seen, a feature of occupational roles in any order. Property classes could not exist solely in terms of economic institutions; they are facts of a political economy. The "bourgeoisie" and the "proletariat" are social categories corresponding with the economic categories of "entrepreneur" and "wage worker." Moreover, as with occupations, belonging to one class or to another may be a prerequisite or a tacit condition for the assumption of selected roles in other orders. The unit of the property class is the family and "the firm" rather than the individual; wealth and family coherence are often, as in latter-day capitalism, most intimately related.

Even the world religions, especially their economically relevant ethics, are decisively related, in origin and development, to specific strata. As Max Weber has pointed out,[2] Confucianism was classically the status ethic of the mandarin stratum, of men educated in literary and secular rationalism, although their "religion" profoundly influenced the styles of life of other strata. Early Hinduism was carried hereditarily by a caste of literati, the Brahmans, who constituted the stable reference group for all status stratification in their society; whereas Buddhism was carried forth by migratory begging monks, and Islam, during its earliest period, by "a knight order of disciplined crusaders." Since the exile, Judaism has been carried by marginal strata of urban plebeians, and led by intellectuals trained in literature and ritual. Christianity, beginning as a doctrine of itinerant journeymen which spread in ancient cities, only slowly invaded rural society. "Paysan," "peasant," and "villain" bespeak of the Christian burgher's disdain for the rustic pagan and villager.

The specific combinations of strata which have embraced religious creeds are by no means accidental, and every change in the socially decisive strata has been of importance for every religion. It is well known that in twentieth-century America the members of various Christian denominations are recruited along class and status lines: Episcopalians and Presbyterians tend to be upper class; Unitarians and Lutherans middle class; revivalist sects, Holy Rollers, Jehovah's Witnesses, lower class. Churches characterized by crowd ecstasy and euphoria seem typical of lower-class groups;

[2] See Chapter IX: Institutional Orders and Social Controls, II, Section 2: Characteristics of the World Religions.

churches emphasizing ritual observances, of higher-class groups. Shintoism is a cult for a warrior nobility. American Catholicism now combines upper and lower classes—the recruitment of high-class persons to augment the urban plebeian Catholics is a recent trend of note.

In the United States today, as in most advanced industrial countries, occupation rather than property is the source of income for most of those who receive any direct income. The possibilities of selling their services in various labor markets, rather than of profitably buying and selling their property and its yields, now determine the life-chances of over four-fifths of the American people. All the things money can buy and many that men dream about are theirs by virtue of occupational level. In these occupations men work for someone else on someone else's property. This is the clue to many differences between the older, nineteenth-century American world of the small propertied entrepreneur and the occupational structure of the new society. If the old middle class of free enterprisers once fought big properties in the name of small properties, the new middle class of white-collar employees, like the wage workers in latter-day capitalism, has been, from the beginning, dependent upon large properties for job security.

Wage workers in the factory and on the farm are on the property-less bottom of the occupational structure, depending upon the equipment owned by others, earning wages for the time they spend at work. In terms of property, the white-collar people are *not* "in between "capital and labor; they are in exactly the same property-class position as the wage workers. They have no direct financial tie to the means of work, much less any legal claims upon the proceeds from property. Like factory workers—and day laborers for that matter—they work for those who do own such means of livelihood, or for public agencies.

Yet if bookkeepers and coal miners, insurance agents and farm laborers, doctors in a clinic and crane operators in an open pit have this condition in common, certainly their class situations are not the same. To understand the variety of modern class positions we must go beyond the common fact of source of income and consider as well the amount of income.

In terms of property, white-collar people in America are in the same position as wage workers; in terms of occupational income they are "somewhere in the middle." Once they were considerably above the wage workers; they have become less so; in the middle of the century they still have an edge, but, rather than adding new income distinctions within the new middle-class group, the over-all rise in incomes is making the new middle a more homogeneous income group. Characteristically, the income pyramids of white-collar employees and wage workers overlap. Thus, the incomes of skilled miners and die cutters considerably exceed those of schoolteachers and salesladies.[3]

Distributions of property and income are important economically because, if they are not wide enough, purchasing power may not be sufficient to take up the production that is possible or desirable. Such distributions are also important because they underpin the class structure and thus the chances of the various ranks of the people to obtain desired values. Everything from the chance to stay alive during the first year after birth to the chance to view fine art, the chance to remain healthy and grow tall, and if sick to get well again quickly, the chance to avoid becoming a juvenile delinquent—and very crucially, the chance to complete an intermediary or higher educational grade—these are the chances that are crucially influenced by one's position in the class structure of a modern society.

These chances are factual probabilities of the class structure. It does not follow from such facts that people are aware of them or in similar class situations will necessarily become conscious of themselves as a class or come to feel that they belong together. Nor does it follow that they will necessarily become aware of any like interests that may objectively be attributed to their condition as rationally expedient. Nor need they define like interests as common interests or organize to pursue them in a movement or in a party. Nor does it follow that they will necessarily become antagonistic to people in other class situations and struggle with them. All these—class consciousness and awareness of common interests, organizations and class struggle—have existed in various times and places and, in various forms, do now exist as mental and political fact. But they do not follow logically or historically from the objective fact of class structure. Additional factors have to be

[3] On compensation by "honors" rather than "wages," on "pecuniary" v. "psychic income," see Adam Smith, *The Wealth of Nations*, Book I, Chapter 10.

adduced to explain why people become or do not become class conscious, that is, raise demands and share articulate hopes and fears in response to special class situations.

There are many reasons for lack of class consciousness. (1) Class situations are not always transparent to the people in them. Lower-class people, for example, may live in a widely dispersed way and thus lack the opportunity to come together in any solidarity. (2) They may also lack leadership capable of articulating their griev-ances. (3) Issues other than those of class may hold the attention and preoccupy the minds of people. (4) We should also remember that what is conceptually available to modern men, trained in economic thoughtways, was not so available to people of past ages. (5) Most people, in fact, tend to identify with "their betters": lower groups see themselves as their educated and wealthy supe-riors see them, and frequently there emerges socially split images among groups which co-operate in functionally different positions in feudal manor, artisan's shop, and factory. (6) Many people may hold certain class situations only in periods of social and economic expansion, migrations, and vertical mobility. Those who rise suc-cessfully by finding themselves in advantageous positions (for in-stance, around 1900, in the oil, the motion picture, and the electrical industries) are apt to ascribe their success not to "good luck," or to "circumstance" but to their intelligence, foresight, and personal excellence, with the concomitant implication that others lack com-parable traits. They consider good fortune as compensation for excellence and, as did the successful of the ancient world, consider themselves as the "darlings of the gods." The implication of this view for the disadvantaged requires no elaboration.

In any case, whether or not class consciousness and class action arise from class situations is a matter of empirical study. The de-velopment of interest organizations along class lines is one of the outstanding trends of twentieth-century society. In all industrial-ized nations labor has developed trade union organizations and co-operatives, and under special conditions, labor parties. Farmers are organized in a "farm bloc," and industrialists are organized in chambers of commerce and join forces in trade associations and the NAM.

3. *The Status Sphere*

Prestige involves at least two persons: one to claim it and another to *honor* the claim. The bases on which various people raise prestige claims, and the reasons others honor these claims, include property and descent, occupation and education, income and power —in fact, almost anything that may invidiously distinguish one person from another. In the status system of a society these claims are organized as rules and expectations governing those who successfully claim prestige, from whom, in what ways, and on what basis. The level of self-esteem enjoyed by given individuals is more or less set by this status system.

There are, thus, six items to which we must pay attention: From the claimant's side: (1) the status claim, (2) the way in which this claim is raised or expressed, (3) the basis on which the claim is raised. And correspondingly from the bestower's side: (4) the status bestowal or deference given, (5) the way in which these deferences are given, (6) the basis of the bestowal, which may or may not be the same as the basis on which the claim is raised. An extraordinary range of social phenomena are pointed to by these terms.

Claims for prestige are expressed in all those mannerisms, conventions, and ways of consumption that make up the styles of life characterizing people on various status levels. The "things that are done" and the "things that just aren't done" are the status conventions of different strata. Members of higher status groups may dress in distinct ways, follow "fashions" in varying tempi and regularities, eat and drink at special times and exclusive places in select society. In varying degrees, they value the elegant appearance and specific modes of address, have dinner together, and are glad to see their sons and daughters intermarry. From the point of view of status, the funeral, as a ritual procession, is an indication of prestige, as is the tombstone, the greeting card, the seating plan at dinner or the opera. "Society" in American cities, debutante systems, the management of philanthropic activities, the social register and the *Almanach de Gotha*—noble titles and heraldic emblems—reflect and often control the status activities of upper circles, where exclusiveness, distance, coldness, condescending benevolence towards outsiders often prevail.

Head roles in any institution may be the basis of status claims, and any order may become the social area in which these claims are realized. We can conceive of a society in which status rests upon economic class position and in which the economic order is dominant in such a way that status claims based on economic class are successfully raised in every order. But we can also imagine a society in which status is anchored in the military order, so that the person's role in that order determines his chance successfully to realize status claims in all, or at least in most, of the other orders. Thus the military role may be a prerequisite to honorific status in other publicly significant roles.

Of course, men usually enact roles in several orders and hence their general position rests on the combinations of roles they enact.

Claims for prestige and the bestowal of prestige are often based on birth into given types of kinship institutions. The Negro child, irrespective of individual "achievement," will not receive the deference which the white child may successfully claim. The immigrant, especially a member of a recent mass immigration, will not be as likely to receive the deference given the "Old American," immigrant groups and families being generally stratified according to how long they and their forebears have been in America. Among the native-born white of native parentage, certain "Old Families" receive more deference than do other families. In each case—race, nationality, and family—prestige is based on, or at least limited by, descent, which is perhaps most obviously a basis of prestige at the top and the bottom of the social ladder. European royalty and rigidly excluded racial minorities represent the zenith and nadir of status by birth.

Upper-class position typically carries great prestige, all the more so if the source of money is property. Yet, even if the possession of wealth in modern industrial societies leads to increased prestige, rich men who are fresh from lower-class levels may experience difficulty in "buying their way" into upper-status circles. In the southern states, in fact, impoverished descendants of once high-level old families receive more deference from more people than do wealthy men who lack appropriate grandparents. The kinship may thus overshadow the economic order. The facts of the *nouveau riche* (high class without high prestige) and of the broken-down aristocrat (high prestige without high class) refute the complete identification of upper-prestige and upper-class position, even though, in the course of time, the broken-down aristocrat becomes simply broken-down, and the son of the *nouveau riche* becomes a man of "clean, old wealth."

The possession of wealth also allows the purchase of an environment which in due course will lead to the development of these "intrinsic" qualities in individuals and in families that are required for higher prestige. When we say that American prestige has been fluid, one thing we mean is that high economic-class position has led rather quickly to high prestige, and that kinship descent has not been of equal importance to economic position. A feudal aristocracy, based on old property and long descent, has not existed here. Veblen's theory [4] was focused primarily upon the post-Civil War period in the United States and the expressions of prestige claims raised in lavish consumption by the *nouveau riche* of railroads, steel, and pork. In a democratic society equipped with mass media we are not surprised to find that many images of upper-status types are diffused. It is also well known that in contrast with feudal elites the American upper classes have not shied from publicity. Society columns and obituary pages chronicle the activities and connections of conspicuous members of the high-status groups.

The prestige of the middle strata in America is based on many other principles than descent and property. The shift to a society of employees has made *occupation* and the *educational* sphere crucially important. Insofar as occupation determines the level of income, and different styles of life require different income levels, occupation limits the style of life. In a more direct way, different occupations require different levels and types of education, and education also limits the style of life and thus the status successfully claimed.

Some occupations are reserved for members of upper-status levels, others are "beneath their honor." In some societies, in fact, having no work to do brings the highest prestige; prestige being an aspect of property class, the female dependents of high class husbands becoming specialists in the display of expensive idleness. But only when those who do not need to work have more income than those who must, is idleness likely to yield prestige. When work is necessary but not available, "leisure" means unemployment,

[4] See Thorstein Veblen, *The Theory of the Leisure Class* (New York: Viking, 1924).

which may bring disgrace. And income from property does not always entail more prestige than income from work; the amount and the ways the income is used may be more important than its source. Thus the small *rentier* does not enjoy an esteem equal to that of a highly-paid doctor. Status attaches to the *terms* for income, to its source and timing of payment. Socially the same number of dollars may mean different things when they are received as "rent" or "interest," as "royalties" or "fees," as "stipends" or "salaries," as "wages" or as "insurance benefits." Men striving for status may prefer smaller salaries to higher wages, meager royalties to substantial profits, an honorific stipend to a large bonus.

Among the employed those occupations which pay more, and which presumably involve more mental activities and entail power to supervise others, seem to place people on higher prestige levels. But sheer power does not always lend prestige: the political boss renounces public prestige—except among his machine members—for power; constitutional monarchs, on the other hand, retain and possibly gain public prestige but lose political power. In offices and factories, skilled foremen and office supervisors expect and typically receive an esteem which lifts them above unskilled workers and typists. But the policeman's power to direct street masses does not bring prestige, except among badly frightened drivers and little boys.

The type of education, as well as the amount, is an important basis of prestige; "finishing" schools and "prep" schools turn out ladies and gentlemen fit to represent their class by styles of life which, in some circles, guarantee deference. In other circles the amount of intellectual skill acquired through education is a key point for estimation. Yet skill alone is not as uniform a basis for prestige as is skill connected with highly esteemed occupations.

All the variables which underpin status—descent, skill (on the basis of education and/or experience), biological age, seniority (of residence, of membership in associations), sex, beauty, wealth, and authority—may be quite variously combined and usually in typical ways. These combinations may be and often are quite intricate. For example, the cross-tabulation of descent, wealth, and skill alone logically yields the following types: where wealth and high birth is combined with skill we may find, for example, the experienced statesmanship of a Churchill; but where there is wealth and high birth but no skill, perhaps a publicized heiress, or an hereditary successor to throne. The self-made man of the nineteenth century in the United States had wealth and skill but low birth; the ignorant Negro woman who suddenly wins the sweepstakes, has wealth, but low birth and no skill.

Sir Walter Scott, a heavily indebted nobleman who did well as a writer, had no wealth but both high birth and high skill. And famous artists, such as Beethoven, or famous scholars such as Albert Einstein, do not have wealth or high birth, but excel in skill. The Russian refugee nobleman who becomes a waiter in a Paris hotel lacks both wealth and skill although he has high birth. Finally, the Jewish Luftmensch,[5] the hobo, the tramp, or the Negro farmhand have no wealth, no birth status, and no skill.

Such a panorama may serve to indicate the manner in which one raises questions and classifies observations about the status sphere of given social structures.

We cannot take for granted that to claim prestige is automatically to receive it. Status conduct is not so harmonious. The status claimant may in the eyes of others "overstate" his "true" worth, may be considered "conceited." If he understates it, he may be considered "diffident" or "humble." The conceited status claimant may of course receive the deference he claims, but it is likely to be "spurious deference" for "spurious claims." His conceit in fact, is often strengthened by flattery, sometimes to the point of megalomania, as with despots in a context of priestly or courtier byzantinism or organized mass adulation.

In cases of mistaken judgment people may give genuine deference on the basis of spurious or pretended claims; there are the false Messiahs, the false prophets, the false princes, and the professional charlatans.[6]

Spurious deference for misconstrued claims may be illustrated by referring to the mock coronation of Christ as "the King of the Jews" with the crown of thorns. Genuine respect for genuine claims needs no particular elaboration.

[5] A man without an occupation, formerly found among Eastern European Jews.
[6] On professional charlatans, see Grete de Francesco, *The Power of the Charlatan* (New Haven: Yale Univ. Press, 1939).

False humility is often transparent as a technique for eliciting deference. We call it "fishing." The bid for good will, with which speakers often open their talks, is often no more than thinly veiled flattery of the audience. Once upon a time kings were flattered; today more often "the people" are. To be sure, such flattery of the people goes hand in hand with open disdain for the European "masses" or the American "suckers." Hitler proved highly successful in allocating to German Gentiles the rhetorical certificate of presumably high birth and ancestral background by calling them each and every one "Nordics."

Thus the extent to which claims for prestige are honored, and by whom they are honored, varies widely. Some of those from whom an individual claims prestige may honor his claims, others may not; some deferences that are given may express genuine feelings of esteem; others may be expedient strategies for ulterior ends. A society may, in fact, contain many hierarchies of prestige, each with its own typical bases and areas of bestowal; or one hierarchy in which everyone uniformly "knows his place" and is always in it. It is in the latter that prestige groups are most likely to be uniform and continuous.

Imagine a society in which everyone's prestige is clearly set and stable; every man's claims for prestige are balanced by the deference he receives, and both his expression of claims and the ways these claims are honored by others are set forth in understood stereotypes. Moreover, the bases of the claims coincide with the reasons they are honored; those who claim prestige on the specific basis of property or birth are honored because of their property or birth. So the exact volume and types of deference expected between any two individuals are always known, expected, and given; and each individual's level and type of self-esteem are steady features of his inner life.

Now imagine the opposite society, in which prestige is highly unstable and ambivalent: the individual's claims are not usually honored by others. The ways in which claims are expressed are not understood or acknowledged by those from whom deference is expected, and when others do bestow prestige, they do so unclearly. One man claims prestige on the basis of his income, but even if he is given prestige it is not because of his income but rather, for example, because of his education and appearance. All the controlling devices by which the volume and type of deference might be directed are out of joint or simply do not exist. So the prestige system is no system but a maze of misunderstanding, of sudden frustration and sudden indulgence, and the individual, as his self-esteem fluctuates, is under strain and full of anxiety.

American society in the middle of the twentieth century does not fit either of these projections absolutely, but it seems fairly clear that it is closer to the unstable and ambivalent model. This is not to say that there is no prestige system in the United States; given occupational groupings, even though caught in status ambivalence, do enjoy typical levels of prestige. It is to say, however, that the enjoyment of prestige is often disturbed and uneasy, that the bases of prestige, the expressions of prestige claims, and the ways these claims are honored are now subject to great strain, a strain which often throws ambitious men and women into a virtual status panic.

As with income, so with prestige: white-collar groups in the United States are differentiated socially, perhaps more decisively than wage workers and entrepreneurs. Wage earners certainly do form an income pyramid and a prestige gradation, as do entrepreneurs and *rentiers;* but the new middle class, in terms of income and prestige, is a superimposed pyramid, reaching from almost the bottom of the first to almost the top of the second.

People in white-collar occupations claim higher prestige than wage workers, and, as a general rule, can cash in their claims with wage workers as well as with the anonymous public. This fact has been seized upon, with much justification, as the defining characteristic of the white-collar strata, and although there are definite indications in the United States of a decline in their prestige, still, on a nationwide basis, the majority of even the lower white-collar employees—office workers and salespeople—enjoy a middle prestige place.

The historic bases of the white-collar employees' prestige, apart from superior income, have included (1) the similarity of their place and type of work to those of the old middle classes which has permitted them to borrow prestige. (2) As their relations with entrepreneur and with esteemed customer have become more impersonal, they have borrowed prestige from the management and the firm itself, and in exclusive stores, from wealthy patrons.

(3) The stylization of their appearance, in particular the fact that most white-collar jobs have permitted the wearing of street clothes on the job, has also figured in their prestige claims, as have (4) the skills required in most white-collar jobs, and in many of them the variety of operations performed and the degree of autonomy exercised in deciding work procedures. Furthermore, (5) the time taken to learn these skills and (6) the way in which they have been acquired by formal education and by close contact with the higher-ups in charge has been important. (7) White-collar employees have "monopolized" high school education—even in 1940 they had completed twelve grades to the eight grades for wage workers and entrepreneurs. They have also (8) enjoyed status by descent: in terms of race, Negro white-collar employees exist only in isolated instances—and, more importantly, in terms of nativity, in 1930 only about 9 per cent of white-collar workers, but 16 per cent of free enterprisers and 21 per cent of wage workers were foreign born. Finally, as an underlying fact, the limited size of the white-collar group, compared to wage workers, has led to successful claims to greater prestige.

4. Class and Status

Status may be said to "overlay" class structures. Each has its peculiarities and its relative autonomy, yet the first is dependent upon the second as a conditioning and limiting factor. One of the great perspectives of social thinking has been the formulation of the transition from feudalism to capitalism in terms of the shift from "status" to "contract," or from "feudal estates" to "class society." One of the aspects noted in this formulation is that, since the great middle-class revolutions, legally privileged and underprivileged estates of feudalism and absolutism have been leveled down, for "equality before the law" meant doing away with legal status barriers. This of course does not mean the doing away with status groups, nor with all grounds upon which status distinctions rest. But it does mean that status dimensions are more closely tied to the economic order and that class dynamics are automatically transformed into status dynamics.

The leading groups devoted to military, political, juridical, and religious pursuits stand out in all societies. So among top status groups are found warriors and priests, kings, lords, and gentlemen.

To these have been added the "merchant princes" and "oil kings" as well as "lumber kings," "railroad czars"—in short, as Franklin D. Roosevelt called them, "the economic royalists." A variety of status groups may emerge on the basis of one class. Upper-class youths may thus be divided into "the smart set" and "the steady conservative set." The smart set may "sow their wild oats," take up eccentric faddish behavior, and seemingly break with the old ways of their steady parents, who may smilingly remember their own "crazy days," and rely on their wellborn children to "find their way" back. The steady set may remain sober in mind and body, take early to correct family routine, and play a quiet game of cards with a moderate drink. Among working classes, one set of men may devote themselves to labor union activities and possibly to politics; they may accordingly feel different from and superior to workers who are nothing but sports fans and movie addicts. When Jewish traditions and cosmopolitan milieu combine, a special group as, for example, the Garment Workers Unions of the Eastern United States may create cultural activities of all sorts which bring special and general public prestige. But regardless of status proliferation, any basic change in class position usually does exert its restrictive or its facilitating influence. If mass unemployment during a world depression reduces income levels, heightens feelings of insecurity, intensifies competition for jobs, reduces family savings and earnings—then status differentiation among the lower classes is minimized, there is no money for educational pursuits and mass luxuries, for leisure-time hobbies, and membership in many organizations.

Industrialization and applied science have increased man's mastery of nature to a previously undreamt extent, but they have also made mankind interdependent, and dependent upon the functioning of the world economy as a sort of "second nature." Accordingly, concern with economic life has become public and the control of strategic economic institutions has given rise to public distinction. Captains of industry have thus attained high prestige positions. The Kaiser was behind the times when he mocked at Mr. Lipton as a "tea merchant" who did not quite qualify for royal friendship. On the other hand, he did seek to "ennoble" Alfred Krupp, the cannon king of the Ruhr, and it was possibly a sign of the times that Krupp felt a noble title could add nothing to the prestige of his name, based on his steel plant and its output.

Power over the political and military, the economic and the religious community brings prestige to those who legitimately make or pronounce the key decisions, or to those to whom the key decisions are ascribed by the community. Such power is today exercised at the tops of large-scale, far-flung, and steeply graded organizations of government, army, church, and business. All the staff members of such organizations are likely to enjoy prestige, whatever prestige the world at large gives to the respective organizations. When the state is highly sentimentalized—usually because the church has been closely allied to state power and the prince once stood at the head of the church—a religious halo is bestowed upon "the state" and upon all who serve it. And when the ecclesiastic structure is the one stable and ancient organization in a history of changing state constitutions, then ecclesiastic prestige may overshadow that of the state, and a cardinal or "prince of the church," holding life-long tenure of office, may rank higher than an ephemeral president of a republic. Big power carries in its train big prestige. Powerful nation-states in the long run get greater prestige for their members than do small states. Thus the American passport secures to its bearer greater respect in the world than the Hungarian passport.

And yet this statement must be qualified, for prestige based purely on power may in fact rest on "fear" rather than on sympathetic respect. Power as such may be sought as an end by many men, but most men sooner or later will ask, power for what? They will not accept power as an ultimate end, and whenever power is "naked" it is likely to be questioned as "abusive." In order to be respected, power must be disguised as estimable ends; it must be thought to serve the alleged ends of justice and freedom and other aspirations. It must be sanctioned and implemented by *credenda* and *miranda* in order to be admired.[7] Only then will it exercise its "spell" over man. Such a spell may be elaborated by specialists, and when the elaborated values are widely shared we may speak of "cultural prestige." Power and culture prestige combined fascinate man and secure the glory of power, or "majesty."

[7] See Chapter XIV: The Sociology of Leadership. Cf. C. E. Merriam, *Political Power* (Glencoe, Ill.: Free Press, 1950), Chapter IV.

5. *The Status Sphere and Personality Types*

Of all the dimensions of stratification, status seems the most directly relevant to the psychology of the person. This is not of course to say that it is the most important; in fact it is so often dependent upon other roles in various orders, and upon other dimensions of stratification, that in most causal sequences status must be seen as a dependent variable. Nevertheless, in its psychological effects and meanings it is "close up" to the person. For the level of self-esteem is rather immediately a function of status position, and the type of self-image as well as styles of conduct defining types of persons may often be most readily understood in terms of the status spheres.

We shall illustrate these general points by a typology of personalities among minority group members. We choose this area because racial and ethnic "minorities," in our scheme, are primarily status phenomena, and, moreover, status phenomena of an extreme enough character to permit rather sharp disclosure of the mechanics of the status sphere as they affect character structure.

A minority group, as we shall use the term, refers to a status group based on descent, whose members are denied status equality with nonminority people, irrespective of individual achievements. In the United States, the Negro, the Jew, and immigrants of various nationality extractions find themselves in this position. There are of course many differences between these varied minorities: Negro status is no mere matter of racial descent, but represents the harsh legacy of slavery; the immigrant's, of nationality origin and the length of time his kinship group has resided in this country; the Jew's status as a Jew is often of mixed basis, including religious, nationality, and ethnic factors.

The major historical basis of status differences between Jew and Gentile is in the religious order. Insofar as civic, military, and political functions required the Christian oath, Jews did not qualify; and in a complementary way, on religious grounds, since the days of the Babylonian exile, the Jewish people have segregated themselves from their social surroundings by rituals of food, costume, circumcision, and holiday. In early periods, all this meant conventional and often legal definitions of Jewish status and of

Jewish styles of life. In the economic order, for example, Jewry has been excluded from all esteemed and established occupations, which the dominant society monopolized. In twentieth-century America, however, many of these occupations are now once more open to Jews, and in addition, the religious and especially the ritualist conduct of Jews has broken down. So, the possibilities for many quite complicated marginal situations for Jews now exist in the status sphere of American society.

The status of any minority is revealed by their exclusion from specific occupations, educational opportunities, social clubs, preferred residential areas, as well as by resistance to their intermarriage with members of the majority society. It is in this situation that the minority child comes to awareness of his status. In time, he also comes to experience its conflict with majority groups as his conflict—as others significant to him reveal hostile stereotypes based on it. Finally, he attempts to come to terms with the status situation in which he finds himself; and in the process he is organized into one of several types of personality. Whatever traits he has as a mature person of minority status will be a product of his status situation and of his cumulative reactions to it and interactions with it.

The points in terms of which personality types may be constructed are, first, the groups in terms of which the minority group man or woman seeks status—his own minority group or the majority society; and the status symbols by means of which he strives to claim status—again, those of his minority group or those of the majority society. In terms of these two points, we can gain a view of four types:

The Symbols and Styles by Which Status Is Sought	The Groups in Which Status Is Sought	
	IN HIS OWN MINORITY	IN THE MAJORITY SOCIETY
Of His Own Minority	I	II
Of the Majority Society	III	IV

Within each of these four situations there are many possible varieties and types of men and women. Perhaps most Jews in the United States, for example, are in none of these situations: they seek status among both groups and with the symbols of both. Still, they are sociologically differentiated by means of the proportion of their relations and roles that are based on Jewish or on

Gentile symbols, and which involve Jewish or Gentile contexts. The compromises are many and result in a range of types from the utterly bewildered, caught in bitter conflicts of self-esteem and guilt, through the embittered and disillusioned, to those who feel secure in strict segregation.

In situation I, in which status is sought among one's minority by means of minority group symbols, we find the ultraorthodox Jew, whose time is spent in a ghetto-like world, who withdraws from and minimizes all contacts with the outside, and has no significant others among Gentiles. Or, he may be a middleman who confines his contacts with Gentiles to strictly segmental business relations; unlike the ultraorthodox, he faces the two worlds but chooses the Jewish as his status area. Socially and psychologically he is unavailable to outgroups.

In situation II we find those personality types that have been formed by identification with Jewry as a whole and who seek status from this identification, but among Gentiles. One finds here resentful, militant anti-Gentiles who in extreme cases may accurately be called Jewish chauvinists. For they ascribe all Jewish ills to the anti-Semitic Gentiles. There is also "the crusader" who is understandably touchy and "out to see that Jewish toes are not stepped on"; and on higher ethical and intellectual planes there is the individual who seeks to build up the culture of his people and their prestige by fruitfully using their cultural symbols in a Gentile world.

In situation III, we find those "emancipated Jews" who use the status symbols of the larger society in order to gain status among their own minority group. In status situation IV are those Jews who successfully escape Jewish status by using Gentile symbols and styles among Gentile groups. Here overreaction is not infrequent; on the one hand, there is "the social climber" who by his conspicuous economic success and sometimes fawning conduct would buy the respect of the majority community and, on the other hand, "the 100 per cent American" who is conspicuously attached in a kind of superloyalty to Gentile ideals and status symbols. And in the extreme, there is the person who chooses not to be a Jew, and who, in completely successful cases, is not a minority type of personality at all; he has left not only minority status but its marginality as well.

6. Power

By definition, all roles that are instituted, no matter in what institutional order, involve distributions of power. But the power dimensions of a social structure involve the power relations of roles in one order with the roles in another order. The power attendant upon one's role in the religious order may not be confined to the religious order. In fact, religious bodies frequently serve as frame organizations, at least for the kinship relations of their members. Where the religious order is dominant among orders, and hence "theocracy" exists, one's religious role will ramify into all other orders, even determining effective power level in economic or political or educational institutions. This matter of the "dominance" of orders will be systematically discussed in the following chapter.[8]

The power position of institutions and individuals typically depends upon factors of class, status, and occupation, often in intricate interrelation.

Some occupations involve formal authority and *de facto* power over other people in the actual course of their work; and certain occupations by virtue of their relations to institutions of property as well as the typical income they afford, may lend social power even outside the job area. Members of other occupations are supervised by other employees, many of them contingent of a managerial cadre. They are the assistants of authority: the power they exercise is a derived power, but they do exercise it.

Entrepreneurial classes, through investment decisions and the right "to hire and fire," hold power over job markets and commodity markets, directly and indirectly. They may also support power, because of their property, over the state, especially the state that is saddled with internal or external debts and in need of good credit standing in the business world. As Franz Neumann has neatly indicated, each of the powers of property may be organized for execution, in employer's association, cartel, trust, and pressure group. From the underside of the property situation, propertyless wage workers may have trade unions and consumers' co-ops which may contend for "more" or for "co-determination"

[8] See Chapter XII: The Unity of Social Structures.

in a struggle with the organized powers of property on labor and commodity markets.

When we speak of the power of classes, occupations, and status groups, however, we usually refer more or less specifically to political power. This means the power of such groups to influence or to determine the policies and activities of the state. Direct means of exercising such power, and signs of its existence, are organizations that either are composed of members of certain strata or act in behalf of their interests, or both. During wartime, even more directly, business executives fill positions in the army and other state agencies, from which they decide, within the law, what the government shall buy from whom at "cost plus." The power of various strata often implies a political willfulness, a "class-consciousness" on the part of members of these strata. But not always: there can be, as in the case of "unorganized, grumbling workers," a common mentality among those in common strata without organizations. And there can be, as with some "pressure groups," an organization defining and representing the interests of those in similar situations without any single purpose or attitude being shared by those represented.

The accumulation of political power by any stratum is generally dependent upon some four factors: will and purpose, objective conditions or opportunities, the state of organization, and the political skill of leaders. Opportunity is limited by the group's structural positions, which is to say, its functional position as a stratum in the institutional structure.

New York harbor pilots or Manhattan elevator boys—not to mention miners, steel workers, and railroad workers—hold in hand more crucial links in the multiple chains of interdependent functions that constitute modern society than do musicians, barbers, textile workers, or small-scale farmers. Obviously, the functional place of workers is not simply a question of skill: to push the button of an elevator and count the floors requires less skill than to play the violin or to operate a barbershop. The question is: What links in the interlocking chains of activity are broken by the group's withdrawal of effort? Strikes in the mining or steel industries are automatically national issues rather than local events. Similarly, coal and steel prices are of national concern, because coal and steel "go into everything" and thus affect the cost of a wide range of commodities. It is during critical strikes and cost-price-profit decisions that formally or legally "private" decisions are revealed to the public as substantively "public" in nature and consequence. Bargaining strength and veto power are wielded by groups and leaders in such command positions. Often the height and significance of such positions become transparent to those who hold them—and to the public—only in crisis. Then men on all sides learn "the facts of life."

The best of opportunity, however, will be lost without the will and capacity to make the most of it. This is dependent upon the group's sense of cohesion, its consciousness and definition of common interests and objectives, and the practicability and skill of realizing them. In these matters the few have an advantage over the many. Both functional position and consciousness interplay with organization and skill; organization and skill, in turn, strengthen or weaken consciousness and are made politically relevant by the functions they perform.

When social structures change rapidly, because of technological or economic shifts, military conquests, or migrations, then those established status positions which are remote from the centers of power are displaced by those that are closely anchored to the sources of power. During warfare, for example, the status of military pursuits is enhanced and with it that of youth: "In the clang and clash of arms, the muses are silent." When he conquered Italy, Napoleon was only twenty-eight years of age. The turnover of generals during World War II—in Germany, the Soviet Union, and the United States—meant a "rejuvenation" of military leadership, though not as drastic as in preindustrial warfare.

The roles geared to the control of the instruments of destruction, administration, communication, and production in stormy periods stand out as centers of power, and accordingly of prestige. The revolutionary "nation in arms" identified its cause with that of mankind, and developed a sense of a universal mission which has justified French imperialism ever since General Bonaparte proclaimed: "Peace to the huts! War to the palaces!"

7. Stratification and Institutional Dominance

We have "abstracted" the dimensions of stratification from more concrete institutional roles in order (1) to be able to discuss separately each dimension and its relations with the other dimensions, and (2) to discuss how, in terms of these dimensions, institutional orders are related to one another.[9]

That institutional order which is dominant in a social structure (power) will usually be the order in which status is primarily anchored and upheld. High class position and preferred occupations will also, given sufficient time, be acquired by those who are "heads" of the most powerful institutional order. This point may be illustrated by brief examination of the stratification systems of the United States, Germany, and the Soviet Union.

I. In the United States, especially during the nineteenth century, the economic order was dominant in the social structure. Capitalist economy and the inheritance of property by kinship groups set the dominant class structure. High economic agents successfully claimed the greater prestige, and were powerful actors behind the scenes, as well as on the stage, of the political and other orders.

A. Increasingly in the United States, class and status situations have been removed from free market economic forces and have been subject to more formal political rules. Over the last twenty-five years the political order has gained increasing weight and influence upon the economic bases of stratification. Governmental regulation of the economic processes has become a major means of alleviating inequalities and insuring the risks of those in lower-income classes. Not so much free labor markets as the bargaining power of political and interest groups now shape the class positions and privileges of various strata in the United States. Hours and wages, vacations, income security through periods of sickness, accidents, unemployment and old age—these are now subject to many intentional political and economic pressures, and, along with tax policies, internal and external loans, transfer payments, tariffs, subsidies, price floors and ceilings, and wage freezes, make up the content of "class fights" in the objective meaning of the phrase.

The "Welfare State" in the United States now attempts to relieve class tensions and build a mighty defense force without

[9] This second point will be discussed more systematically in Chapter XII: The Unity of Social Structures.

modifying basic class structure. In its several meanings and types, this kind of state favors economic policies designed to redistribute life-risks and life-chances in favor of those in the more exposed class situations, who have the power or threaten to accumulate the power to do something about their case. Labor union, farm bloc, and trade association dominate the political scene of the Welfare State, and contests within and between them increasingly determine the position of various groups. The state, as a frame organization, is at the balanced intersection of such pressures, and increasingly the privileges and securities of various occupational strata depend upon the bold means of organized power.

Pensions, for example, especially since World War II, have been a major idea in labor union bargaining, and it has been the wage worker who has had bargaining power. Social insurance to cover work injuries and occupational diseases has gradually been replacing the common law of a century ago, which held the employee at personal fault for work injury and the employer's liability had to be proved in court by a damage suit. Insofar as such laws exist, they shape the opportunities of the worker. Both privileges and income level have thus been increasingly subject to the political pressures of unions and government, and there is every reason to believe that in the future these pressures will be increased even more.

B. There have been changes in the interrelation of status with educational, economic, political, and military institutions.

The drift to bigness in business and to an enlarged and centralized government has meant the rise of the civil service state and of corporate bureaucracies in business. Accordingly, the demand for the expertness of the bureaucratic careerist has been met by an enormous expansion of educational facilities. The college degree has become the ticket of admission to many preferred middle-class job opportunities and their status prerequisites.

C. This trend has been reinforced by the decision of the United States to translate her power potential into diplomatic bargaining strength, by underpinning it with "military force in being." The unified defense forces have made the status rivalry between generals and admirals a mere holdover from the past, and the United States is now a permanently "all-around military power." The educational bonus for veterans has reinforced the weight and the prestige of the military service by the translatability of military credit into educational opportunities which, in turn, serve as a means of social ascent which increases the prestige of the officer corps and veteran into other status channels. During the Civil War, William Graham Sumner could deem himself too good for army service and could have himself bought out of army service by a friend. But in an age of world wars the claim of civilians to status superiority over the military can no longer be realized with comparable success.

D. Since the end of mass immigration and the relative closing off of the nation through a system of quota immigration admitting only "token" numbers of qualified immigrants, the fusion of nationality groups with the main body of the population has greatly advanced. These assimilation and acculturation processes have both permitted and been facilitated by the emergence of mass organizations of labor under the benevolent legislation and administrative policies of the "New Deal." The congeries of craft unions, comprising only 2½ million members in 1933, has been numerically overshadowed by the new industrial unions of both the AFL and the CIO, which have swelled the ranks of organized labor beyond the 15 million mark.

With this, the multifarious "immigrant neighborhoods," with their petty group competitions of ethnic organizations, old world cultural emblems, and patterns of status segregation have been leveled and even superseded by mass organizations along class lines. New and attractive channels for power and status ascent have thus come to the fore. The benevolent support of organized labor by the largest integrative organization of immigrant urban labor—the Catholic Church—has helped in this. So, for some sections of the metropolitan masses, it has become more relevant to status whether the family head is a "union man" than whether he is a "Hungarian" or an "Italian," a "Pole" or an "Irishman." Association with a functional class organization has thus for many overshadowed affiliation with organizations along nationality lines.

E. Yet all this does not mean that status by descent is no longer a factor in American stratification. In a way, a central group of undisputed "old American stock" still finds itself surrounded by a plurality of more recent Americans of immigrant stock. These peripheral groups strive, by assimilation, to slough off behavior items and symbolic practices which permit the central group to refer to them by national descent. These ethnic groups gain or lose status *externally* by the friendly or hostile position of the nation of their descent with reference to America, and their prestige thus rises and falls in accordance with the power constellation of nations. They gain or lose status *internally* by their position in the sequence of immigrant generations; longer residence in America makes for their reception into the undisputed "American" center.

Thus during the late war Americans of Greek or Slavic background experienced prestige increments, whereas Americans of German, Japanese, and Italian background experienced status deprivations—for which they sometimes sought to compensate by professions of loyalty and extraordinary contributions to the war effort. After the war, when the position of China and Japan, of Germany and the Slavic countries, changed, so did the distribution of prestige: German, Italian or Japanese descent no longer was such a status burden, and Slavic or Chinese descent no longer secured the prestige it once did.

F. For upper- and middle-class groups of undisputed "American" standing, however, the background of descent seems to have become a more attractive feature of status imagery and self-stylization. Bric-a-brac, family heirlooms, and furniture rate with pedigree organizations of the sons and daughters of this and that. In eighteenth-century England antiquarianism underpinned a new sense of historical continuities culminating in Edmund Burke's work; in America today the preference of upper middle classes for genuine colonial homes and the interest in "Americana," family heirlooms, and old American glass underlies the renewed interest in the national past rather than the elaboration of the future as "the American dream." "Looking backward" no longer leads to a vision of a future utopia. Courses in American history are increasingly considered obligatory for *all* university students. Members of the living generation come to consider themselves the heirs of an illustrious tradition rather than newcomers and pioneers. The days when the successful businessman could claim status as a "self-made man," rather than an "upstart," may be a bygone phase of American social history. For everywhere established and cultured status groups have ridiculed the parvenu in terms of Molière's model of the *bourgeois gentilhomme*. And, in this respect, American society is being "Europeanized." During the war, Henry Kaiser was hailed as a "dynamic constructionist" in the face of the "Big Five"; after the war he was considered by many highly placed men an intruding parvenu. The status heights are attained by those of established wealth who combine military, diplomatic, and/or top administrative roles with leading positions in the big business community, such as Dawes, Young, Harriman, Hoffman, and Wilson.

II. Status, in due course, follows power. By observing twentieth-century Germany, for instance, we can see how a sequence of political regimes has led to corresponding redistributions of prestige.[10]

A. In Imperial Germany, the Hohenzollern and other princely dynasties, the Prussian *Junker* nobility of military officers, career diplomats, civil servants, and conservative party leaders of the Prussian parliament occupied top status positions. A system of class suffrage guaranteed their monopoly of political power over Prussia and, through Prussia's position, over the confederacy of princely states that was Imperial Germany.

This group was set off from the rest of the nation by membership in a university duel corps, as displayed by facial scar and colored ribbon. Its members held the status of reserve officers, and their caste conventions of dueling and ceremonial beer-drinking, their speech, postures, and mannerisms made them the conspicuous target of caricatures. The conventional demarcations of this status group cut through university staffs, the Protestant clergy, the civil service, liberal professions, and business communities of town and country.

Yet the representative man of this group could not serve as a model to be popularly followed (like that of the British gentleman) in an industrial and urban society engaged in world affairs. Important sections of the business elite, Jewish bankers and Hanseatic merchants, scholars and writers, professional men, and politicians developed status roles of their own. As the Austrian court nobility under the Hapsburgs sought to enlarge their basis by granting spurious titles to newly risen business elites, so the German upper-status groups emphasized bureaucratic rank as status badges. Formal modes of address, calling cards, mailboxes, and even tombstones were used to indicate titled ranks. The correct

[10] See H. H. Gerth, "Germany on the Eve of Occupation," *Problems of the Post-War World*, T. C. McCormick, ed. (New York: McGraw-Hill, 1945), p. 422 ff.

title mattered more than correct initials and served to diffuse this prestige gradation through all public institutions, such as state hospitals and university clinics, state theaters and state opera houses, the business community and the liberal professions. It was characteristic of this status system that all roles were geared to vocational specialization, and that the pride of even the *Junker* was attached both to noble descent *and* to his military, diplomatic, or bureaucratic rank, his academic degree or his role as manager of a farm. Prussian poverty and pride in vocational efficiency never allowed a representative stratum of "cultured gentlemen," courtiers, or bourgeois patricians to emerge as a nationally representative status group.

Below the top layer and its bureaucratically ramified satellite groups stood the broader middle classes of small businessmen, craftsmen, and peasants, and finally class-conscious labor, organized in the largest political party, controlling one-third of the national vote, rallying the largest trade unions and co-operative societies in a Social Democratic movement under the leadership of a socialist intelligentsia, a machine of political professionals and union organizers.

B. After the collapse of Imperial Germany, the flight of the Kaiser and his paladins, and the abdication of the ruling princes, a trade-union leader up from the ranks became the first president of the Weimar Republic. Labor found itself at the top. But the class structure was but little affected by the establishment of the Weimar Republic. The displacement of the feudal status system did not affect the institutional anchorages of class or status. When, by 1925, the upsurge of political reaction had brought Field Marshal von Hindenburg—now in mufti—to the presidency, and the four years of business prosperity brought corporate wealth and the Junker-led farm bloc to the fore, labor lost what prestige it had held in the immediate postwar years.

But the keynote, so far as prestige goes, is that in the Republic no universally accepted status symbols firmly attached to this or that group really emerged. The status sphere was not one unilateral distribution but a plural affair and internally competitive. In the meanwhile, paralleling, as it were, this prestige fragmentation, concentration of power in the economic order went forward swiftly.

C. With the economic collapse and world depression of 1929, with mounting bankruptcies and foreclosures, with mass unemployment and despair spreading through the old and the new middle classes, loyalties to the Weimar Republic were undermined. The "Jews" and the "Marxists" were made scapegoats by the plutocratically financed Nazi movement, which revived pan-Germanic ideologies, raised anti-Semitism to a frenzy, and carried the "unknown" soldier of Austrian descent into the Reichs chancellery of Bismarck's creation.

After Hindenburg's death, Hitler, as *"Führer* and chancellor" with his national socialist party and its octopus-like mass affiliations, organized all institutional orders for total war and aggression. Hitler became the number one recipient of honor and the fountainhead of everyone else's honor. A quasi-military status model of uniformed, party-disciplined Nazis was imposed upon all occupational groups, through regimented mass organizations of youth, women, labor. All of them were headed by the ubiquitous Nazi plebeian and his assimilated types. With the advent of war, the dynamics of status operated in favor of the practitioners of violence, the Gestapo terrorist of the Elite Guard and the army.

D. Under the occupation regimes, after Germany's defeat, the conquerors from West and East naturally overshadowed German society. There were administrative and juridical purges of organized Nazism. In the West the political reorganization has been based upon the bureaucracies of the several states, and rested on a reconstituted bourgeois party of middle-class notables, financed by reconstructed big business. Veteran organizations of officers have emerged, and the general restoration policy under such slogans as the "social market economy," meaning essentially laissez faire, seems to be reproducing a status stratification not so different from the system that preceded the great depression—but, of course, on a generally lower economic level and in a truncated state of 47 million people.

In the East, Germany has undergone a social revolution, involving the communist-managed liquidation of the *Junker* estates, the socialization of strategic industries, the establishment of a quasi-totalitarian one-party state, the displacement of the old bureaucracies by newly trained Communist cadres. The ruling party thus proceeds to manage class and status developments by totalitarian plans—all in the direction of the Soviet model.

III. In the Soviet Union, the economic order is fused with the political order, and subjected to the planned management by political agents. Within the dominant political order, in turn, power, status, class, and occupation have come in large part, directly and indirectly, to depend upon political party membership. In Russia, membership in the Communist party, combined with executive positions, "replaces," as it were, property ownership as a central basis for status and class.

The Soviet system has abolished private property in the means of production and with it the hereditary transmission of power based on property. Stability and the status quo are maintained without these by means of politicized, rather than primarily economically based, ruling groups. As Karl Mannheim has put it, the problems were "how to produce a new ruling group . . . to guarantee a stable social order, how to discover new status defining factors other than income and property, and how to provide new work incentives." The general answer to all three was found by shifting the dominant institutional locus of stratification from the economic to the political order and thus instituting "new power and status" gradations in place of the "old inequalities of wealth and income." But income differentials were introduced and opportunities to save by state bonds were opened up. To these economic incentives were added the rivalrous incentives and rewards of status, as well as coercive punishments.

There are honorific distinctions for the vanguards and stars of various occupational groups. There are "heroes of labor," Stakhanov and shock workers of all sorts, as well as state-honored writers and actresses, composers, schoolteachers and soldiers, and the mothers of many children. Each functionally significant group serves as a base for a conspicuous vanguard of Stalin-decorated "heroes," of this or that routine pursuit brought to extraordinary perfection.

The star performers serve as universally publicized pacesetters; they receive special emoluments in money and in kind, and operate in especially planned competitive fields built into the over-all plan of the managed social structure. Thus a Stalin-honored shock worker may receive a considerably higher income and have higher status than an undistinguished plant manager under whose jurisdiction he works. Individual competition, group competition, and institutional competition are utilized in a planned way to maximize effort and efficiency. The competitively selected winners are received into the ruling party by co-optation—if they did not already belong. Their public prestige is thus partially ascribed to the fact that they are pre-eminent communists or exemplary "Soviet men and women." The party, in the last analysis, sets the tasks, awards the premiums, and in turn cashes in on individual perform-ances.

The party is thus at once the fountainhead and the depository of all prestige and status. Personal merit is premiumed through the "star system," which, with its prestige halo, seemingly spells out "equal opportunities for all," deflects attention from the un-known (and in fact only statistically assessable) differences in life-chances of the various groups.

In any case, differences in status and power, mediated by the one-party state, are definitely established, as well as income in-equalities. The "ruling class" is the Communist party (and its mass of affiliations), a political fact; and not high propertied classes, an economic fact. This system of domination is anchored in large bureaucratic organizations of trade unions and trusts, in addition to the branches of a state apparatus usual in Western democracies. The source of power and its distribution thus has to do with mass organizations which monopolize the means of administration and communication, production and destruction. "The totalitarian party," Mannheim puts it, "is the ruling class in a world of total syndicalization." [11]

8. Stratification and Political Mentality

What is at issue in theories of stratification and political power is (1) the objective position of various strata with reference to other strata of modern society, and (2) the political content and direc-tion of their mentalities. Questions concerning either of these issues can be stated in such a way as to allow, and in fact de-mand, observational answers only if adequate conceptions of strati-fication and political mentality are clearly set forth.

Often the "mentality" of strata is allowed to take predominance over the objective position. It is, for example, frequently asserted

[11] See Karl Mannheim, *Freedom, Power and Democratic Planning* (New York: Oxford, 1950), p. 82 ff., from which we have drawn in this subsection.

that "there are no classes in the United States" because "psychology is of the essence of classes" or, as Alfred Bingham has put
it, that "class groupings are always nebulous, and in the last analysis only the vague thing called class consciousness counts." It
is said that people in the United States are not aware of themselves as members of classes, do not identify themselves with their
appropriate economic level, do not often organize in terms of
these brackets or vote along the lines they provide. America, in
this reasoning, is a sandheap of "middle-class individuals."

But this is to confuse psychological feelings with other kinds of
social and economic reality. Because men are not "class conscious"
at all times and in all places does not mean that "there are no
classes" or that "in America everybody is middle class." The economic and social facts are one thing; psychological feelings may
or may not be associated with them in rationally expected ways.
Both are important, and if psychological feelings and political
outlooks do not correspond to economic or occupational class, we
must try to find out why, rather than throw out the economic baby
with the psychological bath water, and so fail to understand how
either fits into the national tub. No matter what people believe,
class structure as an economic arrangement influences their life
chances according to their positions in it. If they do not grasp the
causes of their conduct this does not mean that the social analyst
must ignore or deny them.

If political mentalities are not in line with objectively defined
strata that lack of correspondence is a problem to be explained;
in fact, it is the grand problem of the psychology of social strata.
The general problem of stratification and political mentality thus
has to do with the extent to which the members of objectively
defined strata are homogeneous in their political alertness, outlook, and allegiances, and with the degree to which their political
mentality and actions are in line with the interests demanded by
the juxtaposition of their objective position and their accepted
values.

To understand the occupation, class, and status positions of a
set of people is not necessarily to know whether or not they (1)
will become class conscious, feeling that they belong together or
that they can best realize their rational interests by combining;
(2) will have "collective attitudes" of any sort, including those
toward themselves, their common situation; (3) will organize them-

selves, or be open to organization by others, into associations, movements, or political parties; or (4) will become hostile toward other strata and struggle against them. These social, political, and psychological characteristics may or may not occur on the basis of similar objective situations. In any given case, such possibilities must be explored, and "subjective" attributes must *not be used as criteria* for class inclusion, but rather, as Max Weber has made clear, stated as probabilities on the basis of objectively defined situations.

Implicit in this way of stating the issues of stratification lies a model of social movements and political dynamics. The important differences among people are differences that shape their biographies and ideas; within any given stratum of course, individuals differ, but if their stratum has been adequately understood, we ought to be able to expect certain psychological traits to recur. Our principles of stratification enable us to do this. The probability that people will have a similar mentality and ideology, and that they will join together for action, is increased the more homogeneous they are with respect to class, occupation, and prestige. Other factors do, of course, affect the probability that ideology, organization, and consciousness will occur among those in objectively similar strata. But psychological factors are likely to be associated with *strata,* which consist of people who are characterized by an intersection of the several *dimensions* we have been discussing: class, occupation, status, and power. The task is to sort out these dimensions of stratification in a systematic way, paying attention to each separately and then to its relation to each of the other dimensions.

The Unity of Social Structures

EVER since men came to suspect that Adam Smith's "Unseen Hand" was no longer the hand of a harmony-loving God, students of society have had to recognize and examine the disunity as well as the unity of societies. In our times, we can no longer assume that friction and strain, tension and stress are on the automatic decline. In fact, their pressure, as we know full well, may accumulate to the breaking point: whole societies may be disrupted, masses of men as well as statesmen astonished, and no hopes exist for a new harmony or "equilibrium."

On the other hand, "common values" held in "harmony" may to some men seem as frightful as great disharmony seems to be to others. For harmony as well as common values may of course be imposed, not by any unseen hand, but by the *hubris* of a dictator. There is a price to pay for harmony, as well as for disharmony.

In the main, however, academic students of society have tended, in one way or another, to place great value on harmony and unity. The unity of a social structure, for example, has frequently been conceived as in some way a "manifestation" or "expression" of an underlying "geist," "theme," or "style." Spengler's "geist" is an outstanding case,[1] and deriving from him—and from Nietzsche—the late anthropologist, Ruth Benedict, who attempted to subsume and understand whole societies as "Dionysian" or "Apollonian."[2] Sorokin's "logico-meaningful" unity, reminiscent of Georg Simmel's formal analogies, is a quite sophisticated example of this type of integration.[3]

[1] Oswald Spengler, *The Decline of the West*, C. F. Atkinson, tr. (New York: Knopf, 1926).

[2] *Patterns of Culture* (Boston: Houghton Mifflin, 1934).

[3] Sorokin's unity, in fact, comes in four major types—spatial or mechanical

There is no doubt but that such morphological notions do often allow us to grasp, sometimes in a suggestive way, the structural features of total societies. The interpretation of variegated details in the light of a general, pervasive principle *is* fascinating and suggestive, and much imaginative work has been done with the aid of such conceptions. But they do present certain difficulties: [4]

(1) Because these "wholes" are often formally composed of quite variegated materials, their construction tends to blur the various parts of the social structure, or at least, does not invite discriminations of variations among the parts. (2) In particular, the interest in such morphological wholes often blunts attention to all those tensions, conflicts, and contradictions of interests and values that may exist in heterogeneous institutional structures. (3) In these models, the linking of one part of a society with another is quite often by analogy, and accordingly, we are distracted from the central task of finding adequate and sufficient *causes* for the various phenomena we observe. Because they allow us to deal, *in the beginning,* with the whole society, such schemes do not encourage us to trace ramifications from one part of the society to other parts.

It is possible to use what is sound in such conceptions of "stylistic" unity—and to control their assumptions—by our notion of symbol spheres. In these terms, what this mode of interpretation amounts to is the assumption of the unity and the autonomy of symbol spheres and of the causal weight of master symbols in ex-

juxtaposition: a random group of people in the street; association due to an external factor: rain drives them to shelter; causal or functional unity: they assemble for a movie; and "logico-meaningful" unity: their underlying commonalities in conduct due, in modern society for example, to the role of money, punctuality, and mechanical movement.

We may also place in this type of theory Morris E. Opler's "themes," which "denote a postulate . . . declared or implied, and usually controlling behavior or stimulating activity, which is tacitly approved or openly promoted in a society." *American Journal of Sociology,* November 1945, p. 198.

[4] Most of these drawbacks also hold of the popular "dichotomy views." We refer to Sir Henry Maine's distinction of "status and contract," which is perhaps the father, even if often quite far removed, of Tönnies' "community and society," Spencer's "military and industrial societies," Durkheim's "organic vs. mechanical," Redfield's "Folk and Urban Society," Becker's "sacred and secular." Often, in fact usually, the dichotomy is also used as a trend model: societies move from status to contract, from sacred to secular, from military to industrial.

plaining the details of individual conduct and institutional structure.[5]

In this chapter, in which we attempt to grapple with the problem of social unity, we shall briefly review those aspects of our model which bear upon the statement and solution of the general problem. We shall present this "review" by setting forth a recommended procedure for analyzing total social structures, and, on a more general level, by advancing four types in accordance with which social structures may be unified. In order, however, that the reader may have in mind concrete materials, we shall begin with a brief account of the integration of Sparta, and end with an account of the disintegration of Rome.

1. The Unity of Sparta

Whenever rigid and militarized societies have emerged in the West, the image of unified Sparta, with its common values enforced by military co-ordination, has been resurrected. Men such as Jean-Jacques Rousseau implemented the revolutionary upsurge of democratic enthusiasm by raising up images of the stern virtues of the Roman Republican and disciplined Spartan warrior. Nazi intellectuals were fond of trying to add a somber glamour to their ranks by providing flashbacks to the stand of the Spartans at Thermopylae.

From the time of the second Messinian War during the eighth century B.C. ancient Sparta was organized as a totalitarian democracy of warriors on a permanent war footing.[6] The original three tribal subgroups, or *phyles*, had been superseded by five *phyles* subdivided into "dining clubs," each comprising fifteen professional warrior athletes. These heavily armed men were in constant training or in constant action, from the time of their initiation into the army at the age of twenty years—which was reminiscent of the bachelor houses of archaic tribes—to the veteran's retirement to his household at the age of sixty.

[5] We have already criticized these assumptions above in Chapter X: Symbol Spheres, Section 4: The Autonomy of Symbol Spheres.

[6] Cf. Our account is based upon Max Weber, *Wirtschaft und Gesellschaft* (Tübingen, 1921), pp. 567 ff. and 591 ff.; and Arnold Toynbee, *A Study of History* (London, 1951), especially Vol. III.

At the head of the political community there stood two kings, hence two royal families, who were accountable to five soldierly magistrates, or ephors, elected to their offices for annual terms by the acclamatory shouts of the lined-up army formations. The kings were annually sworn in by these ephors, who may be compared to the Roman tribune of the people, to political commissars like Saint-Just, who purged the revolutionary French army of unreliable *ancien régime* officers, or to the commissars of the Red Army.

The Spartan army was led in the field by one of the kings, who was responsible to the five ephors, to the point of exile or death, for the conduct of war. Apart from this perilous function, the kings were representative figureheads, restricted to the performance of rituals.

This ruling class of warriors led a rigorous and austere life. Military honor, eligibility for admittance to the crack fighting unit of 300 elite guards, for the ephorate and, after retirement, for the council of elders, formed the goals of their aspiration. To be publicly shamed—and by husky women at that—for having lost one's shield, for having flinched in combat, for not having stood to the last by one's comrade-in-arms and one's homosexual partner was the object of fear. Disputes among these peers were settled by all-out wrestling duels in which anything went—from the gouging of eyeballs, the splitting of nostrils, to the biting of genitals. An ascetic code controlled the personal deportment of these warriors. To say a great deal in a few words and without fuss has become famous as "laconic" speech. Gold and silver were despised, as were all bodily comforts. The famous one-pot-menu of "black soup"—probably made from oxblood mixed with buckwheat—was not enjoyed at Spartan state dinners by Athenian ambassadors.

The two kings, the five ephors in charge of the five *phyles*, a council of elders, and the assembled army thus constituted the political and military order of Sparta, which is known as the Lycurgean system. Its rational features seem to indicate a planful enactment by a series of statesmen rather than a crescive emergence. The fact that Homer has Ulysses's son receive a chariot horse as a farewell present after his visit to the Spartan king, as well as the known differences in dress between nobles and commoners, allow us to infer that this warrior community resulted from the democratic leveling down of an older stratum of charioteering nobles into a homogeneous army of disciplined footmen, who deployed their phalanx in full view of the enemy.

This political-military order was linked to the economic order through the economic role of the warrior's wife. She had to provide for her economically expendable husband who, living in his bachelor club, could not share her table. The warrior needed a land-rent to pay for his equipment and upkeep in the syssitia, or "officers' mess." Upon initiation into the army he received an allotment of land and, being in training, he could not farm it and was obliged to find a spouse capable of managing his farm with helot labor. The helots were the bottom stratum, the conquered population who had been reduced to serfdom. Each year the ephors ceremoniously declared war upon them in order to keep them in their places.

The Spartan bachelor chose his wife from among the young women engaged in athletic contests, which thus served as a bridal show. Exclusion from the ranks of the spectators was a severe punishment for the young man. As the Greeks displayed themselves nude in the sports field—which is unique for any upper class— we may infer that the physical strength and endurance of the amazon rather than presumably superior sensitivity, premarital chastity, or status badges of wealth determined "good looks" in the warrior's eyes. Women had no other educators than men. They were prepared, if need be, to bend a helot to erotic service, or to cut him down if "uppity." In all this, the Spartan farmwife found aid and succor in the activities of youthful bands of Spartan adolescents, who were economically and pederastically attached to the warrior syssitias. They were encouraged to rove the countryside for food. Their generalized other was confined to the warrior community, and, in their chronic fighting relation to the helots, force and fraud were meritorious. To have a dead helot to his credit gave prominence to the member of a Spartan youth gang. What chance would a helot have if a Spartan woman put the finger on him?

The life of the Spartan wife was not easy. Besides her economic role of extracting a sufficient rent for her absentee warrior husband from the land-tilling helots, she was expected to bear and to rear many children, preferably all boys. (In passing we should remark that the father of four boys was freed from all obligations to the state.) As in other ancient societies, infanticide was customary in Sparta. Given the interest of the warrior community in the quantity and quality of population, public officials inspected the newly born and selected those fit for survival. Spartan wives offered themselves or helped themselves to the erotic services of men other than their husbands, if the husbands were not up to eugenic par.

At the age of seven, children were removed from maternal care in the home and enrolled in gangs, which combined children of different ages in such a way that the older led the younger, up to the final hurdle of unanimous co-optation by a syssitia. As at birth, so during his educational career, selective elimination threatened the Spartan youngster. Life in the successive boy-gangs selected and reinforced those traits required by the he-man warrior. Birth and inheritance were not sufficient for admission into this highly organized ruling class. Exclusion and ostracism by one's peer group threatened the boy who was lacking in physique, courage, or astuteness and skill in aggression, in self-discipline or obedience of the austere warrior code of this garrison state. These boys and their gangs were attached to the men's "messes," and formed "fan" relationships with the warriors, which included pederastic practices.

With the old nobility, the old priesthood had gone. Unlike other Greek states, Sparta left no temples or priestly sponsored art to posterity. Priests and poets, artists and philosophers were singularly out of place in the midst of these military professionals, who as is usual for such men, despised intellectuals as at best unmanly "penpushers," and at worst likely to import alien ideas and distract men from the proper business at hand. These warriors, who accepted death in battle as man's usual fate, craved neither salvation for their souls nor spiritual comfort in suffering, for they were proud to "take it" without even the rationale of stoic philosophers. Their motivation and control was a conventionally enforced code of honor, and in this they compare with the Confucian erudite. The difference is that the first was a code for warriors, the second a code for pacifist literary officials.

In brief, then, this is the structural scheme for the unity and disunity of Spartan society: in this warrior democracy, the military and the political orders are fused. The household and economic production are not differentiated, but form one unit. Formally, the military-political controls the economic through kinship relations. For the ruling Spartans, the division of labor thus coincides with sexual differences: women take over the household and farm management; men fight. The wives therefore reside in the countryside among the helot farm labor; the men are concentrated in their garrisoned city. Thus, when a man enters military service he must at the same time enter marriage, in order that his wife may provision him.

In the eighth century B.C., some 8,000 warriors were set up in this way.

But by the fourth century B.C. only 400 warriors were fully qualified for action.

Why? Why did Sparta decline?

Although the warrior allotments were not negotiable, economic and social differentiations did slowly advance. A dowry system seems to have allowed for the accumulation of landholdings, and as the Spartans did not aim at imperialist expansion and territorial gain, they did not compensate for this gradual shrinkage of the economic base for warriors qualified to equip themselves and meet their syssitia obligations in kind or in iron money. During the fourth century, the concentration of holdings was reinforced, according to Plutarch, when legislation enabled "the holder of a family property or an allotment to give it away during his lifetime or to bequeath it by will, to anybody whom he chose." The dependence of the warrior on his wife and her role as "heiress" would seem to account for the high status of women in the end. Arnold Toynbee has also pointed to the demoralization of the Spartan warrior when he attempted to enact leadership roles in wider contexts than those of his native society.

In summary, then, the general reasons for Sparta's disintegration are found in the concentration of land holdings to a point where not enough warriors, given their military tasks, were provisioned. Thus, autonomous processes in the household and the economy ramified into the military and political orders, and undermined them. These processes of quantitative change (fewer but larger economic bases for warriors) made for a smaller army because family size (especially sons) did not increase in proportion to the increased sizes of the holdings.

We have briefly articulated the social structure of Sparta in order —as we have already remarked—that the reader may have in mind some concrete materials. We shall now "back off" from these materials, and consider more abstractly and in terms of procedures, the general problem of social unity.

2. Units and Their Relationships

It is easy to believe that each section of a society is related to every other section, that society is in some manner a whole of busily interacting parts. But this assumption does not tell us very much. As a beginning point it is useful, but by itself it is an uninformative truism. For what it does, at best, is advise us to be on the lookout for specific connections between specific parts and their relations to the whole. Whatever models of integration we end up with, much less whatever theory, there is a descriptive task at hand for anyone who would intelligently describe social structures as "wholes." This task will be governed in the first instance by the units of social structure that are used. So our first question is:

I. *Units:* How shall we *articulate* a society—that is, what unit or units shall we seize upon or abstract as "parts" which we would relate to other "parts"? And, specifically, for any given society, how articulated or autonomous are these units?

We cannot claim, and in this social psychology we cannot attempt, a detailed coverage of world history; we obviously seek to transcend ideographic details and to *use* them in search for generalizations and regularities; so we give up the simple canon of "complete description." We must acknowledge that we have to select, and we must therefore become the self-conscious masters of our canons of selection. What are these canons? We must consciously select a set of units which will enable us (1) to proceed systematically in our descriptions of the internal compositions of each society we would examine and thus (2) give ourselves a maximum chance for comparisons between social structures. (3) Moreover, the unit chosen must not only permit economy of systematic description, but it must be a description adequate for causal imputations. To do this requires that we find a fruitful level of generality, which means a level that is flexible, or that has a shuttle from high to low built into it. (4) Our level of generality must be low enough not only to allow but to invite concrete descriptions, for there is no substitute in "theory" for pains-

taking mastery of detail; it must equip us to see what we otherwise might miss. And (5) it must be high enough to allow comparisons across all known societies. These, along with (6) the requirement that the units be open to psychological analysis, are the
criteria which we have kept in mind in choosing our units and
constructing our scheme of social structure. Our unit, the institutional order (with its subunits of specific institutions and finally
of role), along with the idea of spheres, satisfies in a provisional
way, we feel, these critieria.[7]

II. *Relations:* The second question we face is of more immediate
concern to the problem of integration: Precisely how are these
units interrelated, that is, what is the "dimension," or what are
the dimensions, in terms of which we would relate them with one
another? The relations of our units are conveniently construed in
terms of a means-ends *schema,* which involves the dimension of
power. Thus we are interested in finding to what extent, if any,
events in one institutional order may be considered preconditions
of events in other orders. We are also interested in tracing the
ramifications of trends in one order with other orders, and in understanding how such ramifications may facilitate or limit activities
and policies in other orders. In short, our units—institutional orders
—may be related with one another causally in a variety of ways
and degrees. Given orders may be functionally independent or
dependent of one another.

III. *Procedural Scheme:* Let us make our answers to both of
these questions more concrete, and thus begin to illustrate why
we feel that the scheme invites description of prevailing units and
of the causal relations obtaining among them.

In examining a specific society our first decision has to do with
whether we will use as our prime units institutional orders, institutions, or roles. This decision should rest upon the degree to
which the society is, upon examination, found to contain autonomously existing orders of institutions. Now, our scheme of dis-
tinguishable institutional orders is obviously derived from observa-

[7] The reader may wish at this point to reread Chapter II: Character and
Social Structure, Section 2: Components of Social Structure, and Chapter VII:
Institutions and Persons, Section 1: The Institutional Selection of Persons,
and Section 2: The Institutional Formation of Persons.

tion of modern Western society, and only in a society which has a relatively autonomous development of these functions (or of others) can we best proceed with this unit.

We can conceive of societies (for example, the nomadic sib) in which there is only one coherent institution—in this case, the extant kinship group—which provides in its organization all the roles required to fulfill such functions as are served in the society. In such a case, we should seize upon roles as our basic units which are to be related.

On the next "level," we might imagine a society (for instance a tribal confederacy of nomadic sibs) in which there was more than one institution, but in which these did not differ from one another in terms of function. For example, in this case we have a society in which kinship units also performed all other functions. Accordingly, we should seize upon institutions as the basic units to be related.

We thus have three levels of unit, as it were, to choose among as our first level of description. We say the *first* level of description because obviously in cases where institutions are the units we shall also handle the roles, and where institutional orders have been unfolded as articulate units, we shall also handle the institutions that prevail in each and the kinds of roles that in turn compose them.

Why do we always choose the "higher" of these three units that exist for our first description? Because the roles in which we are most interested are part of an institution and can be understood only with reference to its institutional context; and, institutions, if they are part of an institutional order, can most readily be understood as part of the order in which they occur. This contextual guide-line is important; for example, apparently identical institutions may be found in different orders, but qualitative differences may occur to what, in isolation, may appear to be identical. The monopoly factory in Tsarist Russia differed in origin as well as in its position among the totality of Russian institutions from the factory in 1912 America. In Russia such a factory often results from political concessions to foreign capital; in America, as a more indigenous development of a laissez-faire economy. The "same" institution "means" different things with reference to the order to which it belongs and with reference to the relation of this order to others comprising the social structure of which it is a part.

Because of the usefulness of this simple contextual principle, we are prompted, wherever possible, to proceed in the first instance, on the level of institutional order. In fact, we sometimes do so even when such an articulation of institutions is a purely heuristic assumption rather than a discoverable fact. This means that we might so proceed even in a society in which no functional differentiation has produced identifiable orders, or in which they have been "fused" so closely that the actors do not experience their behavior as placed in different orders. In such cases, obviously the conception of institutional order is an "artificial" imposition. Yet, to distinguish for analytical purposes is not to overlook their unity. Only if we do proceed thus analytically can we understand such a society as, in fact, representing one type of unified integration.[8]

As is well known, each of the institutional orders of the sort we have presented here begins to form and to become autonomous with the Western Renaissance and Reformation. From that time, politics emerges from the all-pervasive religious order, as the prince emerges as a wielder of secular power. Then also, in the symbol sphere, philosophy, science, and art gradually cease to be hand-maidens of theology. Then Machiavelli discerns "pure power problems" of the political man, who treats all life as means of getting, holding, increasing, and wielding power. With the emergence of the factory, i.e., the segregation of enterprise from household during the eighteenth century, the economic order begins to acquire autonomy, the police state increasingly withdraws from the mercantilist intervention in the economic order. Only then could economic science conceive of the economic man—and his rationally expedient behavior in markets—as a suitable model for analyzing the economic order in industrial society. The general process of the unfolding and autonomy of orders perhaps reaches its extreme when in the symbol and technological spheres (which thus made pretenses to be autonomous orders) men speak seriously of "science for science's sake," of "art for art's sake." Thus segregated activities and ends are fetishized.

The problem of the unity of a social structure, especially as it bears upon the unit chosen, obviously differs for differently articulated societies. The first empirical task, in approaching any given society, is to discover the most convenient units that prevail, in

[8] See below, this chapter, Section 3: Modes of Integration.

terms of which the problem of structural unity or integration may best be stated.

Having due regard to this, we will nevertheless assume institutional orders as our unit, and use that unit in presenting our procedural scheme, for this enables us to handle, at least formally, the salient problems of unity encountered in societies that are not articulated into orders. For a society in which all five orders are autonomous enough to permit separate delineation and thus relationships, one must "fill in" the following boxes:

INSTITUTIONAL ORDERS					SPHERES
POLITICAL	1				EDUCATION STATUS SYMBOLS TECHNOLOGY
ECONOMIC	6	2			
MILITARY	7	10	3		
RELIGIOUS	8	11	13	4	
KINSHIP	9	12	14	15	5
	POLITICAL	ECONOMIC	MILITARY	RELIGIOUS	KINSHIP

First, the range and the basic characteristics of the institutions prevailing in each order are determined: 1 through 5. This first task includes a description of the spheres of each of these orders: education, status, symbols, technology.

Second, the relations between each of the orders with each of the others are described: 6 through 15. This second task consists of a detailed tracing of the ramifications and other relations of each order upon all others. So much is basic: Only when this is done on a purely descriptive level do we have (1) a basis for comparing different social structures and (2) a basis for causal imputations in explanation of various roles, institutions, or the shape of the social structure as a whole.

"Ramification" refers to the operation of one order within other orders: or, to the use of one order for the ends of the ramifying order. The "ramifications" of any order refer to its total range of such operations in all other orders. The political order may thus ramify into kinship most closely and brutally when all intimate relations and locales of the kinship unit are used by police agents who see them as "a network of living traps" for the suspect or prisoner of the political order. When political relations—for example, international affairs—are carried on by competing dynastic families, women, as shrewd manipulators of men in the kinship order, may exert considerable influence upon key political decisions. The economic order may ramify into the political, as in modern capitalist societies; for example, as economic institutions, corporations seek to influence the content and administration of laws in order to gain or to retain economic privileges. Their political actions are thus means for an economic end. Ramifications has to do with the relative powers of orders, and the use of one as a means for the other's end.

From the more or less descriptive level, executed as concretely as time and information allow, and with the aid of typologies found relevant for each institutional order, we move by examination and comparison to explanations of the integration of social structures as wholes.

3. Modes of Integration

From a somewhat formal standpoint, we can observe certain general ways in which the institutional orders composing a social structure are integrated. These modes of integration are, for us, analytic models which sensitize us to certain types of linkage of one order with another. They may also, of course, be viewed dynamically, as processes of social-historical change.

By a *milieu* we understand the social setting of a person that is directly open to his personal experience. It is a surface of his daily social life. In his day-to-day life, he acts in a variety of milieus— the home, the place of work, the scene of amusement, the street. In these milieus he of course observes changes, but most people do not often ask why these changes occur. When we do reflect upon such changes in milieus—such as our neighborhood over a thirty-year period—then we must go beyond the milieu itself to explain the change observed in it. And this means that we come upon the idea of *structures*.

By a *structure,* in the present sense, we understand the modes of integration by which various milieus are linked together to form a larger context and dynamics of social life. These modes of integra-

tion may be stated as *principia media,* as middle principles, ena-
bling us to link what is *observable* in various milieus but *caused*
by structural changes in institutional orders. Thus the neighborhood town of 1850, with its well-known milieu, appears in 1950
as a scatter of milieus, none of which is recognizable as the old:
the dirt path is now an asphalt strip, and the railroad connects
the daily work of the inhabitants with the world market.

We have found some four principles of structural change useful
in understanding the integration of a society:

I. By *correspondence* we mean that a social structure is unified
by the working out in its several institutional orders of a common
structural principle, which thus operates in a parallel way in each.

II. By *coincidence* we mean that different structural principles
or developments in various orders result in their combined effects
in the same, often unforeseen, outcome of unity for the whole
society.

III. By *co-ordination* we refer to the integration of a society by
means of one or more institutional orders which become ascendant
over other orders and direct them; thus other orders are regulated
and managed by the ascendant order or orders.

IV. By *convergence* we mean that two or more institutional
orders coincide to the point of fusion; they become one institutional
setup.

It is quite difficult to isolate concrete societies which fully and
exclusively exemplify each of these types of integration because
reality is usually mixed. The integrations of some areas of a society
can often best be understood in terms of one mode of integration,
while other parts can best be understood by application of another mode. Nevertheless, to make clear what is involved in each
type of integration, we can, in a brief way, sketch cases in which
each seems to predominate.

I. *Correspondence.* The handiest case of correspondence is perhaps the model of a classic liberal society, best exemplified by the
society prevailing in the first half of the nineteenth century in the
United States.[9] The meaning of "laissez-faire" for the economic

9 Cf. Charles and Mary Beard, *The Rise of American Civilization* (rev. ed.;
New York: Macmillan, 1933); and A. Lowe, *Economics and Sociology* (London: Allen, 1935).

order is a demand on the part of economic agents for freedom from political dominance. It is paralleled by the religious demand for autonomy from political or state control or even sponsorship of any one type of religious institution; moreover, here too, one Protestant man faced his God, free of any hierarchy of interpreters. In the political area, as in the economic market, there is a free competition for the individual's vote. In the kinship order, also, marriage is a contract between the marriage partners into which they enter of their own free will; marriages are not to be arranged by parental collusion of economic or status sort. Just as free individuals compete economically, so do they in the status sphere: "the self-made man" stands in contrast to "the family-made man" of the kinship order's status sphere, just as a much as to the man who moves on his own across the autonomous economic markets. So status styles are often represented as conspicuous consumption of the self-made businessman.

On the highest level of abstraction, in the symbol sphere, the idea of human freedom, of the spontaneity of thinking, acting, and judging, is proclaimed and elaborated. In particular, the conception of human genius, of the prerogative of free creativity, becomes central, and even sets an ideal model for the nature of human nature. So educators attempt "to make the student think for himself."

The basic legitimation of instituted conduct in each of these orders is very much the same: the free initiative of the autonomous individual for rational and moral self-determination. Thus the symbol spheres of the various orders run in parallel or corresponding fashion. In each order free individuals could institute new organizations according to the principle—or at times even the expectation—of voluntary associations. Independent decision-making and organization thus unify what on the surface might appear as merely the unplanned complexity and enormous variety of nineteenth-century "causes."

The correspondence of diverse and relatively autonomous orders is the outcome of processes in which all significant orders develop in the direction of an integrative principle of competition or laissez faire. In all orders competition means that individuals act in a field of action which impersonally disciplines them for uniform strivings and motives, and in its terms free men find their places. This principle also secured a rather smooth and gradual transferal or shift in power within and between orders. The translation of economic into political power is particularly relevant.

Of course, the model of a liberal society does not contain only elements that correspond to the principle of individual freedom of choice. In fact, definite compulsions are introduced in the political order which, although enacted by free men, nevertheless are compulsions: in Europe (since the time of Napoleon) there has been universal compulsory military service. And there has been compulsory taxation and universal compulsory education up to various standards. In these respects, the modern state has advanced beyond any previously known political controls, for only in modern times, with modern technology and special techniques of communications available, have such large-scale and intensive administrative accomplishments been possible. These, although most important, have been quite uneven in their application, and in the case of property, given its wide distribution, have really been a sort of anchor of the basic freedom. Accordingly, such compulsions are important for the model of classic liberal society as exceptions to the integration of the whole by autonomously choosing individuals.

Many other examples of correspondence come to mind: the occidental feudal principle of an "exchange" of personal allegiance for protection, as displayed in the psychology of vassalship in political, economic, military, religious, and kinship orders with the "lord," in the first four, and, in the upper ranks, with "the occidental lady" emerging in the noble household. The psychological link of personal loyalty and sworn allegiance between lord and vassal allows for the coherent although decentralized domination of rather large territories. And this same mechanism, giving rise in the kinship order to the knight and the occidental lady—the wife of another knight, to whom the knight must prove his love and worth, in vassal-like manner. In the religious order, the Christian knight's orientation was similar: faith and vassalship to Christ, the Lord in whose name he crusaded against heathen and barbarian. Thus, the three orders—politics, kinship, and religion—correspond in the psychology of vassalship under the code of loyalty, love, and honor.[10]

[10] Cf. J. Huizinga, *The Waning of the Middle Ages* (London: Arnold, 1949); H. O. Taylor, *The Medieval Mind* (London, 1938), 2 vols.; and Eileen Power, *Medieval People* (Boston: Houghton Mifflin, 1924).

II. *Coincidence.* We are not aware of any society that is integrated solely in terms of coincidence: different structural and psychological tendencies in each of the different orders bringing about a unified end product. But there are many instances at hand of the partial operation of coincidence as a mode of integration, which represents the unplanned, unforeseen, and "fortuitous" result of institutional dynamics. Every coincidence is of course causally determined, but insofar as causal ascription to material or ideal interests has to be made, such interests might well be heterogeneous, and, being anchored in different orders, perhaps even ultimately conflicting.

The breakdown of feudal codes of privilege and the development of an administrative and legal framework which facilitated the rise of capitalism is an outstanding example. When the absolutist prince breaks the power of feudal status groups he sets up, or at least calls into being, modern bureaucracy. The prince is interested in using his officials in any part of his territory in order to cheapen the costs of his administration, and to rotate officials so as to promote uniform administration and to secure his central control. This interest of the prince, however, is blocked by the legal peculiarities of different regions, cities, and provinces which for the official mean an unlearning of local statute and a new learning.

The bureaucrat, on the other hand, finding extended career opportunities in the increase of his usefulness because of his universal transferability, has a material interest, which fuses with his purely intellectual interest in a rationally consistent set of guiding principles. The official's interest is in legal norms that are consistently applicable as reinforced by the university teacher's interest in systematic organization of his teaching routine, course repetition, and textbook presentation. Hence, for quite different reasons, the interests of the prince, the bureaucrat, and the academician coincide in the direction of a rational systematization and codification of legal rules.

In the meantime, there is another causal series which coincides with these to support this process: in the economic order, the rising entrepreneurial middle class promotes a rational legal order. Due to the expansion of their market operations the entrepreneurs are interested in a homogeneous law, for this would allow them to calculate the legal consequences of their economic actions and the chances of contracts being enforced by court action. This interest of the economic agent in the calculability of law obviously coincides with the interests of the bureaucrat in the rationality and standardization of legal rules, and the interest of the prince in the cheapness of administration and his control over it. A second and allied motive of the enterpriser is an interest in legal security. The arbitrariness of the enlightened despot's "cabinet justice" was, in the eyes of the enterpriser, an irrational, incalculable risk. His interest in security of contract coincided here with the bureaucrat's interest in security of tenure. Hence both the bureaucratic personnel and the middle classes were interested in reducing the element of despotic arbitrariness in favor of fixing and systematizing a set of unambiguous legal norms. This phase of legal history and the coincidence of different orders is the unforeseen, unplanned, and "blind" result of heterogeneous interests; at a later juncture of the historical process, the constellation of these interests naturally breaks up.

A comparable point of coincidence between eighteenth-century despotism and entrepreneurial capitalism in the making may be adduced. Princely absolutism for politico-military reasons sought to increase the tax yield of its subjects by all sorts of mercantilist policy schemes, including subsidized enterprises of privileged persons, technological and industrial training institutes, travels of officials for espying technical advances in Great Britain, in Berlin the hiring out of soldiers to textile manufacturers, in France under Colbert the digging of canals by the army. The subsidized enterprises mostly fell by the wayside (only fiscal porcelain manufacturing establishments such as Sèvres, Dresden, Meissen, and Berlin have remained). And taxes and their princely investment deflected otherwise available private capital into unprofitable, hence uneconomic, channels; these aspects of mercantilism hence conflicted with the entrepreneurial interest. The promotion of technological innovation, however, i.e., the French canals, or later the improvement of the Rhine River and the construction of military roads, under Napoleon, proved invaluable to capitalism, as did the general bearing down of princely absolutism on traditionalist petty routine.

Within a latter-day liberal capitalist society, such as the United States during World War II, the military order wants recruits in order to build an army; educational institutions want students in order to maintain schools as going concerns. These different purposes coincide in army and navy student training programs, in which the armed forces gets men in uniform being trained for special roles, and the educational plant stays open. Like other cases of coincidence, the various groups of people whose institutions have coincided may have set forth legitimations for participation in the same conduct pattern: the war officers believe that it is part of military preparation; the educators feel that, however that might be, it is also good for nonmilitary, general educational ends. And again, as with many coincidences, the results outrun both formal legitimations. Such a program may be seen as part of the breakdown of voluntary liberal education on higher levels and the reaching of compulsory practices into these areas. In order to survive as going concerns the higher-education plants become in many ways ramifications of the military order. Quite a few physicists and atomic scientists were bewildered after the war when executive departments for reasons of security considered the publication of "secrets of nature" as dangerous and possibly disloyal disclosures of "secrets of state."

The most striking and detailed case of a coincidence of orders is provided by Max Weber's work on Protestant religion and capitalist economics, on the role of Puritanism in the character formation of the economic vanguard of modern capitalism.[11]

The theology of Calvinism emphasizes the view that man is evil and that due to the inscrutable will of a stern and hidden God only few men are predestined for salvation. This interpretation of Christianity at once reinforces and resolves intense anxieties in the believer as to whether he is or is not among the elect. Out of this situation two possibilities derive: fatalism or intense activism. Puritanism interprets man's Christian conduct in everyday life as being an indicator though not a guarantee of his salvation chances, so a religious significance is attributed to everyday work. Whereas formerly only certain monastic orders had used work as a means of religious asceticism, now every believer has to prove his religious worth by self-denying work in this world. He must work not for profits, not out of enjoyment of his work, nor yet of its fruits. His

[11] We have discussed this in other connections; see pp. 188 and 234-36.

work must be an ascetic exercise pursued methodically for the sake of the kingdom to come. His work becomes his "calling," and only those who have consistently proved themselves in their callings can claim to be "elected." Those who successfully claim to be among the elect associate themselves in sects, and admit new members, by adult baptism, only after a scrutiny of the applicant's total record of conduct. The earliest sects adopted anabaptism, meaning the rebaptism of qualified adults and their reception into an exclusive, voluntary association.

The economic consequence of such motivation is the emergence of a type of person who, in the economic order, will not readily consume the profits he makes—as an entrepreneur or middleman. Suspicious of ostentatious wealth and luxury, he considers his accumulation of wealth as Christian stewardship. He has only one course open: reinvestment in his business for extended production. This in turn gives the Puritan enterpriser the opportunity to employ additional men, in religious terms to extend opportunities to anguished souls who in an age of enclosures and vagrancy, crave to prove themselves as God-fearing Christians. Thus, the entrepreneur provides institutional opportunities under Puritan control to unemployed and dependent groups. From his perspective, wages increase the workers' opportunities to prove themselves as frugal and sober and hard working. High wages would only constitute temptations to wander from the ascetic path. The worker, in turn, knows that what counts is to prove himself in whatever workaday life God has placed him.

Admission to the elect and recognition by sect members give each member a claim for brotherly help from economic distress which is not his own fault. This relevance of sect membership for credit, based upon religiously trained character, facilitates economic ascent. For the observance of new ethical standards in exchange behavior, of honest dealings, of charging the same "fair price" to all buyers, of avoiding higgling as "idle words," of reliability in the fulfillment of contracts—all this lent business prestige to the sectarians. This prestige, translated into good credit standing, in turn, added to the Puritan business, and at a later time, allowed Benjamin Franklin to state as a rule of experience: "honesty is the best policy."

Thus: The psychology of the religious man furnishes motives for his economic roles. This psychological coincidence may be traced in the kinship order, where unpurposive erotic play and enjoyment is suppressed by a code of sobriety, and in the political and military orders, where the spontaneous release of agression is inhibited. The disciplined attack of Cromwell's Ironsides gave these "men of conscience," who "fought for what they knew and knew for what they fought," the superiority of machine war over the personalist combat of the feudal cavaliers. Cromwell's army was held together after victory, and pursued the routed enemy rather than wasting time in carousing and plundering.

The inner-worldly asceticism does not withdraw from this world but proves itself in the midst of worldly affairs and temptations. It is based upon a religiously motivated character structure integrating the pious man's conduct in all orders of life. In extreme cases, it may lead to complete withdrawal from political and military orders, as is shown by Quakers, Hutterites, and Mennonites who refuse to hold office, will not take oaths, and remain "defenseless."

The importance of such a psychological type for modern capitalism is evidenced by the fact that even after the universal process of secularization and the disappearance of the specific theological symbols—voluntary associations and clubs, fraternal societies and the like—prestige premiums are still placed upon such character traits, which they justify in terms of conventional middle-class morality.

The ramifications of Puritanism, and hence of a primarily religious phenomenon, fed into the great economic transition from feudalism to modern industrial capitalism. The decline of the guild system and of its restraints on competition, the technological and organizational advances of the workshop, were reinforced by the migration of persecuted Protestant minorities who established themselves outside urban jurisdictions. The parceling up of markets by politically privileged monopolies was successfully fought by Puritan businessmen. Thus numerous technological, monetary, and organizational changes in the age of discoveries, and changes in trade routes from the Mediterranean to the Atlantic, found an area of coinciding changes in religion, in personality formation, and in new religiously motivated ways of playing the crucial roles instrumental in the emergence of modern industrial capitalism.

But, in due course, the Puritan businessman experienced what all monastic orders, in their contexts, have experienced in the face of the riches resulting from the asceticism of hard work without consumption of its fruits. The "inner-worldly asceticism" succumbed to the temptations of this world. And repeated vogues of religious revivalism have not changed decisively the big trend toward a phase in which as Weber put it, "Once in the saddle, capitalism could dispense with religion." In short, it could rely on pecuniary incentives for work and openly proclaim "the chase after the dollar," or in the words of the "bourgeois king," Louis Philippe, "enrichissez vous!"

III. *Co-ordination.* In co-ordination unity is achieved by the subordination of several orders to the regulation or direct management of other orders. This in twentieth-century "totalitarian" societies unity is guaranteed by the rule of the one-party state over all other institutions and associations. But these societies also involve correspondence and coincidence.

The general schema—for the integration of Nazi Germany, for example [12]—runs like this: during the 1920's the economic and political orders develop quite differently: within the economic order institutions are highly centralized; a few big units more or less control the operations and the results of the entire order; within the political order there is fragmentation, many parties competing to influence the state but no one of them powerful enough to control the results of economic concentration. So, there is a political movement which successfully exploits the mass despair of the great depression and brings the political, military, and economic orders into close correspondence; one party monopolizes and revamps the political order; it abolishes or amalgamates all other parties that would compete for power. To do this requires that the Nazi party find points of coincidence and/or correspondence with monopolies in the economic order and certain high agents of the military order. In these three orders there is a corresponding high concentration of power; then each of them coincides and co-operates in the taking of power. The army under President Hindenburg is not interested in defending the Weimar Republic by crushing the marching columns of a popular war party. Big business circles help finance the Nazi party, which, among other things, promised to smash the labor movement. And the three types of chieftains

[12] Cf. Franz Neumann, *Behemoth* (New York: Oxford, 1942).

join in an often uneasy coalition to maintain power in their respective orders and to co-ordinate the rest of society. Rival political parties are either suppressed and outlawed, or they disband voluntarily. Kinship and religious institutions, as well as all organizations within and between all orders, are "politicized," infiltrated, and co-ordinated, or at least neutralized and subdued.

The immediate organization by means of which certain high agents in each of the three dominant orders coincide, and by which they co-ordinate their own and other orders and institutions, is the totalitarian party-state. It becomes the over-all frame organization which imposes and defines substantive policy goals for all institutional orders instead of merely guaranteeing government by law. The totalitarian party extends itself by prowling everywhere in "auxiliaries" and "affiliations" to other orders. It either breaks up or infiltrates, and so controls, every organization, even down to the family.

The legal order is reduced to an adjunct of the police state, with its terrorist organizations of elite guards and police forces. The individual has no "constitutional rights" which courts would or could enforce against arbitrary acts of men in high places. The individual does not count; the ruler abolishes "the rule of law" and proclaims "the rule of men." In the military order, the party leader establishes an autonomous bodyguard subject only to his personal command, and the army is duplicated by the elite guard of about half a million men who are sufficiently segregated in composition and command as to be a party-controlled army, existing alongside of the mass army of the nation. The kinship order and educational institutions are controlled through a compulsory organization of all youth in a "state youth," which in turn is controlled by a youth auxiliary of the party. A voluntary mass organization of women controlled through a party auxiliary guarantees control of the management of the household, which in turn steers the consumption of rationed *ersatz*. The state party acquires economic enterprises through expropriation (of Jews and politically disloyal owners). Outstanding examples are the Göring works, the Eher publishing house, the numerous party papers owned by the party, and numerous municipal enterprises and public utilities which either are directly appropriated by the party or are under the management of party members.

A system of state and hence party controlled "chambers" is organized, membership in which is compulsory for all entrepreneurs and corporations. Farming is organized into a compulsory cartel, the Reich's Food Estate. The labor market is controlled through the compulsory organization of all gainfully employed persons in the Labor Front. The free professions in addition to their traditional state control are organized in party controlled chambers of culture, seven of them, under the direction of a propaganda ministry. Thus, with the partial exception of the churches, the symbolic sphere of all orders is centrally managed.

There is more than one official hierarchy, and this fact, through the resultant competition and overlapping of ill-defined authority, allows for periodic purges, as well as quick changes of the official line. This fact also means that the *Führer*, and his inner circle, are relatively independent of the pressure of his own staffs. His personal decisions are ultimate and are enforceable by the effective use of his bodyguard, which reaches into the army and into the police. When most of the institutions in an order cannot be superseded by an organizational monopoly, the state party tries to occupy at least the strategic institutions or to co-ordinate the institutions under a superimposed party auxiliary.

The symbolic sphere of all orders, as we have said, is controlled by the party. With the partial exception of the religious order, no rival claims to autonomous legitimacy are permitted. There is of course a party monopoly of all formal communications, including the educational sphere; and all symbols are recast to form the basic legitimation of the co-ordinated society: the principle of absolute and magical leadership in a strict and unilateral hierarchy is widely and increasingly promulgated.

IV. *Convergence.* Two different orders may coincide, often in completely unplanned ways, to the point of fusion or convergence. In a rapidly expanding society, for example, the frontier zones of the nineteenth-century United States, the institutional articulation of different orders in the East may peter out on the vanguard edges. So, for lack of functional specification, certain Eastern institutional orders converge in the West. The frontier farmer is thus a military agent as well as an economic man, and the household becomes a small military outpost as well as a family abode. "Neighborliness"—or the relations between contiguous kinship units—fills in the gaps of institutions not yet organized. There is no church, there are no police, there are no schools—so, in this kinship-centered society, these functions converge in and are carried by the family. The roles of women as wife and mother come also to include the nurse, the midwife, and the teacher; the roles of men as husband and father, to include the lay religious leader and, if needed, of the vigilante and militiaman.

It should, of course, be understood that in any concrete social structure, we may well find mixtures of these four types of structural integration or structural change. The task is to search within and between institutional orders for points of correspondence and coincidence, for points of convergence and co-ordination, and to examine them in detail. The presence of one type does not exclude the possibility of others. We do not believe that there is any single or general rule governing the composition and unity of orders and spheres which holds for all societies. Reality is not often neat and orderly; it is the task of analysis to single out what is relevant to neat and orderly understanding.

4. Why Rome Fell

Those historians who emphasize the military order as decisive for the fall of Rome have made much of the "invasion of the barbarians" and the allegedly declining military virtues of a Roman mercenary army. Others, especially schoolteachers of the nineteenth century, have found fault with the morality of the ruling stratum before the advent of Christendom; they have made the most of luxuries, debauchery, lack of hard work, and so forth. Anti-Christians, such as Nietzsche, have emphasized the asceticist ideal of the Christians as corrosive of the lordly virtues, and even Gibbon attributed much of the population decline to the spread of monastic celibacy and hermitage life. A Communist historian makes the most of the uprising of slaves in Sicily and Africa, but Nietzsche has made the most of the uprising of the slave in morality. Whereas Toynbee and Rostovtsev make much of the Roman proletariat, external or internal, Friedrich Engels makes much of the alleged inability of freemen to work because of their leisure-class attitude and self-respect in the face of degrading slave labor. Obviously, as one observes the total decline of a civilization as complex as Rome, many causes and aspects can be highlighted. However, it is possible to locate a number of contradictions which cut more and more widely through the Roman social structure and which proved insoluble to the Caesars.[13]

I. The plantation economy of Roman agriculture was based upon slave labor, which did not reproduce itself, as the masters garrisoned the field slaves by sex, interdicting reproduction as an unwelcome risk to their investment. As in the American old South, the plantation economy resulted in deforestation and soil erosion, in extensive cultivation, and in increasingly barren land in Italy and Sicily. The prime objectives of chronic Roman warfare, in fact, were the conquest of rent-yielding land and of slave labor. As prisoners of war became slaves, the military campaigns were in the nature of slave raids. Roman imperialism was economically necessary; the military and the economic orders were functionally linked. As the economy shrank in productivity and production, tax yields to support the military and political excursions also shrank, which in turn, failed to provide new labor forces of slaves.

II. The displacement of the free peasantry by slaves on plantations (the *latifunda*) brought with it a decline of population, and since the defeat of the Gracchi (who for military reasons fought against the extension of the *latifunda* into conquered lands), the army had increasingly to rely upon paid soldiers rather than upon drafted freemen. The decline of agriculture, however, as we have just seen, caused a decline in tax yields, since the land tax, as in all agrarian societies, was the major source of public income. A strain was thus placed upon the state, due to the increasing military burdens accompanying the great expansion and pacification of the empire, and the decline of money taxes. These tendencies were reinforced by the technique of collecting taxes through tax farmers, who squeezed their respective provinces for private profit with a short-run view, considering that "in the long run we are all dead." These private speculative gains, even though partially used to defray the public expenses of office-holding, should the man of wealth later take office, could not compensate for the diminution

---

[13] Our account draws upon Weber's essay "The Social Causes of the Decay of Ancient Civilization," *Journal of General Education* (Vol. V, No. 1, October 1950, Christian Mackauer, tr.). Cf. M. I. Rostovtzeff, *The Social and Economic History of the Hellenistic World* (London: Oxford, 1941), 2 vols.; and Arnold Toynbee, *A Study of History*, Vols. 5 and 6.

of the tax yields from the provinces. In addition, more and more of the costs of a competitive political career were unproductive expenses for ostentatious pomp and luxury, circuses and sumptuous buildings.

III. In due course, the state sought a solution to its fiscal problems by paying officials in kind, and by levying forced labor upon the productive classes of artisans and middlemen. Guild associations were made compulsory and hereditary for certain trades—such as traders shipping grain to Rome—and these associations were obliged to contribute their services, as a joint liability, to the public weal.

Veterans who had served with the colors for a certain number of years received a soldier bonus in land located along the public water mains, military highroads, and—after the defeat of Varus's legions and the stabilization of the frontiers—along the line of fortifications and camps running along the Danube and the right side of the Rhine. These veterans received hereditary and non-negotiable land allotments, which were mortgaged hereditarily and forever with the maintenance services or even with obligatory military services in case of need.

All of this bespeaks of a decline of the money economy and of the fiscal system; as the greater cohesion of the economic order is fragmented, payments in kind replace soldiers' wages and official salaries.

IV. The big consumer cities, especially the city of Rome itself, also represented a financial burden for the state. The bulk of the population, the so-called "proletariat," i.e., "men rich in children," went idle. They were free Romans having the right to vote, who had been displaced from their farms, served in the army, and sold their votes to the highest political bidder. Much of the payment was in bread and circuses, and Roman circuses were anything but cheap.

V. As all these fiscal strains mounted, speculative middlemen and capitalists in the grain trade were displaced, the provision of grain was made a public business, the imperial bureaucracy took in hand the overseas grain shipments and their allocations to cities—in order to control the price of grain and to take the private profit out of the grain trade. This was the greatest blow which capitalist middlemen received in Roman antiquity, for the rest of the much vaunted commerce between ancient trade emporiums actually con-

sisted of luxury trade across the Mediterranean, linked to the cara-
van trade across the Middle East which brought Chinese silk and
tea, spices and other specialties to the West, and whatever gold
the West had to the East, to India, where it was wrought into
temple and princely treasures. "International trade," in short, represented a thin and widely spun network of consumers' goods and not
bulky raw materials or production resources. Given the small size
of the ships, which were unable to sail against the wind and which
were mainly propelled by expensive slave-power, only high-priced
luxury goods could be profitably transshipped.

VI. In the economic order, in summary then, we find an increasing contradiction: land rents diminish with the decreasing
productivity of the land, and the increasing price of slaves as the
frontiers are stabilized and no new slaves brought in. So the costs
of production generally rise, the accumulation of great private
fortunes slows down, and tax burdens become onerous. Given the
liturgical obligations of office-holding, to be voted into office is
like being popularly expropriated, for the elected office holder
had to defray the costs of his office out of his private means.

A "flight from the city" got underway. Those who had landed
wealth and could afford to do so, retreated to their landed estates,
taking their treasures along and establishing themselves in the
countryside and thus escaping the coercive environment of proletarian consumers' cities. The center of gravity of the Mediterranean coastal civilization gradually shifted to the hinterlands;
upper-class families became rusticated and sought to live self-
sufficiently by organizing all essential services in their rural household economy. The thin network of trade broke up; both private
and public economy reverted increasingly to subsistence economy.
Slaves, who could always revolt, required costly supervision and
management, and were accordingly set up as self-motivated workers
who could work their way to freedom by paying off stipulated
annuities, i.e., the slaves were treated as a source of rent rather
than as implements of larger economic institutions. Thus socially
low freemen and socially ascending slaves merged into a homogeneous plebeian stratum—to which Christianity made its greatest
appeal. The larger the city and the poorer the people, the greater
the number of Christian converts. Paul is credited with having
established the first Christian cells in the provincial capitals
of the Roman orbit. This new set of values, coming from the

Middle East, thus met the great needs of a society that was drifting without hope to its ending.

In brief summary, then, Rome in the course of three centuries (from Augustus to Diocletian) disintegrated for these reasons:

The economic order was technologically static because of the undue investment risks entailed by a harshly controlled slave labor force. Slaves who were threshing grain, for example, were forced to wear muzzles in order to restrain their unauthorized eating. The water mill, although known, was never installed. Agricultural production declined: *latifunda* were allowed to run down as their hired managers "worked them out" for short-run returns.

Thereafter there was a search for new land and new labor power, which was realized by imperial warfare and conquest. This, in time, failed to meet the economic demands because, as the conquered territories became more distant from Rome, the fiscal burdens of administration and defense increased to the point where consolidation of the existing boundaries replaced attempts at new conquests. But such consolidations, given point 1 above, were no solution, and attempts to shore up the failing system all proved abortive.

In Rome's unity, the economic and the military were functionally dependent; in Rome's disunity, their developments failed to correspond. And so in the dynamics of the two orders, the scissors opened, until the pivot of the two blades of Rome broke.

The institutions composing a social structure may be unified by *correspondence* (the several institutional orders develop in accordance with a common principle), by *coincidence* (various institutional developments lead to the similar resultant ends), by *co-ordination* (one institutional order becomes dominant over the others and manages them), and by *convergence* (in their development, one or more institutional orders blend).

In describing each of these modes of integration we have given brief examples. But in trying to make clear some of the complexity and variety of total social structures, we have also discussed some of the sociologist's methods of constructing social structures, and, in desperate brevity, we have attempted to illustrate these procedures by describing the structural unity of ancient Sparta and—the classic case of disunity—Imperial Rome.

Neither Sparta nor Rome endured. Regardless of how unified a social structure may seem, its unity is part of history, and history is change. Our examination of the integrations and disintegrations of Sparta and Rome thus point—like all social psychological topics —to the problem of socio-historical change.

PART FOUR

DYNAMICS

CHAPTER

XIII

Social-historical Change

FROM folklore as well as philosophic reflection and esthetic experience we inherit a rich legacy of often paradoxical axioms about change. From an old Roman adage we learn that "Times change and we change with them," but from an old French saying, that "The more it changes, the more it remains the same." In our music the mathematically measurable "beat," the metrical articulation of time, is distinguished from "rhythm," the pulsation of a melodic flow of energy, which has more to do with our heartbeat and the right-left swing of the human gait than with the mechanical exactitude of the metronomic tick-tock.

There is in the Western mind the idea of "Chronos"—the mathematically divisible extension of time as a pure quantitative series of equal measures; and there is "Kairos"—the time for fateful decisions, the climactic moments which alternate with stretches of time during which nothing seems to happen. In the history of social thought we find that thinkers have often been preoccupied with what seems to them the incomparably unique moment at which man faces novel decisions. These scholars have been concerned with those situations in which man finds himself at unknown "forks in the road," where no signposts map out future means and ends.

"History teaches that history teaches nothing," wrote Hegel, the philosopher of the Napoleonic age, who believed that it was impossible to stand in the present and yet penetrate the future. For man's past, by definition, is dead; it has fallen behind in the inexorable march of the world spirit.[1] Other no less powerful minds —Nietzsche and Freud—have sought to master the shock of the new by denying that there is really anything new under the sun. Ac-

[1] G. W. F. Hegel, *The Philosophy of History* (rev. ed.; New York: Wiley, 1944).

cording to them, what matters for man and his life has already happened in the archaic and closed past which still impregnates the present. What lies ahead is always the return of the same.

For Freud, the primeval crime is the son's killing the primordial father of the primitive horde in order to possess the mother. This crime is transmitted through time and repeatedly asserts itself in the changing costume of surface appearances. It is the core of man's constant nature. Lamarckian assumptions concerning the hereditary transmission of once-acquired psychic traits support this notion of constant elements to which change is analytically reduced. The history of the Judeo-Christian religion, for example, is to Freud a text revealing the repeated drama of parricide and original guilt. This fact is revealed in the Freudian process of reducing changing behavior to constant instinct, changing symbolic elaborations to the constant pressure of the guilt complex.

Man's history is thus stripped by the psychoanalyst of presumed surfaces and turned into immutable nature. For, as with Aristotle, change is spurious, and only the constant is genuine. So the burden of the past holds sway over the future. As man's biography, when correctly understood, represents the recapitulation of the initial childhood constellation, so the historic drama of mankind is but the unfolding and reassertion of the initial archaic crime and of its burden.

One wonders why parricide rather than, let us say, fratricide should thus be posited as the primordial theme by Freud; why the story of Oedipus Rex rather than that of Cain and Abel should be seized upon as the mythological axis of human nature. The latter might be as serviceable for a Hobbesian construction of basic human nature as the former. At any rate, anthropologists, especially Malinowski, have shown the limited bearing of Freud's discernment of the Oedipus complex on non-Western societies, kinship structures, and personality formations.

Nietzsche's idea of the Will to Power, and its basic implementation by the psychic resentment of the socially weak against the high and mighty, is out of place when we deal with Buddhism, and holds true only partially for Jewish and Christian traditions. Moreover, it requires an unwarranted reduction of all love to the quest for power, of all giving to getting, of all unselfishness to selfishness.

In a different way, the construction of all human history in accordance with Marx's historical materialism is apt to block open-minded inquiry, for it reduces selected aspects and phases of social history to a series of selected illustrations in proof of the alleged sovereignty of the economic order. It has been established, for example, that the military needs of Christian Europe in the face of the Mohammedan threat from across the Pyrenees made for feudal landlordism with its economically expendable, professional horsemen. And again, it requires a metaphysical affirmation of the "economic basis" as "the real" kernel of social life to construct recent economic changes of competitive war economics in terms of impulses from the economy, rather than from military "necessities" and their technological requirements. At the same time, it is of course obvious that economic and technological conditions limit and facilitate what man can do in the roles and contexts of non-economic institutions.

Such great intellectual constructions are fascinating; the interpretative work of the system builders who would answer the question of "Whither Mankind?" in terms of the hidden labor of "the world spirit," man's "will to power," the "instincts of life and death," or the "productive forces and relations" are intriguing. But the complexity of themes now available in human knowledge has repeatedly proved that all such over-all constructions in their bold emphasis are apt to close rather than to open further inquiry into the rich variety of human thought and experience.

1. Six Questions

Every model of social structure implies a model of social-historical change; history consists of the changes which social structures undergo. When we discussed various institutional orders, and especially their types of integration in Part Three, we had also to analyze social changes. In the present chapter, we will systematize and elaborate the implications of our model of social structure for the analysis and understanding of social-historical change.

I. Our first question is the same as the question posed by problems of integration: *What* is it that changes? What unit is to be observed in change? A conception of social structure as an articulation of institutional orders provides, as we shall see, a set of answers to this question.

II. The second question is *how* this unit changes, which points to psychology as well as to the social sciences in general. It points to psychology for it leads us to seek for the mechanisms which allow the person to redefine his situation, to perceive alternatives, to choose new goals, to raise new demands, to communicate new hopes and fears in the face of challenging tasks and obstacles; in short, to learn new ways of doing things.

The question of how changes occur points to the social sciences in general, for we must ask for the mechanisms which allow newly invented roles to establish themselves in institutional orders alongside previously existing roles and institutions, displacing some, forcing others to adjust, and so on. Borrowing and diffusion, invention and imitation, integration and disintegration, expansion and contraction, acculturation and deculturation, advance and retrogression, and many other such paired terms of social analysis, may prove useful in this connection.

III. We may ask, what is the *direction* of change? At this point, there is a rich vocabulary of value-laden terms, centered around "progress" and "decadence," "integration" and "disintegration," "rise and fall." What from one perspective, for example, appears to be the "decline" of Rome, from another point of view appears to be the "emergence" of feudalism. From the perspective of feudalism, the fact that the Roman *colonus* is tied to hereditary land mortgaged to public services in roadways, water mains, or military fortifications seems like the emergence of serfdom.

IV. What is the *tempo* of change? We are able to discern two different situations in sequence, and the number of discernibly different situations per time-unit may naturally vary. In some parts of some societies, changes may occur in slow-motion, the actors themselves not even being aware of change, which overtakes them unwilling and unaware. In other parts of the society one phase may follow another at baffling speed. It may, for example, be difficult for many Europeans to revise their definitions of the swift redistributions of world power after World War II—until it is brought suddenly into the open by powerful actions.

Psychologically, social changes may thus range from instances of slow-motion which go unnoticed by the participants, to the opposite extreme of historical situations in which the participants take universal change for granted and are surprised at the affirmation of anything allegedly constant other than flux itself. The simple alternative of static v. dynamic accordingly gives way to a series ranging from the relatively constant (for nothing is "absolutely" static) through gradualist drift, deliberately piecemeal and cumulative reforms, through a variety of breaks, discontinuities, and leaps, to total crises and revolutions, with their often incongruous rise and fall of institutions and leaders, symbols and practices.

V. All of these questions about social change, however, even if satisfactorily answered, would not satisfy our explanatory interest. About any given historical epoch we do wish to know what changes, how it changes, in what direction, and at what tempo. But we also wish to know *why* such change is possible and why, in fact, it occurred. Accordingly, we must ask for the necessary and sufficient *causes* of historical change.

VI. We must also answer certain questions which have to do with how "objective" and "subjective" factors in any given historical sequence balance each other. These may conveniently be broken into two questions: (A) What is the causal importance of the individual in history? And (B) what is the causal role of ideas in history? Just as a model of social structure is needed to understand "objective factors," so is a model of character structure and its linkages to social structure needed to understand "subjective" factors.

Under European despotism, historiography was largely court and dynastic historiography; the great decision-makers appeared to be "absolutist" princes and their small circle of generals, cabinet officers and counselors, possibly mistresses and camarillas. Heroized individuals thus appeared to observers as sovereign decision-makers who by "divine grace" or "right" seemed to determine the direction and tempo of history. In his monumental essay on "culture history," Voltaire proposed to pay attention to broad and deep and epochal changes of societies and cultures, and with each periodic upswing of democratic sentiment for the last two centuries his emphasis has been reasserted. It is no accident, incidentally, that whenever great crisis situations bring doubt about "the world we live in" and large scale and protracted warfare among large political units brings statesmen and generals into the center of world-wide attention, the "role of the individual in history" became a topic for discussion. Hegel during the Napoleonic age, and Mommsen under Bismarck, focused on Julius Caesar to illustrate their theories of genius. Sidney Hook under Franklin D. Roosevelt focused upon Lenin and Hitler in illustration of his ideas of event-making and eventful men.[2]

These questions and points of emphasis will be kept in mind as we briefly lay out the existing range of theory, develop a general explanatory model of social-historical change, and consider the dynamics arising from the technological sphere.[3] Moreover, we accept the requirement that a model of social-historical change must enable us not only to understand the units and mechanics of historical sequence, but to locate and to explain, as well as use, other *theories* of social change. As sociology has absorbed much of the old concerns of philosophy of history, a brief reflection on the available theories is appropriate. We can emancipate ourselves only from what we know to be a fetter.

2. The Range of Theory

From a somewhat formal standpoint, theories of social-historical change may be classified into two major types:

I. There are *principled monistic theories,* in which all institutional orders are reduced to one institutional order, and accordingly, a metaphysical accent is placed upon one kind of human behavior and all other institutional behavior is derivative. Vulgar Marxism, many varieties of racial and geographical theories, and vulgar Freudianism illustrate the type.[4]

[2] *The Hero in History* (New York: Day, 1943).

[3] We shall consider the role of "the great man" in history and the character of movements and revolutions below, Chapter XIV: The Sociology of Leadership, and Chapter XV: Collective Behavior.

[4] It is usually the fate of outstanding intellectual work to be banalized in the process of its mass diffusion. Qualifications are dropped in favor of black or white assertions, unsolved intricacies are ignored, open-ended speculations are closed and stereotypes, uncertainties become orthodox credos. So, instead of thinking as did Marx or Freud, epigoni are busy with quotations from their works. All such banalization, we refer to here by the adjective "vulgar."

Vulgar Marxists thus reduce all phenomena to an economic base; economic institutions are thought to be the reality of which everything else is a mere expression. Yet, the fact that religious institutions in Rome draw pilgrims and tourists to Italy and hence affect the Italian currency situation does not make the Vatican an economic institution. Noneconomic institutions are thus "reduced" by analysis to other orders, overlooked, or their causal influence understated. In all such monistic theories there is an implied image of the nature of human nature; in vulgar Marxism, for example, man is seen merely as someone who follows economic interests.

II. There is also *principled and dogmatic pluralism*, which is the more popular theory in current social science. It aims at presumed *a priori* exhaustiveness, and thus tries to explain something as due to all possible causes, rather than by a statement of adequate cause.

We of course assume that social structures are causally bound. Events and transformations, if they are sufficiently known, can always be causally explained. The historical "accident" is not uncaused, but merely, as Sidney Hook once put it, "not deducible from the data of the original system. For example, the breakdown of the rice economy in Japan was determined by the preceding social development; the visit of Commodore Perry by certain political considerations. The conjunction of both was relatively accidental. One event could not have been deduced from the other nor both from a third." [5]

Several factors and mechanisms of social change may of course operate at the same time, and moreover, in various directions. But not all changes are "cumulative," in fact, some are quite jerky and discontinuous. And all phenomena do not result from a great plurality of causes: some are due to unilateral jerks and jolts.

Many thought models of historical change may be useful for discerning types of change in specific historical sequences. Some institutional orders, and no doubt whole social structures, go through what may seem like cycles; other sequences seem linear, while still others seem like the fluctuations of a pendulum. And of course, which model one discerns is in part dependent upon the time-span one uses. We do not believe that any unilateral form

[5] "Determinism," *Encyclopaedia of the Social Sciences*, Vol. V, p. 111. Cf. the remarks on "coincidence," above, Chapter XII: The Unity of Social Structures, Section 3: Modes of Integration.

of change is applicable as a guide to, much less as formal explanation of "history"—even of only Western history. But even though such formal conceptions do not possess explanatory value, it is good to know as many of them as possible. For the plethora of history no doubt exhibits at some time and in some society all of them.

Any one of the institutional orders or spheres, which we have segregated may be (and, in fact, each of them has been) taken as the dominant order from which change springs.

I. There are technological theories of history in which machine industry, scientific enlightenment, and efficiency values are the prime movers—and all else lags behind or adjusts. Naturally, during the rise of industry in the nineteenth century, this process was a major, if not the dominant, experience of Western societies, and so an increasing accentuation was placed upon the technological sphere of the economic order as of crucial importance. We shall presently consider the technological sphere in detail.[6]

II. To construct a theory of history on the basis of the kinship order is to make the growth of population the hub of historical dynamics. Thus Malthus saw a difference between mankind, which procreated according to the Biblical principle of abundance ("Be fruitful and multiply") and the rest of nature, which followed the principle of scarcity. Man's increase is geometric; his food supply only algebraic. Accordingly, the need for food lags behind the growth of population, and this disproportion leads to a growing consciousness of scarcity in the face of niggardly nature. Thus, according to Malthus, if man does not act "responsibly" by curtailing his procreative activity and turn away from Biblical fundamentalism to "adjust" himself to natural scarcity, mass pauperism, infant mortality, and death will effect the appropriate balance between burgeoning population and scanty resources.[7]

When population pressure is posited as the prime historical mover, economists often discern industrial dynamics as one result. The enormous population increase in China since the eighteenth century, under static technological and agricultural conditions, may

    [6] See below, this chapter, Section 3: The Technological Sphere.
    [7] T. R. Malthus, *An Essay on the Principle of Population* (6th ed., 2 vols.; London, 1826).

be referred to as sufficient to disprove the universality claimed for such "laws."

III. Closely connected with technological and population theories is Marx's view, which posits class antagonism as the prime engine of historical change. Of course, Marx's emphasis had its "precursors," and since Marx a broad literature of historical materialist interpretations of various periods has been developed. Thus Karl Kautsky has interpreted early Christendom; Eduard Bernstein, the Cromwellian Revolution; and George Lukács has devoted much effort to analyzing literature in materialist terms.[8]

Today, from East Germany to China, school children learn history from the textbooks of Russian authors. One of these books, which we have had an opportunity to examine, deals with ancient societies, with China, Egypt, the Middle East, Greece, and Rome under the recurrent heading of "slave states." Regardless of whether this or that formulation can stand up, it is characteristic of the emphasis that the religion and literature of ancient China—Confucianism and Taoism—receive three lines, and that in a section on ancient Palestine the Bible is mentioned, as it were, in passing— as if ancient Jewry would merit any attention at all without it.

In such a vulgarized perspective, man's relation to nature is reduced to instrumental and efficiency values, social relations to those of master and slave; and the legacies of ancient civilizations in art, religion, and literature, which astound sensitive minds and motivate intellectual reassessments of their social-historical settings, are pushed to the side and obscured. The humanist horizon, which during the last 150 years the moral and cultural sciences have extended to global scope and prehistoric depth, is reduced, and the thematic range adjusted to the mentality of future production managers. Recent history, which is so important for informed perspectives on the future, is of course rewritten with an artistic freedom beyond the boldest imagination of a Seeley or a Treitschke. Faust's dictum against the historians still holds against such historians as these: "What you call the spirit of the times is in the last analysis your own spirit in which the past is mirrored."

[8] See especially, George Lukács, *Studies in European Realism*, Edith Bone, tr. (London: Hillway, 1950); and the two wonderful volumes by Arnold Hauser, *The Social History of Art* (New York: Knopf, 1951), which pertain to much more than art.

Max Weber has correctly pointed out that in applying historical materialism many authors fail to distinguish between what is economic, what is economically determined, and what is merely economically relevant. Modern social science as a whole has given increasing attention to the economic determination of all sorts of noneconomic institutions and activities. Economic institutions are understood to facilitate and/or to limit religious and artistic, military, and educational activities.

We agree with Weber's evaluation of Marx's emphasis upon the economic order in the modern capitalist era: [9] It is a heuristic choice which holds that the economic order is the most convenient way to an understanding of this specific social structure. So much is fruitful in the Marxist perspective that, although it has not been accepted, much of it has gradually become taken for granted.[10]

In Marx's perspective, the economic order has a unique methodological position among the institutions in capitalist society. For it is the order in terms of which the stratification of the whole society is instituted. Accordingly it is the best point of departure for any realistic examination of instituted stratifications. We also accept the principle of historical specificity, which today means that the problems we face are set by conflicting elements in a specifically capitalist social structure. And we should not forget that Marxist (or Marxist influenced) conceptions of social change have fruitfully corrected those views which dramatize political decision-makers and their work but stop short of asking about the limiting conditions of their power.

IV. E. A. Ross once remarked that the theory of economic determinism needs to be rounded out by a theory of military determinism. There is of course a large literature on militarism which

[9] See the introduction to *From Max Weber, Essays in Sociology* by H. H. Gerth and C. Wright Mills (New York: Oxford, 1946).

[10] The original work of Marx was translated for U.S. academic publics, for example, by Thorstein Veblen, who came to the notion of "lag, leak and friction" between, specifically, business institutions and industrial techniques and institutions. William Ogburn later generalized this so as to take Veblen's leak and friction out of it: the specificity of the tension between business institutions and industrial technology. He generalized it in such a way that he leaves unanswered the question of which elements lag culturally, and specifically why they do. See W. F. Ogburn, *Social Change* (New York: Viking, 1922).

the social scientist ignores at the peril of missing very crucial factors in contemporary change.[11]

Admiral Mahan's essay on seapower opened new and larger perspectives on the great conflict between Napoleon and Great Britain. In brief, the admiral showed that the relative cheapness of sea transport, as compared with the costliness of land movements of mass armies, the cheapness of the blockade plus the acquisition of overseas possessions by Great Britain in her two decades of struggle to down France, in the end proved superior to Napoleonic landpower, no matter how brilliant Napoleon's generalship, no matter how high the morale of revolutionary armies who fought under the sun in Egypt, in the mountains of Spain, or on the snowy plains of Russia. In the contest between a strategy of annihilation and that of attrition, seapower employing attrition proved superior to land power and annihilation. Mahan's brilliant analyses thus brought the economic factor to bear on the contest between sea and land power.

Since then, the world scene has changed, but the general problem has remained. Industrialism has lent greater mobility to land armies. In the railroad age, General Grant understood the condition of victory as he fought for mastery of the railroad lines. And at about the same time, during the war of Prussia and Austria for the hegemony of central Europe, Grant's counterpart in Europe, Hellmuth von Moltke, replaced old-fashioned maps with railroad maps.

Since the end of World War I, a still closer "integration" between industrial technology and the art of warfare has come about. Mass armies are motorized, as is military personnel, in the air and under the sea. Trucks and submarines, tanks and airplanes have reopened the problems of the Napoleonic strategy of annihilation on the European continent. Yet sea power and the blockade weapon, along with superior airpower based on U.S. industry, have proved on a now global scale that Mahan's ideas are still pertinent.

Meanwhile, all single-track theories of war that rely on "one weapon" as the last word—on the infantry or artillery (Stalin), on sea power (Mahan) or "air power" (Douhet, Seversky), on the "superiority" of the defense (Liddell Hart, Maginot) or the

[11] See Alfred Vagts, *A History of Militarism* (New York: Norton, 1937) and *Makers of Modern Strategy*, E. M. Earle and others, eds. (Princeton: Princeton Univ. Press, 1943) and the references contained therein.

offense ("the offensive is the best defense"), on the wisdom of trading time for space and "winning the last battle"—have been proved to be partial, and in some contexts to be fallacious.

The theater of world wars is now the world, and the deployment of means and stratagems is total. Whatever destructive and productive capacities men develop they seem likely to use in war. No fear or warning has ever deterred men from hoping for the triumph of their side by use of "superior" force. Thus during the Middle Ages the pope of Christendom condemned the tactics of the English yeomen who with crossbows ambushed unsuspecting knights. During World War I, submarine warfare appeared to the great naval powers as a criminal breach of all the rules of international law and Christian morality. But in the middle of the twentieth century the dropping of atomic bombs has caused no effective moral upheaval, and since the distinction between combatants and noncombatants by all sorts of weapons of destruction has been eliminated, we may safely expect that men will use all weapons at their command in any war to come.

V. There are thinkers who view ideas as the ultimate core of human will and action and who, accordingly, assume that "ideas," "public opinion," or "propaganda" are the prime movers in history. Arnold Toynbee, for example, in his monumental study of twenty-six civilizations reaches the conclusion that Western civilization is doomed without a Christian revival.[12]

During the eighteenth century, intellectuals experienced the formation and rise of a new mass public for their works, which were distributed by the press, the novel, and pamphlet. Their ideas aroused and inspired those middle-class movements of the Western world that accompanied the industrial revolution, and they came to feel that they were supported by an increasingly broad and self-conscious public. In turn, they legitimated the "rights of man" in the name of "public opinion," which accordingly became the master formula for a complex network of solidarizations in the reading halls and coffee houses, the salons of philosophers and the political clubs of factions. "Public opinion" became a master symbol for the demands of the middle class, and the intellectuals

[12] See *A Study of History* (London, 1951), Vol. VI, p. 278.

experienced their own role in terms of the historical force of ideas. Although he broke with this tradition in the early 1840's, Karl Marx stated, "Theory, too, becomes a material force as soon as it takes hold of the masses." [13]

Out of the experience of modern liberalism there arose the conception that the ideas of "exceptional individuals" are essential in historical dynamics; that public opinion makes history; that history is a sequence of ideas. The classic liberal statement of such an ideological theory of history or of progress is given by John Stuart Mill, who in this respect was influenced by Comte:

"Now the evidence of history and that of human nature combine, by a striking instance of consilience, to show that there really is one social element which is thus predominant, and almost paramount, among the agents of the social progression. This is, the state of the speculative faculties of mankind: including the nature of the beliefs which by any means they have arrived at, concerning themselves and the world by which they are surrounded.

"It would be a great error, and one very little likely to be committed, to assert that speculation, intellectual activity, the pursuit of truth, is among the more powerful propensities of human nature, or holds a predominating place in the lives of any, save decidedly exceptional individuals. But notwithstanding the relative weakness of this principle among other sociological agents, its influence is the main determining cause of the social progress; all the other dispositions of our nature which contribute to that progress, being dependent on it for the means of accomplishing their share of the work . . . in order that mankind should conform their actions to any set of opinions, these opinions must exist, must be believed by them. And thus, the state of the speculative faculties, the character of the propositions assented to by the intellect, essentially determines the moral and political state of the community, as we have already seen that it determines the physical.

"These conclusions, deduced from the laws of human nature, are in entire accordance with the general facts of history. Every considerable change historically known to us in the condition of any portion of mankind, when not brought about by external force,

[13] See his "Criticism of the Hegelian Philosophy of Right" (*Selected Essays by Karl Marx*, H. T. Stenning, tr. New York: International Publishers, 1926), p. 11.

has been preceded by a change, or proportional extent, in the state of their knowledge, or in their prevalent beliefs." [14]

We have already criticized this view in Chapter X: The Symbol Sphere.

3. The Technological Sphere

By the "technological sphere" we refer to tools and machines as well as to the ways in which they are used. In this sphere we find wheelbarrows and prayer wheels, flint knives and rosaries, bulldozers, carbide tipped lathe chisels, plywood, and atom bombs. But beyond these material objects, the term also covers the implementation of human conduct by such tools and machines, which means that it refers to the various skills required of those using such artifacts.

I. *Technology and Institutions.* Many modern theories of social change, as we have seen, stress technological developments, and many statements of the major phases of history are constructed as levels of technology. Classifications of technology may be put in several ways, each no doubt useful for some purposes. In terms of the dominant raw *materials* employed, we have ages of stone, wood, copper, bronze, iron, steel. In terms of the source of *power* that is used, we have men and beasts, coal and steam, gasoline motors and electrical power, and finally, atomic energy. Each of these, alone or in combinations, is a useful empirical classification.

For our purposes, however, we find a third way of classifying technologies more promising: in terms of the institutional context(s) in which they are primarily anchored and the social context in which the use and management of a societies' technology appear to center. All institutional orders have their technologies, the religious no less than the economic order or the symbol sphere. There are techniques for playing the piano just as there are techniques for handling a die-casting or a chalice. The ends to which the techniques serve as a means will obviously be determined by the order in which the technique is instituted. Accordingly, the development of the technical sphere in any order is steered and limited by the ends of that order.

[14] *A System of Logic* (7th ed.; New York: Longmans, 1930), Vol. II, pp. 523-24.

If the end is salvation and Buddhist monks believe that many prayers serve better than one prayer, then the technique of praying may proceed by the construction of prayer wheels. Slips carrying a short prayer are fastened to the spokes of the wheel and one full turn of each prayer-carrying spoke is counted as one prayer in behalf of the salvation seeker. One step toward greater efficiency involves the addition of more spokes built into the wheel, or making it spin faster, and finally instead of man's tired hand, wind and waterpower are harnessed to the prayer wheel. This increased prayer output ramifies into a sort of salvation economy. Rivers and streams are valued according to their water flow, for swift currents make for more prayers in one's lifetime. The owners of fortunately placed prayer wheels thus have an abundance of prayers to their credit and may come to feel that they actually have surplus prayers, that is, more than is needed for their salvation. They may then respond to their less fortunate brothers by transferring surplus prayers to their credit.

In modern society, technological spheres range from simple gadgets to complex machines. Kinship roles are modified by the level and type of household technology available, especially in cellar, bathroom, and kitchen. Military roles now involve quite elaborate machines and techniques: modern war technology is not imaginable without a fusion with industrial technology. In the religious order, there are above all great cathedrals, with their pulpits and altars; and in many religious units, more elaborate and specialized implements of worship. In the political order, in addition to palaces and parliaments, there are flags, seals, and files, which implement roles technically and symbolically.

But it is in the economic order's units of production that modern technology is centered and anchored. Indeed, so much is this the case, that most theories of technology as the prime mover and shaker of history tend to shade, often imperceptibly, into an economic determinism.

Now, however accurate the quasi-identification of technology and economy may be for modern history, we run the risk of unwarranted historical generalization when we take it as a universal fact. There has been no steady onward push of technology in the course of world history. It is well known, or should be, that between the third millennium B.C. and the eleventh century A.D., no basic technological developments occurred in the West. In fact, only the earliest river-valley civilizations of neolithic Egypt, Sumeria, China, and the West's modern era (especially the eleventh century and then from the sixteenth to date) have witnessed striking technological progression.

In our formal model of social-historical change, and the role of technology within it, we must remain carefully open-minded and historically specific. The technological sphere is not self-determining; it is not autonomous; it does not develop "all by itself." On the contrary, to be part of history, technology must be instituted—it must involve men in skilled roles—and it may be primarily instituted in orders other than the economic. Today we observe in leading industrial societies a shift in the center of technological initiative and guidance from the economic to the military. In contrast to the nineteenth century, nowadays military, as much as economic, orientations and goals determine how technology progresses; which features of the culmination of invention and material uses will be pushed further, and which held back; which roles in which orders will be implemented by technology and which will not; and thus what social effects technology has. Thus atomic power is being developed for propelling a submarine, not an ocean liner. In modern war, as we have already remarked, all orders and spheres—including the technological—tend to become ramifications of military and political orders.

Due to religious constraints, technological implementation of the household—from kitchen utensils to drawing room comfort—is not found among the Old Order Amish. But the very same religion, in its inner-worldly asceticism, places a premium on active technological ingenuity and inventiveness in the sphere of production. Early in the eighteenth century the ancestors of the Amish along the Rhine invented crop rotation and the winter feeding of livestock (clover); later, as the Pennsylvania Dutch, they astonished their neighbors by putting artificial fertilizers on their fields. Today the Amish install telephones outside their homes in the yard or workshop for business calls, but they will not use them for social calls; they install electricity in their carpenter shops, but they will not wire their homes; they accept the internal combustion motor when it is used in a tractor, but not in a private car. They accept technology only in production, not in consumption.

In the classical Oriental civilization, priestly and quasi-religious bureaucracies have guided technological developments. In India and in Egypt there were colossal temples and pyramidal tombs; and in China, in addition to the Great Wall, there were the Imperial Canal and other irrigation projects, instituted and governed politically, upon which the economy depended.

In the Mediterranean epoch, technological advance was anchored in and restricted to the military, religious, and political orders and the realm of consumption. But in the production zones of the economy, technological advance was deterred. Thus in ancient Rome, the hand and stone mill was never displaced by the water mill, despite the fact that the water mill had been described by Strabo. The risks of slave labor on the plantations, the constant danger of rebellious sabotage, made more complicated and costly machinery unprofitable. The Romans never learned to make effective use of more than two draft animals, for they never learned to hitch teams head-to-tail; hence large teams could not be used for draft work, and the *Quadruga* drawn by four horses hitched shoulder-to-shoulder was more for show than for efficiency. On the other hand, descriptions by Caesar, as well as by others, reveal that the Roman legions were capable of using fairly complicated siege machinery and of great engineering feats in military highways and bridges. And the Romans developed an extensive and colossal technology in the sphere of consumption: aqueducts, complicated circus buildings, and hot water in bathrooms.

Whereas in the case of the Old Order Amish technological advances for four centuries remained strictly confined to production, in ancient Rome technological advances were confined to consumption and warfare, and did not influence the technique of production. Therefore, it may be said that technological spheres do not advance simply on the basis of available knowledge of technical possibilities, but that institutions must raise effective demands for the incorporation of technical implements.

There is no automatic causal relation between the technological sphere and any institutional order, and there is no automatic harmony among the technological spheres of different orders. It has been repeatedly observed during the last fifty years that technological advances of progressive munitions makers have been blocked by the conservatism of military personnel. Alfred Krupp's fight against the Prussian officer corps for the introduction of his superior products was successful only after a German ship carrying the older guns had been sunk by a vessel making use of Krupp guns. The biographies of Count von Zeppelin or Alfred Nobel provide similar illustrations, as do those of Samuel Colt and Billy Mitchell in America. Were military chieftains as conservative as the plantation heads of old Rome, we might conceive of a social structure in which disproportionate technical advances worked in favor of the economic, and to the disfavor of the military. But military conservatism is not the whole story. We meet just as frequently with military demands for technological advances. The development of the medieval gun foundry, the tank, the radio, as well as the subsidizing of modern aeronautics and the production of underwater vessels and atomic energy plants, would probably have been greatly delayed without the demands of war.

II. *Skill Levels and Role Changes.* The technological sphere of an institutional order determines the levels and types of skill required for the enactment of its various roles. As technology and technical roles change, so do the required skills. If we take the role as our unit of change, and focus upon its skill aspect, we are able to understand, up close as it were, the social implications of technological change.

A. Technology may force the formation of new roles as well as the obsolescence of old ones within an institution; it may also prompt the instituting of educational spheres for training the players of these roles.

B. Technology may determine the adequate criteria to be used for the selection of persons to enact the roles it has prompted or reshaped.

C. Finally, technology may split one role into two or more roles, or force the convergence of many complex roles into one simplified role. These positive and negative effects upon required skills and upon the selection and formation of persons to exercise them may, of course, occur in given institutional contexts, and accordingly their "timing" will vary.

In a market for skilled labor, those persons who are playing skilled roles for pay and who cannot effectively claim scarcity value for their skill may gain permanent roles only after they have successfully filled provisional ones. On the other hand, those who, on the basis of the irreplaceability of their skills, monopolize key positions may haggle and bargain for job security as a condition of their employment. This is typically true of eminent scholars or die-casters, highly paid executives or professional soldiers, diplomats or administrative officials.

Loss of skill may result in loss of the role requiring it; such loss of adequate skill may be due to bodily injury or aging or to technological innovation. If institutional demand for certain skills should decline, due to technological or economic changes, intensified competition for the shrinking opportunities may lead to loss of skills by those who have no opportunity to practice them. This is one of the consequences of mass unemployment during business depressions, or of defeat in war, with the discharge of military professionals. After some time, such competitively disadvantaged actors may lose their hopes of ever marketing their skills and so of returning to their former roles; if this should happen, the objective relinquishment of the role is subjectively completed.

Specialization of skills is involved in specialization of roles. What was formerly done by one man may, in a division of labor, be divided, and two men perform it. A new skill role thus develops. In the mass production of music for motion pictures, the role of the composer is split into those who think up tunes, those who arrange accompanying chords, those who make the instrumental arrangements, and so on. Institutional mechanics may also take the opposite course, by setting up a demand that one man combine two skills in one role. One man now does what was formerly done by two. Thus a household, finding itself in economic difficulties, may save money by replacing its gardener and chauffeur by one person who takes care of the lawn and also drives the car, or the roles of maid and cook may be merged.

Technological changes thus eliminate and create roles; in fact, entire institutions, with their varying roles, may be eliminated by the introduction of new techniques. Such changes naturally involve hopes and fears which must be understood in their precise role context. New roles which carry higher status or income or power create and channel ambitions and hopes. The contraction of roles in any institutional order tends to produce scarcity consciousness and insecurity feelings on the basis of which one may observe heightened competition among job holders who seek to displace one another. Or, in contrast, the pressures may call forth solidarity sentiments in defense of jobs which the threatened workers or military men have come to consider as "theirs" by right of years of service. Anxieties or frustrations aroused in this way may appear in other contexts of the person as aggressions. Thus the anxieties of small manufacturers originating in the technological sphere of an economic order may cause cumulative hostilities which may be "free floating" or which may be expressed in the political order or in family life, in mass spectator sports or in a seat on the aisle in the dark of a movie. To the extent to which the helpless person, under the guidance of a severe generalized other and lack of insight, suppresses such hostilities, he may develop guilt feelings and hence punish himself. In extreme cases, such "masochist" tendencies to self-punishment may tempt a desperate man to suicide, or, by a curious inversion of cause and effect, it may compel the actor to "ask for it" by committing a crime. The new transient role, that of the criminal, "makes sense" to him. Technological changes, understood sociologically, may thus have many complicated consequences. But then no causal sequence in a social structure, when adequately traced, is simple.

Although technique is not linked exclusively to economic institutions, since the seventeenth century, science, technology, and economic institutions have become firmly linked. Since then, the technique of production has circumscribed the limitations and possibilities of all technical implementation. Without the modern glass industry, astronomy could not have its giant telescopes; without the production of photographic equipment, modern microscopic observation would be impossible. Without the skill of the carpenter, the occidental violin would be impossible; crafts and skills are thus necessary preconditions for the development of instrumental music. Whatever else his music may express, Bach composed *The Well Tempered Clavichord* to prove the adequate range and possibilities of the instrument when tuned in this way.

The priest and the artist as well as the die-maker must acquire facility with routines—routines which are required for adequately handling the instruments each uses. Insofar as imagination is technologically oriented, it is to be found in all spheres of social life. There are musical "inventions" just as there are electrical inventions. There may of course be differences in tempo between the development of human skill and the production of instruments. A new instrument is a challenge to old skills: it was thirty years after the perfection of the violin by Stradivari and Guarnieri before Corelli invented and established the role of the violin virtuoso. But the reverse may also hold: human skills may confront problems the solutions to which become possible only if suitable technological inventions are available. Beethoven's compositions and style of performance demanded that the piano pedal be developed. He did not develop his technique of composition because the concert grand piano had been invented; the concert piano was promoted by Beethoven, who told the instrument makers what he needed. Sometimes skills lag; sometimes technologies do.

W. H. E. Lecky wrote: [15] "The causes which most disturbed or accelerated the normal progress of society in antiquity were the appearance of great men, in modern times they have been the appearance of great inventions . . . The leading characteristics of modern societies are in consequence marked out much more by the triumphs of inventive skill than by the sustained energy of moral causes." This might lead us to believe that "the inventor" as a type of man has in modern times replaced "the great man" of antiquity. Such an inference would be incorrect. For the inventor— as a free-lance man combining industrial ingenuity and scientific ability—was, in fact, a short-lived type, existing between the era of static technology, which ended in the eighteenth century, and the era of bureaucratized science and bureaucratized industry of the twentieth century. The origins of the inventor lay in the Renaissance of Leonardo and of experimental artisans; his end was already adumbrated in the early nineteenth century, for example, in Balzac's image of David Séchard.[16]

III. *The Autonomy of Technology.* We have remarked that technology does not advance automatically, of its own force; that before technology can effect historical changes, institutions must raise effective demands to incorporate it; that institutional orders vary in this respect; and hence that the technological spheres of different societies are differently anchored. Nevertheless, does not technology have some causal autonomy? Does it not exert a long-run causal force, even if unevenly, upon human institutions everywhere, at all times? These are the rhetorical questions of "technological determinism," perhaps nowadays the leading theory of social change, and there is something to them.

[15] See his *History of European Morals* (New York: Appleton, 1929), 1897, Vol. I, pp. 126-27.
[16] See his *Lost Illusions* (Temple ed.; New York: Macmillan, 1910), especially Part II.

One aspect of the conception of technological development as autonomous deserves particular attention: many discoveries have not been made out of regard for any usefulness. Of course they have been adapted with great ingenuity to given demands, but the discoveries themselves were the results of combinations playfully made out of the existing stock of technologies and ideas. It is the impact of one discovery or invention upon scientific workers in other contexts of discovery that forms the internal interaction of the quasi-organized workmanship and idea-ship of science and technology. It is this "immanent logic" of playful or systematic combinations that is concretely meant by the "idle curiosity" of the scientist, or the pursuit of science for science's own sake.

Now the phrase, "science and technology," stands for an intricately specialized division of labor. Agents well entrenched in the given institutions—modern manufacturers, for example—constantly scan the world scientific output for items useful to their own marketable product. Other agents—those of the military order of the victorious nations of World War I—rested on their oars and had to have some technologies useful to their ends forced upon them by the new model armies of the defeated. But, according to the theory of the autonomous technological continuum and the logic of combinations, neither manufacturer or general can go further than the continuum permits. Of course, by supporting or failing to support the work, they can slow it up or speed it along. Atomic energy research, for example, had quite different settings in the United States and in Hitler Germany. Whereas President Roosevelt promptly responded to Einstein's letter in 1939 and was ready to set aside substantial funds and facilities, Hitler proved less available to the counsel of physicists who were of course unable to guarantee results within six months, as he demanded. Hitler operated in a context of "autarchy" and scarcity; Roosevelt, as far as resources for military requirements are concerned, in an economy of comparative abundance.

In and of itself, the technological continuum is socially, economically, and morally blind; it is no Messiah; it has no other aim then to allow man to implement any given end he may have, with less physical effort in a shorter time. "Radio" can broadcast music or it can teach that the world is flat. But institutions are not blind. The institutional "market" for science takes up the discoveries of science at various stages of the ongoing process of science, and turns them into commodities, weapons, and tools. Oil men gave geologists a hearing, Franklin Giddings [17] once remarked, because geologists make money for them. And there is often a great institutional gap, especially in mature capitalist societies, between scientific discoveries and their public use: legal and business institutions often hold back this "rational" and apparently easy transition. And if we consider "technological unemployment" in the long run as "irrational," surely we have learned that what is technically efficient and economically profitable is not necessarily socially rational. Science is not automatically "at the service of mankind."

But that does not mean that profit-making or war-making or monopolist restriction of invention and frozen patents, "set the ends" of science and technology. There has been, in modern times, a complicated interplay between industry and technology, business and science. Both sides of the interplay reached their modern scale and tempo together. New industries grew from a complex of inventions, and industries have subsidized the development of new leaps forward in technical skills and big gadgets. Inventors have made money-makers possible; money-makers have subsidized inventors, and exploited their work.

Necessity or purpose is the mother of adaptive inventions; but invention is also the mother of necessity. There is nothing in the logic or in the course of science that dictates that its results will be used for any particular end, or indeed that it will be used at all. The growing points of the technological continuum may or may not coincide with the growing points of institutional demand. Both shift, pass one another, coincide for a moment, move on.

The person may become attached to the skill aspects of his roles in such a way that his feelings transcend the orienting function of the institution of which his role is a part. Such internalized standards are involved in all "craftsmanship," and groups, such as the guild, may have ethical and status codes which keep standards of skill high. Craftsmanship also refers to the joyful experience of mastering the resistance of the materials with which one works, or the solution of self-imposed tasks—an experience that might occur

[17] *Civilization and Society* (New York: Holt, 1932), p. 164.

irrespective of the opinions of other persons or of any rule that exists.[18]

The technological sphere has an inner dynamic just as all spheres do, but the chances that technological advances will be instituted by given institutions are not determined solely by the state of technology. They are also determined by the premiums which given institutions place upon the incorporation of such advances. The technology of any given time is a necessary condition for the technical dynamics of an institutional order, but not a sufficient cause for their explanation. In order to have a steamboat it is necessary to have a boat and a steam engine, but to institute a steamboat in the economic or military orders, the boat must be recognized as a serviceable means to the ends of these orders. Napoleon, we recall, refused Fulton's offer.

4. Social-historical Change

By social change we refer to whatever may happen in the course of time to the roles, the institutions, or the orders comprising a social structure: their emergence, growth, and decline. Our model of social structure thus provides us with several interconnected units, each of which may undergo quantitative as well as qualitative, microscopic as well as macroscopic, change.

When we focus upon the concept of role as the unit of social change, we ask how many people play a given role and, at what tempo is one role displaced by another. The first point of observation may be illustrated by the decrease of independent producers in certain industries. The displacement of one role by another may be illustrated by the shift from entrepreneurial to managerial roles in the economic order.

The institution may be taken as the unit; again the number of

[18] One economic aspect of this technical quality is that only relatively wealthy patrons can pay for handicraft; the masses have to do without them. High standards of skill demand long years of apprenticeship, hence the social exclusiveness of the guilds, the worker insisting upon controlling his product from raw material to its completion. Thus we find helmet-makers, sword-makers, shoe-makers, glove-makers. Industrial technology follows a different principle of specialization. In its course from raw material to finished product, the product passes, as it were, through numerous plants, and one firm, such as General Electric, may produce more than 30,000 differently priced products by incorporating a great variety of skill groups in one enterprise.

any given type of institution—churches or sects, factories or farms—as well as the types of institutions that most generally prevail. Thus, individual enterprises in the economic order are replaced by corporations; and there is a decline of independent entrepreneurships.

We may use the institutional order as our unit of change, and thus speak of the changing numbers of institutions of given types that exist in that order, the types of institutions that have become dominant or secondary within an order, and finally, the shifting relations of this order to other orders. If there are disproportionate changes of one type of institution within the order, as over against another, we might observe a shift from quantitative to qualitative kinds of changes. Thus, when the small independent enterprise is displaced by the giant corporation as the dominant institutional type, the whole order, as it were, has undergone a basic change.

The social structure itself can be "overturned," as in total revolution or other epochal transitions. This means that in each institutional order we observe a shift, not only of personnel, but in the type of institution that prevails. It also usually means that the orders composing the social structure, the way in which they are articulated and related, are recomposed so that a new social structure emerges. And most important, such revolutions mean that the legitimations and their ideological elaboration change.

Microscopic and macroscopic changes may occur inside the social structure as a whole, inside given orders, or inside institutions, and these changes may occur at disproportionate rates, in quantitative and in qualitative ways.[19]

[19] Of course, other units of change may be chosen. For example, perhaps the simplest observable change is the purely quantitative increase or decrease of the biological units composing a society. An increase in the average weight of a newly born infant, or of the height of the average man, is not, of course, in and of itself social change, but neither is it a purely "natural process." Such changes can often be ascribed to changed social conditions, such as standards of living or effective diets. Socially conditioned biological changes of this sort, in turn, become socially relevant; the size of army uniforms must be changed, school benches become cramped or obsolete.

Only insofar as social actions are oriented to biological data are such data of direct sociological account. In Germany, for example, kinky hair has not been of public concern, but under Nazism, the distribution of blond hair and blue eyes became relevant, spurious status premiums having been ideologically placed upon them. With the motorization of the modern army,

Many changes in society may be tabulated as changes in quantity. A price curve symbolizes the changing prices which at different times result from price-fights between buyers and sellers competing in, or monopolizing, specific markets: such curves present in concise brevity the points at which on-going interest conflicts were settled by compromise. Any occupation may increase or decline in its membership; and in like manner, the number of institutions in any order or structure may wax or wane.

Such quantitative changes often have qualitative aspects. If the same number of persons live in a scatter they will behave differently and feel differently than if they live huddled together. In the family and in the factory, an increase in the number of actors who are playing given roles will affect all the actors. A small nation of 1 million differs from a large nation of 100 million in a quantitative way, but also in its qualitative position among nations: only large nations are "great powers." The same positional difference may hold for institutions within any order: The Roman Catholic Church is a church of the Western World; the Norwegian Lutheran Church is confined to one nation.

The uneven growth of institutions in the same order changes the composition of that order.[20] If such a structural change occurs with a corresponding change in the composition of other orders, we may speak of proportionate change; if it occurs without such correspondence, we may speak of disproportionate changes between these orders. There may be disproportions in the growth of roles within an institution; or of different types of institutions belonging to the same order. Laissez-faire capitalism is based upon a large number of small competing enterprises; monopoly capitalism results from the disproportionate growth of certain enterprises which finally transform given industries into a handful of great enterprises.

In Germany, during the 1920's, the economic order was increasingly dominated by monopoly corporations, but the political order disintegrated into a competitive scatter of parties, which were superseded during the great depression by the Nazis. Such

flat feet become of less relevance than they were for walking armies. See Chapter III: Organism and Psychic Structure, Section 1: The Social Relevance of the Organism.

[20] See Karl Mannheim, *Man and Society in an Age of Reconstruction* (New York: Harcourt, Brace, 1940).

quantitative changes in one order, without corresponding changes in other orders, may provide the recomposed order the opportunity to exert increasing influence within a social structure. If such influences are lasting, and no correspondence takes place, the position of the order within the social structure often changes significantly: the social structure is recomposed.[21]

It is typical that in the process of institutional recomposition, actors interested in the advancement and expansion of their own orders, will subjectively experience other orders as an encroachment upon their interests. The rise of economic liberalism, in opposition to the prerogatives of the mercantilist state, may again serve as a brief illustration:

The mercantilist prince used part of his tax-income to benefit certain manufacturers through subsidies, tax exemptions, and charters, guaranteeing to such establishments a production monopoly and/or a market. Such privileged enterprises typically handled luxury products for court society (chinaware, tapestries, silver), as well as military provisions. In the meantime, middle-class industrialists, especially their vanguard of textile entrepreneurs, produced for civilian mass consumption. From their point of view, mercantilist enterprises and state-managed enterprises (for example, spinning in prisons) constituted unfair competition, facilitated through what seemed to them an uneconomic investment of the taxes they helped pay. For such taxes raised their costs of production and hence restricted their sales. Insofar as taxes upon the rest of the population served state mercantilist activities, they drained off purchasing power which otherwise, as consumers' demands, might encourage nonmercantilist enterprise. As production for profit on the basis of calculations of costs and prices is identified with rationality, so mercantilist tax policies and other interferences in the economic order appear as an irrational encroachment of the political order upon the economic. From this irrationality, the bourgeoisie wished to be freed. Hence, "control of the budget" became their battle cry and the first princely prerogative which, by their parliamentary parties, they sought to curtail.[22]

[21] See Chapter XII: The Unity of Social Structures, Section 3: Modes of Integration.

[22] They may succeed in these aspirations without recourse to violence as in the case of England's Reform Bill of 1832, or in the face of such aspira-

To analyze historical change, we have said, requires that we find out what it is precisely that changes, how it changes, in what direction, at what rate of speed, and why. These apparently simple questions, as we have seen, involve many contentious theories. There are no satisfactory over-all answers, but there are general ways of questioning which we find convenient to map out in terms of our working model of social structure.

We cannot accept any universalist theory of history based on any one institutional order or upon the type of personality prevalent in it. At any given historical time the precise scope of each of the institutional orders—and their relations to all others—must be determined. These weights and relations are empirically open questions, and we should keep them open, in such a way as to enable us to construct any given epoch in terms of *its* dominant mode of historical change.

There are many examples of how given institutional orders are variously involved in historical change. The shift from war to peace, or from peace to war, obviously sets different relations between the military and other institutional orders.

The shift from peace to war in industrial nations tends to make the military order supreme, and hence gives the expert in military administration and violence at least veto power over anything he fears might impede the war effort. It also alters status relations, for prestige seems always to cluster around that order which is most authoritative. The supremacy of the military order tends to raise the prestige of the armed forces.

Since modern war requires mass armies, it entails the removal

tions, the political order may prove to be inelastic, and agents of the status quo may threaten to maintain and enforce their prerogatives violently. Then a disrupture of the social structure becomes possible, and in such crises, the middle classes may establish armed forces of their own. Against the divine right of kings, they posit the "sovereignty of the people" or of the nation. If the king is successful in restoring his authority, disarming the insurrectionist forces, expelling, arresting, or otherwise punishing the intellectual, political and military leaders, then we speak of putsch or rebellion: the European "revolutions" of 1848. If, however, the insurrectionist forces are successful, seize power and establish a new political constitution (with or without the old king) we may speak of political revolution: The English Revolution of 1649, the American Revolution of 1776, the French Revolution of 1789.

For further remarks on revolutions, see Chapter XV: Collective Behavior, Section 4: Revolution and Counterrevolution.

of large numbers of men from gainful employment (or from unemployment), and from the kinship order. Thus, there are fewer husbands available; many families are without fathers, many mothers without sons, many girls without boys. An increasing number of women assume employment roles formerly enacted by men.

The war effort provides the framework for all orders; the expansion of any order is encouraged only to the extent to which such expansion may contribute to victory. Technological development follows this pattern: uniforms and soldier's diets, microfilm correspondence and motorized army chapels, barracks and bomb shelters undergo intensive and extensive development. But durable consumers' goods—houses and motor cars, refrigerators and television—are out for the duration. There are heavy jet fighters, but no civilian helicopters.

The great elasticity of modern social structure is indicated by the rapidity with which institutional orders may be recomposed and millions of people accommodated to the recomposition. The disciplinary aspects involved are important psychological features of such processes. They involve new rules and regulations, enacted and decreed, which are enforced by various agencies, and channeled through the mass media, as well as educational, religious and other institutions. Consumption patterns are adjusted to rationing and price control, priority and war production; the free job mobility of workers and of people in "defense areas" is legally curtailed; compulsory labor service, civilian defense and national youth organizations are successfully introduced. Millions of people are evacuated from metropolitan areas, school children segregated from their families. And in so far as men identify with the "will to win," the executive-enforced codes lead to new conventions which underpin them.

When we try to answer questions about the transformations of a total society, we must realize that every social area is connected, directly or indirectly, with every other, in short that institutions and roles are interdependent. But we must also realize that that is not saying much: we must find a "way into" these many interconnections. The easiest "way in" involves examination of those institutional orders in which roles are implemented by control over things that require joint activities: the means of production and communication, the means of destruction, the means of administration, or in other words, the economic, the military, and the political order.

The economic order is the starting point for the analysis of roles connected with the level of technology, the degree of specialization of labor, and the class structure of the respective society. It offers us an approach to the big structural dimensions of a society.

The political order, with its various specifications of executive functions, offers us an approach to distributions of power and prestige and, via the staff-enforced distribution of "rights" among all members of the society, especially to "property rights" in which we find a convenient linkage between political and economic affairs.

In interpreting contemporary social change, we have found ourselves more and more interested in those roles and technologies that involve violence and which involve economic production. Like many other observers we believe that revolutions in these orders are now crucial to the course of world history. Tools and arms, industrial machines and military weapons, factories and armies, skill levels and practices of violence—how these interplay with each other seem to us most immediately relevant to the course of twentieth-century societies.

When we consider types of change characterizing an entire social structure, we already have at hand modes of integration. For correspondence, coincidence, co-ordination, and convergence, as we have noted,[23] are not only useful in analyzing integration, but also sequences of historical change; in fact, these modes of integration appear, in dynamic perspective, as principles of social-historical change.

The problem of a "theory of history" is neither one of monistic hunches or principled pluralism, but rather a search for the causes of specific historical sequences: those causes which according to experience and the conventional standards of scientific evidence satisfy our curiosity. In any given historical epoch, we must discern shifts within and between institutional orders, and then we must search for their adequate causes. The mode of historical change characteristic of a given epoch will thus be more or less an inference from the types of integration which prevail in the social structure we are examining.

[23] In Chapter XII: The Unity of Social Structures, Section 3: Modes of Integration.

CHAPTER

XIV

The Sociology of Leadership

AN adequate model for the analysis of leadership must enable us to understand Nicolai Lenin on his way to the Finland Station, as well as the girl next door who advises our daughter on make-up; what happened to Rousseau's ideas and how Tolstoi's general commanded; why a radio songstress influences the intonations of a million high school girls, as well as what happened when Stalin met Ribbentrop. It must enable us to understand those epochal turning points of history in which some individual seems to be the pivot, as well as the trivial, casual, day-to-day influences of everyday life: the genius who is worshipped from afar as a hero, the opinion leader who lives next door.

Leadership, most broadly conceived, is a relation between leader and led in which the leader influences more than he is influenced: because of the leader, those who are led act or feel differently than they otherwise would. As a power relation, leadership may be known to both leader and led, or unknown to either or both; it may be close-up or long-distance; it may occur at a single crossroad in the lives of both, or only in the life of the follower, after the leader is long dead; it may affect only a momentary decision, or it may dominate the life of the led.

How can we sort out all these rather vague phenomena of leadership in order to gain a view that is at once empirically adequate and analytically suggestive? Along what dimensions can we simplify what is involved into types which can then be studied systematically? To understand leadership, we must pay attention to (1) the traits and motives of the leader as a *man;* (2) the *images* that selected publics hold of him, and their motives for following him; (3) the *roles* he plays as a leader, their salient characteristics, and how the leader reacts to them; and (4) the structural *con-*

texts in which his roles, as well as those of the led, are involved. We must analyze each of these aspects of leadership in order to group their possible ranges; and we must systematically relate them—in order to understand their logically possible connections in various types of leadership.

It may not be fruitful to treat all situations of *power* as involving leadership; perhaps we should delimit leadership to certain kinds of *authority*.

A bicyclist may adjust to the movements of the motorist, but the power of the motorist over the bicyclist does not bespeak of "leadership." It is also true that not all men who are interested in having their way are also interested in having others follow them. And, in turn, the weak man may accommodate to the moves of the strong lest he be crushed, but not in order to follow his lead. Coercion of the weak by the strong, whether physical or economic, does not constitute relations of leader and follower, although such relations may emerge from originally naked power situations.

To be called a leader one must wish to have his way accepted, and the direction of the follower's behavior must be in agreement with the leader's own course. Where the led accepts the leader's "right" to influence his course of conduct we attribute not merely power but "legitimate power" or "authority" to the leader.

There are of course all sorts of constellations of authority and power relationships. Should we call a patriarchal father the "leader" of his family? Should we consider a railroad official who advises us about which train to take a "leader"? Not every "superior" is a leader in that he "leads us on" to some goal, and not every ruler has a goal or need have one, beyond maintaining existing routines. Yet to limit "leadership" in some such way would mean to eliminate attention to traditional leaders as well as to underlings who merely execute the will and intention of policy-makers who actually "lead on."

1. The Leader as a Man: His Traits and Motives

It is more fruitful in the beginning to study the social roles of leaders in various contexts than the individual traits of leaders in social isolation. The traits so far discerned by students of leadership are either so formal as to be useless and unrevealing, or, if specific, as varied as the different groups led by the leaders. Some putative traits have been supposed to be organic, so that history is reduced to nature, society to biology; others have been, supposedly, socially acquired. We now know that the first is a fruitless error of reduction and the second inadequate sociology—unless the search for leadership traits is closely united with depictions of the roles of leaders in different groups, in particular with the way these roles select, reinforce, and form the traits of leaders.

This is not to say that there are not personality traits, and even types of personality, historically associated with different leadership roles. It is to say that these traits and types can be generalized out of their contexts only when the personal demands of one leader-role are quite similar to those of another. When this is so, then individual traits and capacities may have carry-over value.

The army sergeant and the industrial foreman; the government official and the corporation executive; the labor leader of a certain type and the personnel manager of a certain type—men enacting these roles may interchange roles the more easily because of the formal similarity of the demands and recruitment patterns involved, and hence, of the types of men recruited and formed by them. But to so relate individual traits and leader roles, we must pay attention to the institutional dynamics affecting roles: both armies and factories are hierarchies requiring morale builders and human whips; public administration no longer represents "pedantocracy" or business corporations a series of "ventures"; the modern union comes to perform many pacifying, integrating functions similar to the personnel department of the company. As the functions and relations of institutions shift, so do the roles of their leaders—making individual character and personality traits more or less, as the case may be, transferable from one institutional context to another.

It is the same with the motives of leaders as with other traits: motives vary by type of role, indeed, motives are often understandable only as part of the role itself. The gratifications that roles provide—prestige, authority, income, or realization of superego ideal—become the motives of men to enact the role. Motives for leadership are thus as varied, on the one hand, as human motivation itself, and on the other, as the contexts of leader-roles.

Motives for leadership may be given in terms (1) of the subjectively intended aims of the leader, hence in terms of his overt vocabulary of *personal* values and goals. These may, in turn, be imputed to (2) covert psychic "needs" or aspirations in terms of

Freudian or Nietzschean mechanics, compensation, displacement, and so on, or to (3) objective social forces and opportunities, requirements and contradictions.

The points we wish to make in this connection are, first, that many motives of many types of leaders may be linked in the superego to articulated "causes," and second, that these motives and causes may or may not have to do with denied expediences, frustrations, or deprivations. Mere calculations, disguised as "gratifications," are not all there is to the motivation of leaders. The prophet Elijah shuns income, forgoes existing opportunities for prestige, and plays out his role even while he hates its demands—he served only "his God." And the point, made by Sombart, and again by Lasswell, that if a Prussian university had given Karl Marx a secure post he might not have been launched on his revolutionary career, seems to us unfounded. There is no evidence to suppose that this young doctor of philosophy wished to become a professor; moreover, as his brother-in-law was the Prussian minister of the interior, he might well, if he wished, have been appointed. The case illustrates this point: We can often explain the motives of leaders as due to superego formations, to the embracing of a cause, with no reference to personal frustrations and expediences.

We should study the traits and motives of leaders in close connection with their roles, appropriately related to their social-historical contexts. An extremely important aspect of this context is the more or less immediate followers of the leader and the images they hold of him.

2. *Images of the Leader and Motives of the Led*

Since there can be no leader without the led, in order to make a transfer from one context to another, the leader, regardless of his traits and motives, must be able to engage the loyalties of those in the new context. The relations of leader and led have often been put pragmatically in terms of the needs of the led. But we are by no means ready to accept such easy formulae as "the leader satisfies the needs of the led" or "the leader articulates what the led want and cannot articulate or don't know how to get." All such formulas, as well as Max Weber's more sophisticated typology of legitimations, we may approach generally in terms of the images which the led hold of their leader. The question of leadership, as Max Weber set it up in terms of authority, is the question of why the led follow. Weber answers the question in terms of three types of legitimation: [1] charismatic, traditional, and legal. These represent formal reasons for more or less voluntary obedience, the first, charismatic, because the led impute to the leader extraordinary personal qualities; the second, traditional, because they feel that the leader has always been followed and rightly so; and the last, legal, because they feel that the leader has attained his position according to legal rules which the led accept. This classification is quite useful; but as an over-all model it is, of necessity, highly formal and leaves untouched many aspects or dimensions of leadership to which we should like to pay systematic attention.

Images of instituted leaders, especially those images that are relevant to why they are followed, vary by institutional order. In fact, as part of the symbolic features of institution, these images justify the leader's roles, and often the role of its occupant. If he is a legitimate leader, he rules, as in Saudi Arabia or a modern totalitarian party, by virtue of the charismatic gifts claimed by him and imputed to him as a presumably extraordinary individual; as in patriarchal family or peasant village, by virtue of wealth, customary family repute, and the presumed or actual wisdom of "the grand old man." Or, as in the constitutional state, by virtue of having met legally enacted qualifications, including that of being "duly elected or appointed." These images uphold the leader's authority among the institution's members—they are the formal motives for their obeying him. They are his formal claims to leadership, which, when he has internalized them, are, with individual variations, his motives as a leader.

Any institutional structure needs to regulate the generalized others of its members. One of the functions of the leader is to import larger codes into the subgroup which he leads. The "leader" is a mediator between the members of his group and the larger social structure. As the responsible head of his family or of his enterprise,

[1] *The Theory of Social and Economic Organization*, Talcott Parsons and A. M. Henderson, trs. (New York: Oxford, 1948), Chapter I. See also Chapter VIII: Institutional Orders and Social Controls, I, Section 1: The Political Order, and Chapter X: Symbol Spheres.

for example, he is to some extent held responsible for what goes on in his family or business; he represents family members, employees, and their conduct before out-groups, especially before larger and more powerful frame groups—the police, the church, the state. The father is thus responsible to the public school teacher for the behavior of his children.

Such a representative position exerts pressures upon the subgroup leader to build into the "generalized other" of the subgroup members elements of the generalized other of "frame groups"—of the state, of the church, and of wider status group codes. Thus he is made the "transmission belt" for the importation of larger group values and codes into the little universe of the subgroup. The father, for example, has to install in his family value preferences which will assure that his daughters will have the properly delimited preferences for acceptable husbands.

This position of the leader toward the outside has a further aspect: the leader may be proud of the attainments of his group members. The father of a family, for example, is credited by outsiders with the successes of his children, receives congratulations for the successful marriage of his daughter or the brilliant achievements of his son. He is held responsible for what goes on in the unit he leads, and he is blamed and credited for the successes and failures of its members. Thus, the deference which leaders receive in their roles as leaders is sometimes quite elaborate (gun salutes, flag hoistings, and other pompous ritual) because through them their group is honored.

This deference often refers to the role rather than to the man who plays it. The man may not personally be highly esteemed for his style of acting out the role, but nevertheless the role is ranked high as being the vessel of the cumulative prestige of the entire group which he leads. We must distinguish between prestige attached to roles and personal esteem bestowed upon role-taking men. Accordingly, different constellations are possible: a role with high prestige may be filled by a lowly esteemed man (Harding); a high-prestige role may be filled by a highly esteemed man (F. D. R., Wilson, Washington); a low-prestige role may be filled by a highly esteemed man (Al Capone); or a low-prestige role may be filled by a lowly esteemed man (a "lazy" ditch-digger).

Of course there may be shifts in these evaluations of men and roles. At the beginning of his *State and Revolution* [2] Lenin has a nice commentary on the changes in attitude towards the revolutionary: "During the life time of great revolutionaries, the oppressing classes have visited relentless persecution on them and received their teaching with the most savage hostility, the most furious hatred, the most ruthless campaign of lies and slanders. After their death, attempts are made to turn them into harmless icons, to canonize them, and surround their *names* with a certain halo for the consolation of the oppressed classes and with the object of duping them, while at the same time emasculating and vulgarizing the *real essence* of their revolutionary theories and blunting their revolutionary edge." With appropriate modification, Lenin's statement may be extended to the iconography of certain Tsars in the Soviet Union since the 1930's. It is well known that Stalin has adopted Peter the Great as a somewhat distant "colleague," or possibly "precursor." And at Teheran, when Churchill presented Stalin with the honorific gift of His Majesty's sword, Stalin, in appreciation of the distinction, took it in the style of Tsarist protocol by kissing the sword. One task a leader performs for his group is to provide "official" sanction to the definition of the group situation in social space and historical time.

Images of leaders are not, of course, always adequately adjusted to the objective significance of the leader. But, in fact, such adequacy of image to man during the man's lifetime may occur: perhaps it did, positively, in the case of Goethe, "the poet-prince" and, negatively, in the case of the late United States Secretary of Defense Johnson. There are inflated images—small leaders with big images; and deflated images—big leaders with small images. These latter are often known to us by their later ascendancy: recall Mozart, buried among the paupers; or Shakespeare at such low ebb in the eighteenth century.

There are of course all sorts of "incongruities" of image and man; for example, one cannot attribute all the consequences which followed Columbus' "discovery" of America—including the rise to world power of the United States—to Columbus' greatness as a man. His relatively low intelligence and poor nautical leadership, his religious superstition and irregular ways with money, provided

[2] Nikolai Lenin, *Collected Works* (New York: International Pubs., 1932), Vol. XXI, p. 153.

more or less good reasons for his being jailed by his king. "Greatness," as Wilhelm Lange has indicated,[3] is more often an attribute of a man's image, held by various publics who "need" to worship the majestic and fascinating, the energetic and the mysterious, the sublime and the overpowering than it is an attribute of a man or of an objective assessment of the historical consequences of his role and deeds. The elaboration of images of Columbus was determined by factors having little or nothing to do with the work Columbus did; in fact, they have obscured the ramifications of his action, which, by the way, Columbus himself never got quite straight.

-We do not believe that the uniqueness and irreplaceability of great men can either be proved or disproved. We cannot, for example, prove or disprove the argument that had Napoleon not arisen to act as he did, another man or men would have so met "the demands of the hour." What has endured from the Napoleonic context are the legal code and centralized administrative system, and Napoleonic strategy and tactics as military models—all borrowed in accordance with his model by other nineteenth-century societies. On the other hand, the historical process of Western society did not, as it were, require Napoleon's enterprise to conquer Russia; that, so to speak, is part of the "overhead" of Napoleon's deeds.

The idea of genius, or of the great man, has to do not only with the man and his work, but also, and often more importantly we think, with his images, with his fame. It is sometimes quite a problem in particular cases to weigh the two, but that is what must be done in each case. We shall have more to say about this general problem of great men presently.

Among leaders there is self-advertising, in which the leader's self-image is advanced by his own posturing; and there are famemakers, others who advance the leader's image. But regardless of *how* they are diffused, self and other images may conflict or coincide:

Napoleon, as well as Goethe, held strong self-images, and so did others of them. But some scriptural prophets deemed themselves unworthy and were detested by contemporaries. Some leaders whom others esteem highly esteem themselves very little: public images are inflated in comparison with the insufficiency feelings

[3] *The Problem of Genius,* E. and C. Paul, trs. (New York: Macmillan, 1932).

of the leader. And there is the opposite: leaders whom others esteem very little but who esteem themselves very much, whether due to quiet pride (Kierkegaard) or bombastic vanity (the German Kaiser).

All these possible images of the leaders are of course relevant to their motives and to the motives of the led. Today both images of the leader and motives of the led are subject to intensive manipulative cultivation. Images and reality are often so closely joined as to make difficult their analytic separation; in fact, they pass from one to another. But the immediate context of leader, led, and image can best be set forth in terms of the functional demands of power-wielding roles.

3. Three Functions of Authoritative Roles

Regardless of who wields it, and of why others follow it, authority seems to have three major functions to which we should pay close attention.[4] (I) There are the imagery, the *representations* of power, the pomp and the circumstance, the handling of the flag, the scepter, the crown, the Presidential smile, the tireless, glad handshake, and the master formulas, "in the name of the king," or "in the name of the people," in terms of which orders are given. (II) There is the *legitimation* of power, an ideological elaboration and specification of the representation or halo; the "miranda" is elaborated into "doctrine," to the simple piety for emblems is added theology. (III) There is *decision-making* and the management of the instrumentalities of power, of staffs, allies, followers, enemies, and neutrals, in order to put decisions into effect.

Both representation and legitimation are at once possible aspects of the leader's role and important features of the authority-context in which he plays it. When we say that they are aspects of his role, we point up the fact that he may modify or even create them; when we say that they are important features of his context, we point up the fact that they lie in the context in which he acts and must be carried by the led and, in fact, form their reasons for fol-

---

[4] For distinctions of the functions of authority, see C. E. Merriam, *Political Power* (New York: McGraw-Hill, 1934) and *Systematic Politics* (Chicago: Univ. of Chicago Press, 1945); H. D. Lasswell and others, *The Language of Politics* (New York: Stewart, 1949), p. 9 ff.; and H. D. Lasswell and A. Kaplan, *Power and Society* (New Haven: Yale Univ. Press, 1950).

lowing him. His decisions and managements also have this dual reference to his own activities and the context and motives of the led. It is for these reasons that the concept of role is so important in the study of leadership.

If we cross classify the presence or absence of these three functional demands of power-wielding—representation, legitimation, and decision-making—we get eight situations:

		REPRESENTATION			
		YES LEGITIMATION		NO LEGITIMATION	
		YES	NO	YES	NO
DECISION-MAKING	YES	1	2	3	4
	NO	5	6	7	8

(1) Some leaders successfully combine all three functions: Lenin and Mussolini, Peter the Great, Shih Huang Ti, the "First Emperor" of China. Napoleon proclaims among his representations "the rule of the genius," gets the Pope himself to come to Paris to anoint him, marries a Hapsburg princess to tie himself in with dynastic and Catholic legitimations, sets up a new army model, a new code of laws, new internal administrative and educational systems. In terms of these three functions, Napoleon is a total leader.

(2) Other leaders may carry representations of power and wield power, but not be active developers of legitimations. Cromwell, "The Lord Protector," for example, leaves the theoretical work of legitimating his rule to others, among them, for a while, John Milton.

(3) Machiavelli, as a political secretary of the prince, manages affairs and is an active creator of legitimations, but does not embody or display the representation of power. Leaving that to the prince, he works out a legitimation for and enacts the role of "the political man" who with rational efficiency tries to win, hold, and increase power for power's sake, reducing all other values to instrumentalities for that immediate end while, at the same time, of course, having in mind the more distant goal of the unification of Italy.

(4) The American political boss neither represents nor legitimates power, but actively makes decisions and manages their enactment. He gives up honor and doctrine, if necessary, for power.

(5) The polar opposite type of leader who does not manage decisions at all, but legitimates and displays representations is difficult to illustrate, but perhaps the Romantic poets symbolize the French Revolution to an English public and elaborate one strain of its doctrinal legitimations. Also, John Reed operates in America with reference to early Russian Bolshevism. And, in classical Rome, the poet Vergil, as a member of the Roman ruling class, writes his *Georgics* and *Aeneid* at the request of what moderns might now call a propaganda industry.

(6) The "ruler" who displays representations and nothing else is more frequent, for example, all the cases of charismatic children: the child king of Egypt, the Dalai Lama of Tibet, as well as kings, queens, and rulers who are "mere figureheads." Also, Tolstoi's general has as his role "appearing to be in supreme control" of the chaos of the battlefield. Since unplanned events decide his armies' dispositions, he is primarily a representational leader.

(7) The pure case of the ideologist, who only legitimates—as did Rousseau for the French upheaval, Marx for the Russian Revolution, or Milton for Cromwell's regime—exists wherever a man's thought is used by power wielders, but who does not himself display power or wield it.

(8) The man, finally, who neither legitimizes, displays, or wields power is, of course, no leader, although, as in the case of Edward VIII, who fell down on all three functional role-demands and abdicated, he may have been expected to enact at least the representational role.

These three functional demands of power wielding, and the types of power wielders they invite us to examine, have primarily to do with large-scale institutional contexts. By itself, the eightfold typology is not an adequate model of the analysis of leadership; it is merely a descriptive range of what leaders may do. We want to spell out in more detail the possibilities of leadership roles in connection with a range of types of contexts in which they may occur.

So, rather than attempt to construct our model purely in terms of traits or personalities of the leader, or in terms of the motives or reasons of the led, we do so with reference to the role-demands on the functions of leadership, as begun in this section; and with reference to institutional contexts and dynamics back of these roles, as presented in the next two sections.

4. Contexts and Roles

By definition, all institutions of any permanence involve leaders; for institutions, as we have noted, are constellations of roles graded in authority in such a way that the members look to the occupant of the head-role to guarantee, externally and internally, the total role constellation. Externally, the instituted leader, or his agent, applies sanctions against those who fail to meet instituted expectations, ranging from the lifted eyebrow of the club leader to the death penalty imposed by the state. Internally, the members incorporate the institutional head's expectations as a more or less crucial component of their particular or generalized others, and then punish themselves when they are out of line. For it is not only that the patriarchal father, as Freud has shown, is thus incorporated into the "original" superego; all instituted heads may be so incorporated, and, in fact, incorporated in their own psychological right.

Types of instituted leaders are as various as the types of institutions they lead. The patriarchal father and the gerontocratic elder, the pope and the parish priest, the army captain and the trade union leader, the school master and the corporation manager—each plays a role more or less in accordance with the expectations institutionally exacted of him as the head. The types of men recruited for these roles and the effects of enacting these roles upon their character structures also include a wide range of possibilities. But as men they are selected and formed as leaders by the institutional contexts in which they play their parts.

This depiction of the instituted leader rests upon the assumption that such leadership is role-determined. It is normally the instituted context in which he leads that selects and forms him as a man, that more or less sets the role he plays, that provides images of him which justify his authority and motivate men to follow him, and him to lead. Some writers, for example, Richard Schmidt, refuse to call such institutional heads leaders, but refer to them as "agents of authority," and to their followers as "subordinates." We do not see the full justification of this, although it does suggest three important points: first, it points us to the crucial distinction between role-determined and role-determining leadership; second, to the fact that the role-determined, the instituted head, may be more or less determined; and, third, that he is probably more determined when his institutional sphere is stable, less determined when his sphere is breaking up or at least changing rapidly.

The institutional head as such does not usually satisfy our image of "the leader" because we often think of leaders as men who create not only their roles but the institutions in which they will play them. This does not mean that such leaders stand alone before institutions; they also have a context or else they could not be leaders. But the prime context of the role-determining leader is the movement or the party, which is at once an instrument of leadership and an immediate context of the roles which its leaders are to play.[5] One of the major aspects of a leader's role in a social movement is to establish his role, as he organizes the internal structure of the movement and tries to advance its power relations with the institutional structure and with other contending movements.

It is probably not wise to split "institutions" from "collective behavior" and conceive of the first as stable and controlling, and the second as dynamic, and, as it were, intrusive. The bureaucratization of modern government, of corporate business life, the spread of totalitarian, one-party states may be more dynamic than all the riots, mobs, and crowds of the last fifty years put together from all over Western civilization. And in these institutional processes new roles have come about, as well as role-determining men of enormous consequences for modern historic change.

The lead roles of many institutions are prescribed, hemmed in by rules of recruitment and office conduct; but in many "instituted" contexts, the role of the leader is less set, more open to variety of elaborations by different leaders. Moreover, in the latter the allegiance to the leader is less set, and must often be won and held by the leader, whose relations with the led must thus be structured by the leader himself.

The context is less a structure than a milieu, and as a milieu, more open to the leader's structuring. When, in due course, the movement is more firmly instituted, then the leader may not have to remold in this way the new members who are selectively recruited; in addition, the deputy leaders, staff members, the movement's old timers may do this job, for there is then hierarchy and

[5] For a discussion of movements and parties, see Chapter XV: Collective Behavior, Section 3: Movements, Parties, and Pressure Groups.

and specialization of roles for different levels and types of leaders. But leadership in this context very often must begin by the necessity of the leader's attracting and holding the voluntary loyalties of the led.

What is needed is a statement of the phases of leadership, as it moves from a small, informal circle around a leader, through innumerable transitions, to a prescheduled role in an institutional order firmly set into a social structure. No formal, universal scheme seems worthwhile: the phases vary by epoch and institutional setting. As the contexts become less formal, the nature of the leader's role usually becomes more personal, but not always: there is the style of playing highly formal roles in highly formal and personalist manners.

The way movements and parties, as major contexts of leadership, are related to institutional orders shapes the way leaders in the one context are related to the second. The party or movement, in attempting to influence decision-making, may (1) put its leader in the lead-role of the institution, as in modern constitutional parties and the state; (2) change the institutions and thus its lead-role, and then put its leader in; or (3) create a new institution and install its leaders at its head.

In terms of leadership, there is, first, the conquest of leading positions, by revolutionaries or reformers; second, the holding and the routinization of these positions in the generational sequence by (a) customary rights and rules of precedence and successorship, and by (b) enacted rights which supersede personal ways of doing things and give issue to impersonal rules and regulations. It seems rather clear that the chance of role-determining leadership is maximized in the first phase, in which men's traits are more important; whereas in the later phases, recruitment patterns are more important.

There are contexts, which deserve detailed descriptions, other than those of institutions and movements.[6] But these are perhaps sufficient to indicate this fact: in examining this range of contexts we do not find a correlation with the possibilities of role-determining rather than role-determined leaders. But we do locate the zone in which role-determining leadership seems to have its major

[6] See Chapter XV: Collective Behavior, Section 2: Aggregates, Crowds, and Publics.

chances: it is the zone of all those types of voluntary associations which are not (yet) firmly a part of more established institutional orders and spheres.

5. Role Dynamics and Leadership

To ask whether leadership is a function of the traits of the leader or of the motives and images of the led is not a fruitful question. The answer, of course, is that it is both, but that is an answer that does not help much. It does help, however, to conceive, as we have, both the traits of the leader and the motives of the led as part of the role which the leader plays. Then we may restate the question in these terms: Does the leader determine the role he plays or does the role determine the leader? This should, of course, not be taken as a general question to be answered in general, but as a question leading us to precise examination of concrete cases. The general answer is that different leaders are quite differently related to the roles they play.

It is not true, as Theodore Newcomb would have it,[7] that "all leaders are motivated to take whatever kinds of roles are called for (or are permitted) by their position in the role system." It is precisely their positions and the demands upon their role that leaders sometimes put into question. Nobody "called for" (or permitted) General Napoleon to chase Parliament home on the 18 *Brumaire,* or later to transform his consulate into an emperor-ship. Nobody called for or permitted Adolf Hitler to proclaim himself "Leader and Chancellor" the day President Hindenburg died, to abolish and usurp roles by merging the presidency and the chancellorship. Far from being utterly dependent upon a "role system," the leader may smash it and set up another in which his role is differently structured. In fact, such social destruction and creation is what is typically involved in one major type of "great leadership." This is not to say that it is not socially determined; it is to say that there are often temporal lags between the deter-mination and the shift in leadership.

This is a complex question, which is to say that it is difficult to identify the keys which when properly ranged and interrelated

[7] Theodore M. Newcomb, *Social Psychology* (New York: Dryden, 1950), p. 656.

might best lead us to observation of the determining factors in any given case. But here are three attempts to sort out such keys:

I. *Flexibility of Role and Reactions of Leader to It.* From the side of context: the roles of leaders may be quite flexible or quite rigid in the latitude they allow the leader; [8] moreover the leaders recruited for these roles also vary widely in the personal way in which they enact them. In terms of these two factors—the flexibility of the role and the reaction of the leader to it—there is clearly a range. At one end is the role-determined leader: the role is rigid and the recruited man fulfills it exactly as required, in the image of the punctilious bureaucrat. At the other end is the role-determining leader: the role is flexible and the man enacts it in a highly personal style, exceeding what is expected, making the most of his opportunities.

The President of the United States, for example, has more latitude in the way he plays his role than the bureaucratic chief of a unit in a division of a department, or the palace-confined Mikado under the Shogunate before 1868. The president can take his role big or little in all three aspects of authority. If he takes it big, as Franklin D. Roosevelt or Wilson did, he can modify features of the instituted role, as well as create new lead-roles in the governing structure as a whole, which action in turn selects and forms new types of men as leaders around him. He is more than a creature of authority: in all three aspects of leadership, he is to some extent a role-determining man. If he takes it little, as Harding did, enacting it in an understated way, he can sit back and take it easy, performing the expected actions but not creating any new ones.

[8] This scale of roles includes each of the three major functional demands on leadership: *Representation* functions may range from the hierocratic rigidity of court ceremonial under a theocratic emperor, as in Oriental despotisms and ancient Roman Caesarism, to the studied informality of the British king at a Boy Scout jamboree and the personable horseplay of Franklin Roosevelt with liberal intellectuals. *Legitimation* functions may be strictly orthodox, as in the case of Stalinism's invention of "theoretical heresies," or Confucianism's hatred of all salvation religions, to the free market in ideas where rival definitions of democracy itself are tolerated as legitimate within the limits of national loyalty. *Decision-making* finally may range from a Leadership Principle, as with Hitler, with the "authority of every leader downward and responsibility upward," to a maximum sharing of all decisions and participation of virtually all citizens.

He is, then, a symbol of authority ("guardian of the constitution") and a role-determined man.

Whether a man takes his instituted role big or little depends not only upon what he as the occupant brings to the role but also upon the institutional context of the role. "Great leaders" may create new roles or expand old ones; they are likely, as Hegel already knew, to emerge when the societies they lead are at points of epochal structural transition. For then flexibility of role and creative reactions to it are most likely to coincide.

The possibilities open to the leader vary with the flexibility of the role-demands; if they are inflexible, so long as he stays within the role he must play it as expected, although he may fall short; if the role is flexible, he will have more difficulty meeting it exactly, less difficulty making the most of it.

This scale, constructed from flexibility of role and reactions of leader, has implications for the imagery of the leader: the role-determining man, since he modifies a received role of decision-making, may be more likely, as part of that modification, to shift the imagery and legitimations of the authority he wields than is the role-determined man, who in the extreme case finds an imagery and legitimations already there, and merely continues to enact their requirements along with other features of his received role.

II. *Modifications of Functions and Scope of Role.* A social structure is composed of various institutional orders, each objectively oriented to more or less dominant ends, the political, economic, religious, kinship, and military. Now, the head of an institution within any order may expand the scope of his command by creating new features of his role or creating virtually new roles, by (1) expanding the functions of the institution of which he is head, or (2) combining previously separate roles into one head role, or (3) by combining roles across institutional orders. The contrary is also true: the leader may shrink in scope and power if (1) his institution shrinks in size or leverage in the social structure, or (2) if the leader's role is split, or if (3) a new institution arises to compete with an old one.

Leaders, then, who take a role that is instituted to serve some function may modify the role, the function, or both.

John L. Lewis, as president of the Committee on Industrial Organization within the AFL, increased the scope of his role as chairman and the function of the organization, turning it from a Committee to a Congress. So did Franklin D. Roosevelt as President of the United States: he expanded the role of the President as well as the function of the executive branch, and, in fact, of the government as a whole.

Lenin, with his conception of a party of professional revolutionaries, greatly reduced mass-oriented activities, the winning of mass membership to the cause, in favor of very strict standards for smaller circles of full-time members. In this way, by his party of experts—rather than of experts, amateurs, and sympathizers—he centralized command in the hands of professionals, gained speed in shifting strategy and tactics, and gained greater security for conspiratorial work; in short, greater revolutionary efficiency.

In the face of an ever-growing complexity of a bureaucratic state apparatus of experts, the absolute monarch in the early modern period was reduced in role to the position of an amateur depending upon the advice of his experts. The function which he served increased, but his role was reduced.

Finally, both function and role may be reduced: the king may come to rule, but not govern; the king of prerogative may be reduced to a king of influence, in short, a figurehead having officially representative functions and, if capable, wielding unofficial influence.

These expansions or contractions of function and of roles may come about by the merging or the splitting of existing roles, and in either case, of course, there may be an increase or a decrease in power:

If, for example, the supreme priest and the emperor merge into one role, as in Caesar-papism, the new role carries increased power by the merger. So Peter the Great reorganizes the Russian Church and appoints the chairman of the synod; or in modern coalition warfare, a supreme command is established; or the president assumes war powers in a "constitutional dictatorship."

The merger of roles may also mean a decrease in power: in wishing to do much, the leader becomes an amateur who blunders. In different ways, both the German Kaiser as diplomat and *Der Führer* as supreme commander may be examples.

If roles are split or divided into specialties, power may increase for one of the roles: the most obvious case is the creation of staff roles and delegation to them of various aspects of power wielding.

The role left is that of co-ordinating the divided roles. So the premier, as chairman of a cabinet, presides over a committee of policy co-ordinating ministers, who in turn are served by various department heads. Specialization of functions in this way is an infinite variety, and forms, in fact, the major subject matter of much of descriptive political science and institutional sociology.

Roles may also be divided and their power weakened; for example, when empires are decentralized so that the center is weakened—as happened in the rise of British colonies to dominions, or Alexander's governors to satraps, or repeatedly in the Chinese empire in which the original functionaries of the central authority developed into warlords and governors in their own right.

It is worthwhile to systematize such possibilities because to do so alerts us to the range of role dynamics possible in any social-historical situation we may wish to analyze. The major point is that the leader's creation of roles can only be understood in the full context of social-historical dynamics. For the institutional context not only provides an apparatus for leadership, but sets the scope of the command and modifies the reasons for men's allegiance to it. The "great leader" has often been a man who has managed such institutional dynamics, and thus created new roles of leadership.

The rise and decline of institutional structures involve the rise and decline of leaders. Thus, in the latter evolution of capitalism, the appointed manager of the large corporation supplants, in some part, the self-made entrepreneur of his family enterprise. And this shift in key economic institutions, and hence in their head roles, ramifies into other institutional areas—the political sphere, the status hierarchy, and even the kinship order, as selected family circles rise to the top.

When capitalism came to Japan, it came as corporate capitalism, without any individualistic epoch; and it found a point of coincidence with already existing feudal kinship units; the leaders of these top cousinhoods, with their sib loyalties, expanded their roles to include the management of corporate enterprises.

In the transition from peace to war, large numbers of men are transferred from economic and kinship institutions to the military order. The expanding military order tends to override the demands of other institutional orders; its symbols of legitimation become master symbols of political decisions, and it borrows or appro-

priates the symbols of other orders, especially the religious and
political; its leaders become more powerful in deciding the pace
and shape of the total social structure. It is, today especially, obvious that such structural shifts do not guarantee the emergence of
role-determining men adequate to the contextual demands and
opportunities.

III. *Creation of Roles in and out of Contexts.* We may finally
consider whether or not the leader creates the role he plays, that
is, modifies existing roles as virtually to reconstitute them, or
merely assumes an already existing role and enacts it within the
generally expected limits; and whether the individual finds an
available institutional context for his role, or is limited in his
playing of it to small informal groups, but mainly among a public. If we combine these two, we get three possible types of leaders:
A. the routine institutional head "the routineer"; B. the creative
institutional head "the innovator"; and C. "the precursor."

A. The routine leader creates neither his role nor its institutional
context, but merely steps into a pre-existing setup containing the
lead-role which he plays. The role to be played is already available and the leader comes to it merely to enact it within the generally expected limits. Such leaders are usually formally or hereditarily recruited, and need not create loyalties to their leadership,
for they are already available in the context of the role which is to
be played. The leader may, of course, enact the role rigidly as it is
set up. Or, he may, although within the general expectations,
personally stylize his enactment of it. But, in general, the major
problem of such leadership is the problem of the recruitment
pattern.

B. The innovating leader, within an existing institutional context, creates a new role and then plays it. The leader here elabo-
rates a role to the point that it no longer is recognizable. He may
expand it by creating new features of it, or by merging two or
more existing roles. In either case, he monopolizes functions of
leadership within the existing context. He may split an existing
role into two and only play one of them, delegating or giving up
the other. Any number of mechanisms of creation are possible, and
any number of reasons for their creation. He may be figuring out
new ways to satisfy expectations or sensed wants of the group in

context, or he may create a new role and by so doing create new wants at the same time as their means of realization. This kind of leader may be formally or informally recruited, and he must create or transfer the loyalties of the led to the new role which he has created for himself.

C. The leader as precursor creates a role, but there is no institutional opportunity for him to play it. So Thomas Münzer, left-wing leader of German Protestantism, is to be hailed later by Marx and Engels as a visionary of communism. So Rousseau remains a leader only in symbolic context with publics, for the time is not yet ripe for action.

Such leaders are usually self-appointed and their performance of their roles as decision-making leaders is imaginary. They are preparing themselves, by pre-enactment, for the day when appropriate contexts may be available. By those who "take readily to existing roles," many such men are judged as crazy, or at least out of joint with their times. But such internal preparation is often part of the leadership phenomenon of the prophet type. If they are successful as leaders, they come in time to represent to smaller inner circles and later to larger publics and then to movements and parties, certain values or models to be imitated and with which to identify. In the meantime, they are abstracted from such contexts and are leaders only in their own minds, and symbolically, but not in terms of power, to publics who hold images of the man with the new role he cannot yet play as a symbol of a context not yet existing. Such leaders are of course self-recruited and must create loyalties among those they would lead.

It follows from this scheme, as well as from our descriptions of the several contexts of leadership that, if we would understand any given leadership phenomenon, the following are important questions to raise:

1. Context: In what context does the leader arise? How is it structured? Did this particular man "create" it by modifications of existing contexts, or did he simply become a leader in it as it existed?

2. Role: What are the salient traits of his role as a leader? In what social orders and spheres does he lead others?—only in opinion, or in activity as well? Did he invent this role? What modifi-

cations, if any, has he made in it, and how? Has he elaborated it as he received it, constricted its scope, amalgamated other roles with it?

3. Man: How did this man come to be in this role? How was he recruited for it? What character traits were relevant to his assuming or inventing this role? What traits are relevant to his continuing to enact this role?

4. Images: What images do those he leads have of him as man and as a leader? Why do they obey him? What techniques does he use to diffuse this image, these legitimations?

CHAPTER
XV

Collective Behavior

NO ONE observing the awful turbulence of twentieth-century history can believe that all human affairs are neatly contained within institutions, or that existing institutional orders necessarily endure. Wars and revolutions have turned over social structures; dictators have risen and fallen within great nations, and even within regions of great nations. Masses of men—as well as small conspiratorial groups, alienated from institutions, and living, for a while, outside stable and stabilizing institutional structures—have smashed whole societies, and promptly built vast new domains. In various ways, in various countries, some periods of history have seemed to proceed by plots, others by polemics. And now no one can believe that all social conduct is ordered within institutions, or that what is now instituted has always been or always will be.

Within and between institutional orders and their spheres is the problem area known loosely to sociologists as "collective behavior," which, in current usage, includes everything from totalitarian one-party states to the ephemeral mob that hangs a colored man for allegedly looking too closely at a white woman; from quiet little groups of neighbors who go bowling together, to religious sects and to fads that appear and disappear in Southern California.

There is no problem area for which both deficits and assets have been so often remarked. If this area contains "mass phenomena" associated with the breakdown of social order—hysterical rages and euphoric ecstasies, during which men act as they never did before and never will again—it also contains those associations which are acknowledged to be major seedbeds of free men of Western nations.

The prototype of modern voluntary associations, as Max Weber has shown, is the Protestant sect, which is "a union of specifically qualified people" rather than an established and compulsory institution. Such associations, when secularized and diffused in various strata, form a pluralist field of units within and between which the individual, for his own self-esteem, must "put himself over." In the process of doing so, he is naturally stamped by the values and models carried by the associations. In such free associations, moreover, the individual can obtain his anchorage and make his stand against "majority domination." And in these smaller circles there occurs a social selection and training of leaders for larger tasks.

1. The Structural Contexts of Collective Behavior

The range of phenomena in this area may best be stated in terms of the degree of explicit organization: at one end of the scale there are what appear to be purely spontaneous activities; at the other, there is a merging of "collective behavior" with institutional organization itself. Ephemeral crowds spontaneously releasing a pent-up tension, as well as tightly organized class and status parties calculatedly making their way within and between major institutional blocs; a barely discernible drift from year to year in the shade of lipstick color, the shift in the atmosphere of street throngs, as well as the farm bloc representative arguing and entertaining— all these belong to the domain of "collective behavior."

Some of these phenomena are already institutions in the same sense as a family or a church; others do not display such structural characteristics at all. But as we examine such activities and social forms over longer spans of time, there does seem to be a sort of drift exhibited by all collective behavior, if it endures beyond the momentary, towards institutionalization. Furthermore, all forms of collective behavior, no matter how momentary, are related to various institutional orders and spheres: they cannot be explained without reference to them. For institutional structures are the precipitants and the foci of collective behavior of every sort; they are the larger frameworks within which such behavior arises and through which it runs its course.

But this does not mean that collective behavior does not modify (sometimes, as in revolution, grievously) the institutional structure. It does mean that the interplay must always be closely examined, and the specific contributions to history of structural shifts as well as of the more fluid, amorphous forms of social dynamics carefully weighed. It is not fruitful, as we have already noted, to conceive of social structures as somehow inert and static, and of collective behavior as providing the dynamic. Such a conception, in fact, is a triple misconception: of the nature of structural change, of collective behavior, and of the typical relations between the two.

It is in epochs of transition, like that of the waning Middle Ages or of the French and Russian revolutions that the established institutions of society lose their hold over their members. Internally, pressures seem to pile up, and externally misgivings and public criticisms are rife. Codes and norms are no longer accepted unreflectively and without dispute, and to an increasing number of persons they may prove to be unworkable.

Every society in such decline provides us with the indexes of its coming apart. When the privileged feudal nobles of Europe closed their ranks by demanding more rigid tests of "blue blood" descent; when the guilds jealously closed their master positions against the increasing pressure of journeymen and apprentices, by demanding a "masterpiece" and by adding an obligatory year of itineracy; when there were not sufficient churches to absorb the students of theology who, as intellectual vagrants, joined the itinerant artisans; when the various intellectual groups organized by "nations" at medieval universities engaged in heightened group competition for church prebends—then established institutional arrangements were on the decline.

Although the specific indexes of disintegration vary by societies, all such epochs of transition may be formally characterized by the fact that old institutional orders, for a variety of reasons, lose their hold over their members. Conduct deviates from the sanctioned norms, and newer ways of doing things are no longer felt to be sinful or criminal. In fact, quite a few men may accept the new as the only possible way of getting things done. Uninstituted or loosely instituted men make their appearance but find no place in the old order. Old ways of conduct with their conventional, legal, and ideological elaborations are available to fewer people, and those who cannot follow these ways lose their stake in the old order, and with it they lose their identifications and loyalties, without, however, promptly finding new ones. Such social transitions may be long endured, or passed through swiftly.

Western medieval society knew a partial breakdown of its instituted ways during the pestilence, and during the threatened conquest, when Mongolian armies penetrated to the gates of Vienna,
and disciplined men on swift horses struck terror to Christian
hearts. Since these times the word "horde" has remained in all
Western languages. It is during such periods of transition—when
old institutions break down and new ones are not yet available—
that mass movements and collective forms of behavior are likely to
appear. In them and in terms of them new forms of organization,
of leadership, and of conduct are developed. So there is the enlightenment movement of the Renaissance, the North Alpine Reformation, the emergence of the counterreformation of Catholic
revivalism. And, in this broad perspective, is not our time of wars,
revolutions, and slumps comparable?

In such periods sensitive minds usually experience stress and
strain, and formulate problems long before broad masses of men
experience them consciously or act collectively in response to the
mounting tensions accompanying what Weber called "times of
distress" or Émile Durkheim called "anomy," that is, a state of
"normlessness." Then occurs in intellectual circles trial and error,
criticism and countercriticism, self-searching and doubt, skepticism
and enlightenment, desperate attempts to revive and to reaffirm
what proves in the end to be outlived and hollow. Words and deeds
fail to jibe, and boredom overcomes many who feel weary of un-
inspiring days. Others crave forgetfulness and intoxication, and
still others see the day of judgment on a sinful age which thus
comes to its doom.

The most ambitious effort, since Le Bon,[1] to use concepts of collective behavior in an explanatory way is that of the late Emil
Lederer, who sought to interpret nazism as "an attempt to melt
society down to a crowd."[2] For him society is organized into a
pluralism of interested groups, each of which is more or less
homogeneous and thus partial, yet capable, especially if small, of
supporting reasoned opinions and reasonable actions. But the crowd
or mass is amorphous, emotional, given to sudden outbursts; it is
not articulated but fragmented, and it is without goals of its own.

[1] Gustave Le Bon, *The Crowd* (new ed.; New York: Macmillan, 1925).
[2] *The State of the Masses* (New York: Norton, 1940), see especially pp. 28,
45, 50, and 66.

Hence it is ideal material for strong leaders and is, in fact, according to Lederer, for nazism the "permanent basis of a political system." Before our times, up to 1914, the economic theory of history, Emil Lederer believed, was approximately correct: political orders corresponded in due course to economic development, classes were the units of history-making; and *groups* rather than individuals entered the nineteenth-century political order. The "present crisis," however, "is not a manifestation of class struggle but a substitution for society of institutionalized masses," at the center of which is a corps of violent gangs who turn all discussion groups into demonstrative political crowds. These crowds, in turn, have no tradition and no connection with other parties; they dominate the streets, and as they mass the citizenry they dominate the political minds of men and women. So, the real opposites today are "states based on stratified society" (which may be "progressive" or "reactionary"), and "states based on masses." In this view there was in nazism only amorphous mass and ruling party, and no other structures.

This theory, which we believe mistaken, confuses the deliberate breaking up of autonomous associations standing between the state and the various strata of a society with the dissolution of such a society into a mass. It overlooks the continuing fact of propertied classes in German society and their strengthening by Nazi policies. It is true that strata and organizations, especially those of labor, were smashed and atomized, but this was accomplished by bureaucracies which prowled out from the top, intervening to coordinate almost every institutional order and sphere, and regimenting voluntary associations into compulsory cartels and "Labor Fronts." Each of these sectors was controlled by reliable party personnel in charge of a thoroughly organized, propagandized, and terrorized society. Whatever spontaneity or "sudden outbreaks" occurred were less a result of spontaneity than of the managed or manipulated discharge of mass fears and trained hatreds under the oppressive weight of the ruling structure which thus consolidated its domination and ensnared the underlying population.[3]

Adequate explanation of "collective behavior" usually requires that we pay attention to three sorts of phenomena: (A) the larger

[3] For an excellent criticism of Emil Lederer, see Franz Neumann, *Behemoth* (New York: Oxford, 1942), p. 365 ff.

framework of institutional structure; (B) the more or less structured and managed associations, movements, or parties; and (C)
collective behavior on its own "spontaneous level."

2. Aggregates, Crowds, and Publics

Ever since Le Bon, the term "masses" has been used to cover a
great variety of processes and phenomena, and accordingly its
meaning is not always clear. In various forms and with various
qualifications, Le Bon's ideas have been used by Ortega y Gasset,[4]
Emil Lederer, E. A. Ross,[5] and Karl Mannheim, as well as a host
of less eminent writers. Such terms as "mass society" or "mass
movement," "mass media" or "mass publics," "mass sales" or "mass
demonstrations," "mass orgies" or "mass spectacles," and so on,
are indicative of the very wide range of phenomena covered. We
shall use the term "mass" simply to signify large numbers of men,
and distinguish, for convenience, aggregates, crowds, mobs, and
publics.

I. When people exhibit like behavior, when they "go in various
directions" and do not share any goal, we may speak of an aggregate, or of an aggregation. *Aggregates*, as in a street scene,
are simply people in the same locality but not in communication
or live contact with one another; such regularities as they display
are due to common stimuli, such as stoplights or signals of police-
men.

Among these there is no joint or common motivation, no leadership, no common focus of attention, no sense of cohesion binding them together. Thus do automobile drivers return on Sunday
evening to the big city, or masses of women go shopping during
the seasonal sales or holidays, or masses of employees go to work
or leave for home in the daily ebb and flow of the metropolis.
Everybody acts for himself, competing for scarce parking space
and economic bargains, and all these aggregates of drivers and
shoppers, commuters and transients—by their parallel behavior—

[4] José Ortega y Gasset, *The Revolt of the Masses* (London: Allen, 1932).
[5] See his great books, *Social Control* (New York: Macmillan, 1904) and
Social Psychology (New York: Macmillan, 1908).

exhibit uniformities of conduct to which traffic regulations, advertising campaigns, radio warnings, and so on, address themselves.

II. When such aggregates, in physical proximity, find a common focus of attention they may become a "crowd" or a "mob." Thus crowds of spectators gather around the scene of a traffic accident, or form casual audiences around Sunday speakers in Hyde Park, or slowly mill in the streets, watching mobs (which are crowds in action) of hoodlums beat up Negroes in "race riots," or watching stormtroopers and Hitler Youth details hunt down and beat up Jews in Berlin's boulevard cafés. In such situations, the focused attention of the massed spectators readily lead to shared responses, ranging from the encouragement of mob activities, through sullen silences, to hisses and boos of protest.

The people in a crowd are in contact with one another, but usually in a random way: they are unco-ordinated and mill about. *Mobs* are crowds that are actively oriented by emblems or slogans to some goal. Crowds as such have no shared ends, no leaders; mobs are crowds that are incited to specific action by self-appointed leaders or "rabble-rousing" shouters. Such spontaneous collectivities seemingly represent ephemeral, transient outbreaks of tension. They provide outlets and targets for psychic forces not placed socially in a more usually legitimated ways.

Back of the crowd, and especially of the mob, there is the larger social context, which usually generates conflicts, hatreds, fears, and tensions, to which the mob now gives vent. Old expectations guiding the usual role conduct of the members have temporarily collapsed, and the mutual, immediate expectations of the crowd are focused, or even fixed, upon the leader, who thus takes over. This is more easily accomplished if the usual roles and expectations of the more routine areas of life become ambivalent or surcharged with psychic and emotional elements.

Mobs may act before friendly or before hostile crowds of onlookers. Accordingly, the relationships between active mobs and spectator crowds vary greatly. Mobs may emerge spontaneously from an excited and milling crowd when self-appointed leaders incite the crowd to action. Usually in such cases, mobs of youths come to the fore and in a loose gang formation swing into action. A broadening field of many gangs and mobs may come to the fore, under the eyes of wildly cheering masses of spectator crowds. Again organized gangs like those of the Russian Black Hundred or the Hitler Youth may terrorize the community by their program activities, and attract crowds of more or less friendly, more or less excited, spectators who may themselves be drawn into the fury of sadistic street terrorism.[5A]

There is a fluid transition between the aggregate masses of men in the street, the spectator crowds, and the wildly moving mobs which may emerge spontaneously or who may follow the lead of organized terrorist squads under central direction. In our century we are no strangers to the mob directed from radio-equipped staff cars and motorcyclists who provide disciplined cohesion for active knots of scattered people throughout metropolitan areas. In such cases, running battles with the police, swift changes of the point of attack, retreats and provocative feints, a devastating, simultaneous sweeping down on carefully mapped-out targets in selected cities throughout a nation—what all this reveals is a virtually warlike discipline. So in the November days of 1938 in Nazi Germany were synagogues burned, Jewish businesses destroyed and looted, and Jewish homes raided. The intermingling of collective behavior and officially organized action, of cloaking the machine-organized terrorism by alleging that irresponsible mob activities, motivated by "righteous indignation," is the cause—is revealed in Goebbel's contradictory formula: "the organized spontaneity of the people."

The mobilization of massed aggregates for less violent action may also be a response to the policies of specific institutions. Thus the shopping sprees and bargain counter crushes of metropolitan housewives are responses to advertised sales. The rush hour traffic of millions of employees are results of the definition of the working day in factory and office; the rush of the voters to the polls results from the definition of voting times and the exhortations of political parties and mass media. Thus, the policies of various institutions —religious, political, economic—are likely to call forth unorganized, although patterned, mass behavior of predictable volume and regularity.

[5A] Chicago Commission on Race Relations, *The Negro in Chicago* (Chicago, 1922); Gerald Brenan, *The Spanish Labyrinth* (New York: Macmillan, 1944); Franz Borkeneau, *The Spanish Cockpit* (London: Faber, 1937).

III. *Publics* are composed of people who are not in face to face relation but who nevertheless display similar interests, or are exposed to similar, although more or less distant, stimuli. The public of a leader may be the only context of his leadership; he offers himself, or at any rate is available, as a symbolic model. The best formal definition of the political public is that recently given by Hans Speier: a public exists whenever people outside a government have the right to give public advice and criticism to the government.[6]

This obviously ties the concept in with the notion of institutional structure, specifically with the state. The leader in such a context is one who can mediate, as it were, between public and state. Such leaders often coincide or are closely related to leaders of movements and parties.

But there is a distinction between three types of public which we must recognize, especially in view of the rise of mass media of communication and the frequent impossibility of realizing in fact the formal right stated in Speier's definition:

(1) In simpler, early-modern times, the public might be adequately imagined as a "primary public": circles of people in discussion with one another. This is what the older literature of public opinion—using the term as a legitimation of democratic forms of government—meant by "the public": discussion groups confronted by issues. And it is further imagined that for every live issue there is a self-activated public. The leaders of such a public are informal "opinion leaders" who guide opinion in their informal spheres, refract media communications to others, and make legitimate the influences from other sources.

Speier, in his definition, has tried to save this aspect of the notion of public at a time when democratic institutions are externally under attack and internally decaying. He does this by explicitly linking the notion of public to the power structure, and more importantly by formalizing the conception of public in a statement of a right rather than of a going fact. This becomes clear when we seriously ask, Who can lead public opinion today? What are its leaders like? What are their chances to fulfill the role assigned to them by this definition?

(2) At other times, such public as exists seems to be adequately described as a set of "media markets": people reached more or less

[6] *Social Order and the Risks of War* (New York: Stewart, 1952), p. 323.

regularly by a given medium of communication. On such markets, no informal leadership as in the primary public seems possible: the only "leaders" who can arise in this context are those in charge of or with ready access to the mass channels of communication.

(3) Moreover, as we know from totalitarian societies, the older primary publics may be infiltrated and regimented by organizations. From the aggregate activities of multitudes of migrants and spectators, buyers and sellers, voters and readers and radio listeners— we may distinguish mass audiences and mass publics recruited by the sale of tickets of admission. If such mass organizations as trade unions, book clubs, educational institutions, army units, churches, parties, or civic organizations "book the show" or sponsor the publication, we may speak of "organized publics and audiences." This pattern would seem to be on the ascendancy in industrial nations during the twentieth century. A whole technique of "audience building" has emerged. The availability of masses at factories and in office buildings and public conveyances provides opportunities to co-operate with religious or political or cultural organizations, by offering employees or passengers as "captive audiences." In totalitarian regimes this availability of people in masses is seized upon by the ruling party during propaganda campaigns to regiment crowds to demonstrations, to endorse government policies by plebiscite and to discipline men to follow the party line. The techniques Americans know as commercial advertising have been centralized and co-ordinated by the single-party state, which thus—through its mass organizations, publicly owned enterprises, collective farms, public carriers and conveyances, mass media, schools, and ubiquitous "agitators"—reaches into every nook and cranny of the social structure.

What happens to men in crowds and mobs?

Negatively, the norms and motives which they have incorporated as features of their instituted roles collapse. If this is complete, or at least extreme, the result is panic or ecstasy. Internally, the generalized other no longer works as it did, and, in extreme, the *person* is unavailable. Out of fear or out of ecstatic joy, man is "beyond himself." This is the key psychological meaning of "anomy"— the situation of normlessness.

Positively, behavior is then more open to two sources: the contents of the unconscious become the leading predispositions,[7] and the individual is sensitized to others immediately around him. The established person—in short, the more routine self-images and conscience—are minimized; the features of the psychic structure, maximized. Mass panic is thus the extreme opposite of institutional order. And if we take seriously the term "crisis," as applied to institutional orders, we mean a collapse sufficient to put men into panic.

Now, movements may accomplish the same process as crowds, but more gradually; it is, in fact, within the context of a continuing movement or party that crowd phenomena are more likely to occur, and when occurring, to have more lasting psychological effects. Many collective phenomena which appear "spontaneous" may in reality be adroitly managed or manipulated, and all of them, in their causal explanation, rest in one way or another upon going institutional structures.

Men in power, especially if they obtained institutional power by means of a movement in which the masses played a part, may try to keep them, as J. B. S. Hardman put it,[8] "in a state of suspended mobility, immune to the solicitations of the opposition and yet potentially" ready, when necessary, to support the authority. Contenders for power and office appeal to the aggregate masses (which as such have no common goals or loyalties) in an effort to identify themselves with the interests and sentiments of the masses, and at the same time to bargain with or threaten concessions out of existing authorities. Masses may be transformed from "a state of passive, if intensely nervous, suspension to one of aggressive activism . . . ," into not a mob but the violent yet structured point of action for a movement that has prepared for the day and hour.

On the other hand, when the structural framework is weak, crowd behavior may even shape the policies of instituted leaders. Thus, of one of the crises in the Middle East during the early fifties, Anne O'Hare McCormick wrote that foreign policy is now being made in the streets.

---

[7] See Sigmund Freud, *Group Psychology and the Analysis of the Ego,* J. Strachey, tr. (London: Internation Psycho-analytical Press, 1922), p. 9 ff.

[8] "Masses," *Encyclopaedia of the Social Sciences,* Vol. X, pp. 198 and 200.

3. Movements, Parties, and Pressure Groups

No one has yet classified in an adequate way all those types of
voluntary institutions or associations, which lie between the family
on the one hand and the state and alliances of states on the other.
But it does seem, as we have already indicated, that it is in this
zone that leadership of the most interesting sort arises.[9] It arises
here because this context permits the invention of leader roles and
the expansion of the scope of existing roles by leaders. Here we
find the attempts to co-ordinate, in Nazi-like manner, by interlocking memberships and the infiltration of leaders into key roles of
other voluntary institutions. Here we find parties that are the organs of a movement becoming so dominating as to eliminate other
parties, and turn the movement into an extension and instrument
of the party. Here we find several movements represented in one
party, as in major political parties of the United States; as well as
several parties within one movement, as in European labor movements. Obviously such intricate overlapping provides opportunities for modification of roles and functions at the hands of those
who would lead.

A movement attempts to change institutions, from the outside,
from the inside, or from both. Like institutions, movements are organized enough to permit a turnover of members without loss of
identity as movements, and their members are more or less aware
of themselves as having common interests and/or principles. It
recruits members, usually from selected class and status levels,
who are more or less ready to act in certain ways, and it lends to
them its orienting aim: in some way to change some institutional
setup. Whether based on interest, on principle, or on both, people
are united in voluntary associations in a more or less energetic
struggle for power, which, so far as the leadership is concerned,
means power of an instituted sort for the leaders.

There are many variations and overlaps between movements,
parties, and pressure groups; clean-cut definitions are more likely
to be arbitrary limitations than helpful descriptions. Party programs, Heberle comments,[10] are more likely to consider several

[9] We have discussed this in Chapter XIV: The Sociology of Leadership, Section 4: Contexts and Roles.
[10] Rudolf Heberle, *Social Movements* (New York: Appleton-Century-Crofts,
1951).

important issues; pressure groups, only limited, specific issues. Parties, as Schattschneider puts it,[11] try to mobilize majorities; pressure groups to organize minorities. Such a distinction seems more or less adequate for Anglo-Saxon countries, but not for movements such as the Catholic center party in Germany, which as a principled "minority party" had no chance to win a "majority" and hardly was so optimistic as to feel that such aspirations made sense: they never polled more than 20 per cent and generally hovered around 15 per cent of the total vote.

There may exist strict "class parties" who advance merely their specialized demands, attract only a following of special interests and orient their platform only to them, and without any particular ideological generalities for a "cloak"; otherwise they are organized like any other party with parliamentary party, machine, and press. Schattschneider in his definition unduly generalizes the United States model, which in many ways is unique. There have been special status group parties—in Hungary, Austria, and Germany— of agrarian nobles, who proudly called themselves small but strong.

Moreover (if one wishes to speak of "majorities-minorities") a "pressure group," such as the German Trade Unions under the Weimar Republic, may be an enormous affair, as opposed to the state party of bourgeois liberalism.

Pressure groups are associations which use political means for the promotion of strictly economic, usually class, interests; parties do the reverse; even declared "class parties" use economic means, as well as political, for both economic and political ends. "Labor parties" generally differ from bourgeois "class parties" in that they aim by reforms or by revolutions to attain a new social structure, hence not at "getting out of capitalism" what they can get, but transforming capitalism in one way or another.[12] The party structure of the United States, in spite of the heterogeneous composition of each party, would seem at least temporarily to drift toward class alignments: "the vested interest" *v.* wage earners, family farmers, and new and old middle classes in the big city.

It should be clear that all sorts of interrelations, and hence opportunities for leaders to elaborate their roles and expand the

[11] E. E. Schattschneider, *Politics, Pressures and the Tariff* (New York: Prentice-Hall, 1935).

[12] Cf. C. Wright Mills, *The New Men of Power* (New York: Harcourt, Brace, 1948).

scope of their commands, exist in the context of voluntary associations.

Movements are composed of people who are attempting to change their position with reference to the personnel or the structure of institutions. The people involved need not share common values; and they may be quite variously motivated in such a way as to converge or coincide in the movement's direction. But whether or not the people involved are conscious of common ends or are propelled by similar motives is not necessary to their definition as a movement, but must be determined in any given case.

Thus the European crusade represented a movement having quite heterogeneous sources, motives, and objectives: [13] there was Pope Urban II's desire to integrate the Greek and Roman church with himself as head; there was the feudal lord's willingness to make war, which was their trade, and which, for all warriors, was a supremely prestigeful activity; there were the new lands to conquer and fiefs to be established for noble scions; there was the desire of the trading classes, especially of the Italian cities, to benefit from shipping services and the luxurious plunder of the East; there was also the spiritual interest of all Christians to conquer the Holy Land from the Mohammedans; and in the asceticist atmosphere of the age, there was the desire of men and women to do penance by the long, dangerous pilgrimage, and thus to save their souls.

Movements may be located in any one or in several of the institutional orders. If their orientation has primarily to do with the personnel, structure, policies, or symbols of the religious order of institutions, they may be understood as religious movements; if they seek to influence state power, who wields it and how, they are political movements. If they seek to change the status system or the class structure we may speak of status movements, such as those of youth, women, and the aged, or of class movements, such as those of middle classes, farmers, and labor. Movements may be specialized by institutional orders and spheres, or they may include several or all orders within a social structure.

The great ideological movements of liberalism, nationalism, and socialism have generally tended to operate in a total way: their

---

[13] See "Crusades," *Encyclopaedia of the Social Sciences*, Vol. IV, p. 614 ff.

goals and policies have to do with extensive modifications of the structure of all orders and spheres—religious and political, kinship and economic, military and technological, status and educational. In liberalism, for example, we speak of "economic liberalism" when referring to "Manchesterism" and free trade; of "political liberalism" when referring to constitutionalism v. despotism; of "cultural liberalism" when referring to the symbol and educational spheres, to the elaboration of personality models in the arts, and so on.

Movements may also be classified in terms of how far-going their aims may be: if they seek to modify existing arrangements, we speak of reform movements, if they seek to change the structure and the ruling legitimations of institutional orders, we speak of revolutionary movements.

Therefore, in examining a social movement one may first locate it at each phase through which it runs, within institutional orders and spheres, and within classes and status levels—in terms of at least three aspects: (1) its professed goals and policies, whether they are reformative or revolutionary and what their specific contents are; (2) the recruitment and composition of its members and leaders; and (3) its objective functions; that is, one must ask *cui bono?*—to whose benefit does its existence and operation redound?

4. Revolution and Counterrevolution [14]

As the term implies, a revolution may be generically defined as a qualitative turnover of institutional orders. Movements or parties which aim to transform and replace the legitimations and institutions of an order, or of several orders, may be called revolutionary. With such exceptions as "industrial revolution," the term is usually used only for relatively rapid transformations. The scope of such movements may be delimited in terms of which orders the

---

[14] For good introductory accounts, see Crane Brinton, *The Anatomy of Revolution* (New York: Norton, 1938); L. P. Edwards, *The Natural History of Revolution* (Chicago: Univ. of Chicago Press, 1927); E. H. Carr, *Studies in Revolution* (London: Macmillan, 1950); Edmund Wilson, *To the Finland Station* (New York: Harcourt, Brace, 1940); but above all, Leon Trotsky, *The History of the Russian Revolution*, Max Eastman, tr. (New York: Simon & Schuster, 1936); Franz Borkenau, *The Communist International* (New York: Norton, 1938); Franz Neumann, *Behemoth* (New York: Oxford Univ. Press, 1942); Alfred Meusel, "Revolution and Counter-Revolution," *Ency. Social Sciences* (New York: Macmillan, 1937), Vol. VII, pages 367-76.

movement is aimed at: it is "partial" if it operates only in some orders, it is total if it aims to transform all orders. It is probably only with the advent of modern, extensive techniques of communication, domination, and manipulation that total revolutions become possible. The Russian is thus more "total" than the French revolution. We may also define the scope by determining whether the movement comes to operate in more than one natural unit. We do not wish to include the occurrence of violence in our definition of revolution, although it is an historical fact that most revolutions, both ancient and modern, have involved violence, on behalf of the status quo as well as against it.

For full-scale revolution there must be more than a change of values; the ruling structure and its legitimations must change. Thus, without revolution, men of various classes and with definite aims and policies may come and go in cabinets, but a state run by cabinets may endure. Revolution involves a turnover in personnel; but such a turnover is not by itself a revolution. A circulation of elites is not enough; there must also be a restructuring of a system of domination and authority.

A revolution, loosely conceived, appears as a profound change in a social structure occurring suddenly and with violence. But it is sudden only in its appearance to the unprepared. And it is not always "with violence"—even in the political order; moreover, the major violence involved is usually an effect of the success of the revolution, when the new regime comes to grips with counterforces who would by violence defend or restore the old structure.

If law, in practice, is what the courts are likely to enforce, and if the courts are of the established order, revolutions are of course, "illegal"—being beyond what courts can enforce. But revolutions, if successful, establish new legal orders. It is, in fact, a definitive characteristic of revolutionary transitions that they mark a gap in legality: old legitimations and laws no longer can be enforced; new ones are as yet not established.

From the point of view of the old regime a revolution is an illegal or a "criminal" change in the conditions of legality. From the point of view of the new regime the agents who enforce or try to enforce the old legitimations are "criminals."

In "palace revolutions," usurpers—often from within the ruling stratum—displace the ruler (King Farouk of Egypt, 1952), or his legitimate successor (Edward VIII, 1936), or the entire dynasty

("The Glorious Revolution," 1688)—without changing the master symbols. And by the so-called *coup d'état* rulers may change the political system and the legitimation formula, as did Napoleon III in 1851, or Hitler upon the death of Hindenburg.

If in a political order changes in the legal order of private property rights, as from one class to another, are instigated, which in turn lead to qualitatively new institutions coming to predominance in the economic order, we may speak of political and economic revolution. In the status sphere of the political order, revolution occurred when the Constitution of the United States outlawed titles of nobility and disclaimed any citizen who accepts a title from another government. This blow against descent prestige cleared the way for the estimation of men on other terms: effort, personal merit, election to office or wealth. The Jacksonian era carried through this status revolution, for many of the phenomena associated with Jackson's administration are more properly considered matters of status than of economics.

The experience of classic bourgeois revolutions was theoretically formulated by Marx, who saw the connection between the economic and the political order in terms of class struggle. This struggle was anchored in the economic order, but culminated in a struggle of the ascending middle classes for the state. The political revolution was thus explained in terms of changes in the economic order. Such economically anchored political revolutions, guided by class parties, bring about a new correspondence between the economic and the political orders. Previous disproportions between the two orders are eliminated in favor of the ascendant class in the economic order. Such political revolutions are usually preceded and accompanied by ideological and status changes: the newly established authorities claim status for themselves and for their supporters. The political symbols turn over. Roundhead and *sans culotte* replace long curls, wigs and breeches. Monuments of old Tsars and generals are torn down, new heroes monumentalized; old street names and old flags, old emblems and oaths give way to new ones. Into the bonfires go the cultural symbols of past power as the zeal of the iconoclast has its heyday.

So during the heroic period of Puritanism, Cromwell's army proclaims itself an army of saints. Inspired soldiers, "the agitators," mount pulpits without waiting for ordination. Puritan bibliocracy is thus established. Similarly, in the French revolution, every deputy of the revolutionary parliament is sworn in with his hand upon Rousseau's *Contrat sociale*. During the climax of the revolutionary enthusiasm the cult of the goddess of reason is proclaimed and in majestic public demonstrations a nude virgin on a flower-bedecked float symbolizes the new deity of political enlightenment. Revolutionary operas glorify the new regime, David stages and directs the festival, immortalizes the revolutionary hero (Marat's death). The new class abolishes old customs, creates new forms of exuberant mass enthusiasm. The ceremonious minuet—the show dance of the elite—is swept away by the uproarious passionate whirling of waltzing masses. Then this exuberance is tinged with proletariat vigor when in 1830 the cancan, with its high kicking becomes publicly acceptable.

Broad masses expand and, under the impact of enthusiastic revolutionary terrorism, old status groups go into hiding and exile, maintaining their esteemed self-conceptions through snobbish derision of the vulgarity of the political parvenus. They compensate for their loss of power by strictly emphasizing the symbols of status, the good name of the deserved ancestors, the well-mannered and soft-spoken conventions of the educated, the refined tastes of the sophisticated. Marginal figures from these upper groups who shift political sides are the most hated of men. Intellectuals (ministers, artists, political secretaries) who theoretically elaborate the nostalgic hope for a return of the "good old days" are cordially welcome. Refugees who have found asylum at foreign courts call for war against the revolutionized country and hope for the return of the lost holdings. And to the extent to which the new order relaxes in zeal and watchfulness, conspiratorial activities increase among the deposed.

New leaders of a counterrevolution are appraised as past experience is rationalized. New theories are developed which dispute the legitimacy of the revolutionary regime and debunk, psychologically, theoretically, and politically, its new measures and styles of life. So after the first revolutionary shocks have been overcome, fatalism and defeatism tend to wane and give way to political plotting, inspired by the observation of incipient cracks and points of strain in the new structure. Out of informal gatherings grow nuclei of political and perhaps eventually military organizations. Their leaders play on the sentiments of the disappointed, woo the good will of foreign governments who may hesitate to grant recognition to the revolutionary regime.

In brief, the forces of reaction organize for counterrevolution. One member or another of the ranks who side with the revolution, feeling the pulse of impending crises, may—as did Talleyrand—change horses and exploit his official position in the new order for political intrigue in favor of a "restoration." By counterrevolution we mean the organized and successful endeavor of previous ruling groups to re-establish themselves in power in the name of the old or newly wrought legitimations.

The defeat of such attempts constitutes the supreme test of the new regime: it is at this point that we find the organized use of revolutionary terror. Political enemies, actual or suspect, are outlawed, their property confiscated, their families executed or expelled, their friends hunted down. The secret police operates in the midst of wild rumors, harsh denunciations, veiled threats. If the incipient counterrevolution cannot be nipped in the bud, military emergencies and states of siege are proclaimed. If the army is politically suspect, the revolutionary vanguard organizes a new revolutionary army controlled by "political commissars" (Saint-Just, Cromwell's agitators, the Commissars of the Red Army). If the counterrevolution should succeed, a still stronger terrorism is organized. Revolutionary leaders and fighters may be shot en masse ("The ten thousand" after the French Commune of 1871, the White Terror in Hungary after World War I).

In all cases there is a rapid turnover of prison populations. The release of prisoners may be equivalent to the Christian glorification of martyrs. Schiller, the court intellectual of Weimar, argued that "man is free, even if born in chains," which may hold for the inner spirit of the intellectual; but for political movements, man is free only when his chains are broken. The storming of the Bastille on July 14, in itself a political bagatelle, has become the date for the annual celebration of the French Revolution. The chorus of the liberated prisoners in Beethoven's *Fidelio* is the revolutionary symbol of political liberation and freedom.

It is convenient to grasp the psychological and ideological aspects of revolutionary movements by focusing upon their definition of historical time and reality and upon their conception of freedom.

As Karl Mannheim has demonstrated,[15] these aspects of mentality allow for a convenient approach to some of the underlying and implied categories through which the revolutionary actor's experience is structured, but which are themselves rarely experienced self-consciously.

I. *Time:* As the charismatic leader and his followers are not bound by communal traditions nor by a legal order, but rather are the initiators of radical beginnings, they experience their time as a crisis. They feel detached from what appears to them as old and dead, although they live in the midst of such death. An epoch is coming to an end, a time is ceasing, the old book is closed. But new gates are opening and they feel themselves at the threshold of a new epoch, and from this their enthusiasm springs. Moses sees but does not enter the new land. The transition from Pharaonic bondage to this new and liberated land is on the way, Christ acts "to fulfill the time" and his birth marks the beginning of Occidental Christendom's history. So the France of 1789 and the Russia of the October revolution attempt to institute new calendars, which begin with their deeds. The leader as well as his followers thus experience their time as the beginning of all time. Karl Marx's dismissal of the last 2,000 years of history as mere "prehistory," and Engel's expectation of the "leap into freedom" indicate the temporal discontinuity experienced by revolutionaries. Not the gradual transitions of a continuum, but the historical hiatus, expressed by many and various symbols, is typical.

II. *Reality:* The charismatic experience of reality shows the same abrupt dichotomy radically separating the black from the white, the dead from the living, and light from darkness. Schiller, as a revolutionary enthusiast, cries out, "And new life springs from the ruins . . . ," an image to be found in many paintings of the period: young mothers and babies playing amidst broken and ancient columns, or, indeed, hanging diapers on them. Traditional forms of life and conventions appear as hollow and doomed; they are as masks of death itself: they are visualized as threats. Institutions, however outwardly firm, are built on foundations of sand. If the doomed aristocrat, in a fleeting moment of self-consciousness, cynically shrugs his shoulders and mutters, "After us, the

[15] See his *Ideology and Utopia*, Louis Wirth and Edward Shils, trs. (New York: Harcourt, Brace, 1936).

deluge," the revolutionary group is full of hope in feeling itself embarking upon a new era. The heir to the past feels that he would make the most of what is left of the old time; the charismatic actor feels that all can be had if what is left would but fall. Facing up to what blocks his way, he is eager not to support but to push over what is already tottering. "And what is this class struggle? It is overthrowing the Czar, overthrowing the capitalist, destroying the capitalist class. . . . We subordinate our Communist morality to this task. We say: 'Morality is that which serves to destroy the old exploiting society and to unite all the toilers around the proletariat which is creating a new Communist society.'" [15A]

A keen sense of a new unheard-of mission inspires the charismatic leader and his followers. Feeling at one with the rush of time, his days are not counted; he sees his days to come. For him there is no end in view; the new reality appears to him under the aspect of infinity. The optimistic image of the new age of harmony, the golden age, the end of darkness, the rising sun, spring, and the end of winter—these celestial allegories and symbols express experiences of a discontinuous reality. Or, there may be organic symbols: the image of the pangs and travails of birth, which Marx uses often, lends itself readily to this experience. Optimism, of a previously unheard-of surge, lifts up the followers of the charismatic leader. With eyes fixed on the distant yet foreshortened goal, they move ahead with the certainty of the sleepwalker, often immunized against the costs of blood, self-sacrifice and terror which the deliberate destruction of the old entails.

III. *Freedom:* These experiences of time and reality dovetail with those of the freedom which is to come through detachment in action. Freedom means liberation, and with the increasing size and power of the charismatic following, freedom is felt to increase. For freedom is seen and felt to be a sharing in the expanding movement of the leader. The enthusiasm of the faithful follower is experienced as essential to freedom. Loyalty to the leader and to new actions increasingly widen the gap between what is to the follower the restraint of a doomed world and a series of obstacles; so the charismatic groups in active pursuit of their resolution experience this resolution as providing a new freedom for all. Their

[15A] Nikolai Lenin, *Collected Works* (New York: International Pubs., 1923), Vol. XVIII, p. 322 ff.

enthusiasm is aggressive and inclusive. They wish to embrace and incorporate all things.

It is this sense of an expanding generalized other which inspires their sense of "mission." Hence this experience of freedom is far from a privatizing of the person. On the contrary, freedom as the withdrawal into privacy is derided as indifference, egoism, and selfishness. Freedom for what? is answered by the charismatic group in charismatic action. The leader challenges the old: in Christ's phrase, "it is written, but *I* say unto you." To the extent to which it binds followers, the leader's word also dissolve their bonds to outsiders.

It would be futile to go beyond some such statements as these, which cannot fail to be relatively abstract, as the symbolic context of any charismatic revolutionary group is of course influenced by the era and the society in which it emerges. Yet these somewhat general comments may suffice to characterize the directions which detailed studies of different types of revolutionary movements might have to consider.

The proletariat play a part in all the classic bourgeois revolutions; actual fighting forces are usually recruited from among its ranks, but they are not necessarily led by wage workers and their aims are often different.

We understand by "proletarian revolutions" those which aim at the conquest of the state for the declared purpose of abolishing big private property in the means of production, however indistinct, confused, hazy, or romantic this implied goal may be in its varied formulations. The insurrection of the Paris proletariat in 1830 is thus the first autonomous revolt of the proletariat. Similarly, the revolution of 1848 and the establishment of the short-lived Paris Commune, the revolution of Germany of 1918 in part, the October revolution in Russia in 1917, China in the forties are outstanding examples.

These revolutions are historically specific in that they are *planned*. Modern revolutions involve specific problems of ideological and political organization, political strategy and tactics and insurrectional technique. It is with reference to such questions that different proletarian parties emerge. A staff of leaders is typically recruited from outside the class for which they speak but with which they identify; they have included aristocratic intellectuals and officers (Bakunin, Chicherin, L. Renn), bourgeois intellectuals and Maecenases (F. Engels, Paul Singer). The party fund which helped the Russian socialists to hold their historic 1903 party congress in London, at which the Bolshevist party under Lenin emerged as the "majority," was financed by Lloyd George. Schoolteachers and seminarists (like Mao Tse-tung and Joseph Stalin), self-educated migratory journeymen (Wilhelm Weitling, Eugene Debs), and *déclassé,* plebeian intelligentsia (such as Lenin), the numerous party secretaries, radical journalists (like Lincoln Steffens), runaway students (like John Reed) have also entered revolutionary parties.

Those strivings which eventuate in revolutions have historically been conceived as national in context and origin. Twentieth-century revolutions, however, are characterized by the fact that they occur in the wake of military defeat and subsequent military interventions. Lenin is the author of a special elaboration of this fact and, based upon it, of a set of tactics to "transform imperialist war into civil war" by "revolutionary defeatism," and "the dictatorship of the proletariat," which legitimates the establishment of the vanguard's power.

There is one fact about the course of one of these modern proletariat revolutions, and its ensuing counterrevolution, that is so psychologically striking that we must attempt to understand its wider psychological meanings. We refer to the "confessions" of the old Bolshevik vanguard during the thirties.

The brilliant intellectuals, primarily of middle-class background, who in 1917 led the Bolshevik revolution succumbed to brutally efficient administrators, primarily of such background—rising from peasant milieu through party schools and up the bureaucratic ladder—that to them the telephone was a prime symbol of power. The old polemic leaders did not last in the era of bureaucratic plots, but the mediocre, as Victor Serge has written, reconciled their convictions with the situation in which they found themselves: "long live our beefsteak, long live our chief, *we* are the revolution . . ."

Since 1917, some twenty-seven men have at one time or another been members of the Russian Politburo—the top power unit of the U.S.S.R. Lenin died of natural causes in 1924, ending by his death the period of the old Bolsheviks; from then until 1938, when the last big purge trial ended, is a transition era. The third era, from 1938 to date, is the era of the entrenched Stalin administration. Nineteen of the total of twenty-seven are no longer members of the Politburo: eight were executed, two murdered, one was a suicide, one was just dropped, and seven died of natural causes.[16]

The remarkable psychological aspect of this shift has to do with the "confessions" of the old Bolshevik vanguard. They "confessed" to actions which there is reason to believe they did not commit. Why? They had been members of the party for major portions of their lives; they had given up all else for party work. Their circle of significant others, in brief, was confined to party members, and the party formed, as it were, the only social locus of their generalized others. So, it may be that their confidence in themselves, in their ability to think and decide, was tied to their faith in the party, the I and the Me having no clear-cut border-line in their conscience. Therefore: no thought, no feeling, no consciousness outside the party. In liberal terminology, their commitment was not provisional or partial; it was permanent and absolute. And since they had no social anchorage for individual behavior outside the party, their last individual act was to sacrifice themselves for the party.[17] One thing we have learned by the Soviet shift "from Lenin to Stalin" is that ideologies can blind as well as guide thinking, feeling, seeing, remembering.

5. Anticapitalistic Movements and Parties

There have been some four general movements in the twentieth century which have so overshadowed other movements that in Europe their struggles and victories and defeats, their reforms and revolutions, have made up "The Social Question." In intellectual circles, their debates and issues have formed the live content of political discussion. In the world scene, their rise and fall have been the keys to world wars and international tensions. They have

[16] These figures are drawn from George K. Schueller, *The Politburo* (Stanford: Stanford Univ. Press, 1951). But compare Paul Scheffer, "From Lenin to Stalin," *Foreign Affairs*, April 1938, pp. 445-53.

[17] See Philip E. Mosely's "Freedom of Artistic Expression and Scientific Inquiry in Russia," *The Annals of the American Academy of Political and Social Science*, Vol. 200, November 1938, pp. 254-74; and especially F. Beck and W. Godin, *Russian Purge and the Extraction of Confession* (New York: Viking, 1951).

each striven to operate in all institutional orders, although the political and economic areas have been their central locales, and they have each been an opposition movement, especially in the economic order—for all but one of them have been generally anti-capitalist.

We can describe them systematically, as we can describe any movement or party, by examining their (1) ultimate goals and (2) typical ways of attaining them, (3) their immediate expectations and (4) demands, (5) their general conception of history and (6) the organizational levers they would use, (7) their dominant mode of action and (8) the composition of their predominant membership, (9) the types of leaders and staff they have displayed and (10) their objective political results.

I. *Anarchism and Syndicalism*—as displayed by Spanish and Italian anarchism, by France's syndicalist movement and in the United States by the IWW; by Russian nobles, like Bakunin and Kropotkin, by nihilism and earlier in what is known as Blanquism —are now largely insignificant as political movements. As movements, they are now significant for us only as precursors in this or that detail of doctrine or technique for later, more successful movements. The historical aim of these movements has been a stateless society or congeries of societies composed of free brethren, which they sought to attain by "propaganda of the deed" (Bakunin), the promulgation of the "myth of the general strike" (Sorel) —by, in short, a spontaneous insurrection of the exploited. They have been eschatological, expecting an immediate and universal crisis in public affairs, and so they have demanded action—immediate and direct. For them all history has been full of evil power, for all power is evil, the existing state being an incarnation of sinful exploitation, and civilization a great progress towards a hubris of the powerful. In the course of history, the state is doomed. The organizational levers with which they would cause its downfall have been loose federations of sectarian type under charismatic leaders, as with Blanqui's especially, small and vigorously disciplined fighting clubs. They wished to engage in individual terrorism, in nihilism, in the propaganda of the deed; or, as in Barcelonean syndicalism, in strikes of spontaneous masses; or in Blanquistic *coup d'état*. They have recruited both men and women, especially people working in small sweatshops, as among Swiss watchmakers or French embroidery workers, or as in the United States, among various types of migratory laborers in the western states. Their leaders have been seen as extraordinary men and women and as both high- and low-brow intellectuals.

II. One may define *socialism*, generally, as the demand for a planned economic order, producing for use rather than profit, and subject to central administration and budgetary accounting. This involves the fusion of economic and political orders by the extension of democratic practices to the economic order, which, in turn, makes for the elimination of property and income class privileges in favor of economic equality. As a movement, socialism must be divided into at least three types, the first two of which—"social democracy" and "left-wing socialism" we shall describe together.

Social Democrats combined their parties in the Second International; its outstanding examples are the German Social-Democratic party operating up to the Nazi era, and reconstituted in Western Germany since 1945. Left-wing socialism has been represented by the Austrian Socialists under Otto Bauer or by the left socialists in Italy under Pietro Nenni. Both types have aimed at a Socialist economy, by which is meant one in which no private property in the basic means of production exists, and in a democratic political order; and both would achieve these ends by the constitutional means of parliamentary democracy. They would win over the exploited classes by their political program and propaganda, engage in election fights as a duly constituted party, and would maintain this organization continuously by linking party with trade unions and consumer co-operatives, as well as other affiliated associations. With these organizations they would come to state power and so enact their program. Their immediate demands have varied according to the going situation, to which they would rationally orient their tactics. Originally, the demand of the Social-Democrats was the universal and equal franchise, for with this gained, they supposed, their movement would flourish; later, their demands were put into detailed petitions and bills for attainable legislation in favor of the underprivileged and in defense of democracy. Left-wing socialists have shared these demands, but to them have added possible coalition with Bolshevik parties and the formation of semimilitary party auxiliaries, for left-wing socialists would not shrink from the use of violence in order to achieve or to defend a democratic order. Thus, in the thirties, when central European democratic constitutions were being smashed, the Austrian socialists' military wing fought back with machine guns to be put down by Dollfuss' howitzers.

Social Democrats have conceived of history as a gradual progression in the direction of the enlightenment of the masses, of rising living standards, and, in the international area, of peaceful compromises among labor governments. Left-wing socialists have foreseen breaks in history and, in viewing the past, have glorified the revolutionary traditions of various proletariats. Their organizational levers have been pretty much confined to the party, but those of the Social Democrats have also included varying constellations of parliamentary factions involving party, trade union, and co-op, with an over-all trend towards the ascendancy of trade unions over parties. The Social Democratic dominant mode of action has thus been the building of mass organizations and the mass indoctrination of party press, the electoral campaign and the lobbying for legislation, and has not failed to include formation of coalition governments with nonsocialist, or "bourgeois" parties. The left-wing socialist's activity has strongly emphasized disciplined party formations with total, or even totalitarian, organization of wage workers, and has moreover included lower middle-class movements. The backbone of the Social-Democratic movement has been the unions of organized labor. Left-wing socialism has enrolled the same elements, as well as descending middle-class elements. The types of leaders and staff ascendant in both types have included parliamentary demagogues, and party and trade union officials.

III. All socialist movements are anticapitalist, and they have aimed in their ultimate visions at a classless society in which power and "politics" would be abolished in favor of the technical and rational planning of society. *Bolshevism's* political and economic results have, in fact, been the rise to complete power of the Bolshevist party, the abolishment of private property in the means of production, a planned war economy, in a totalitarian state, dominating the "Third International" and later the Cominform in varying ways outside the Soviet Union. The means with which it would gain its ultimate end, which resulted in the present Russian state, was revolution, and as a movement its immediate expectations and tactics have been oriented to the presumed presence or absence of a "revolutionary situation." It has therefore raised detailed "shock demands," which are intended to attract and unite under-privileged classes and groups of all sorts, and which have often been slanted and timed so as to be impossible of fulfillment short of revolution. Its conception of history has been that of a dialectical struggle of the world bourgeoisie and the world proletariat, and its organizational lever has been a small, select party of active and disciplined revolutionaries led by skilled and dedicated profes-sionals. Their leaders and staff have historically thus included revolutionary intellectuals, both low- and high-brow, but they have tended, outside of Russia, to be unstable, and in and out of Russia to be punctuated by purges from the top. The modes of Bolshevist action have included all those practiced by left-wing socialists and Social-Democrats, as well as active preparation for uprising, and various types of illegitimate, illegal activities. The membership recruited for the Bolshevik movement has consisted mainly of men, especially of highly skilled groups of the unem-ployed, labor youths and a radical intelligentsia. It has consisted of a hard, persisting core of veterans, and a larger membership that has been unstable and peculiarly high in turnover.

IV. *Fascism,* as in Italy and Germany, has not been an anti-capitalist movement, although its rhetoric has borrowed heavily from Marxian vocabularies. It has been, in its composition and aims, an antilabor movement of chauvinist middle classes, a mili-tary bohemia of officer veterans, and elements of the metropolitan dregs. In its results it has been a totalitarian imperialism of mo-nopoly capitalistic base with modifications and extensions of big business, jurisdictional areas, social controls, and personnel. Fas-cism's ultimate aim has been world empire; its dominant means, world war; its immediate expectations, the crises of parliamentary democracy and existing capitalistic economies. Its promises and demands have been: power to us, and then we'll detail the pro-grams—all other demands set forth by its leaders have seemed to be a conflicting but Machiavellian hodge-podge of incitements. Its conception of history has been of a process of racial pollution and decadence of nations, which may be saved by racially pure elites; all history is thus seen as a circulation of elites and a suc-cession of empires. The fascist lever of organization, the totalitarian party and its innumerable officials, have included semi-military auxiliaries—as with Bolshevism. This rather miscellaneous party has been led by *Führer, Duce,* or *Caudillo*—and in accordance with the leadership principle, merged with and upheld by bureaucratic machines under military discipline.

Collective behavior—a phrase that refers to the revolutionary overturn of social structures as well as the peaceful milling about of casual street throngs—is obviously a catchall for various phenomena that do not readily fit into conceptions of institutional order. And yet, none of these movements, parties, crowds, aggregates or publics can be understood or explained without sensitive reference to the social structure that is their context. For collective behavior, after all, is the behavior of the same people who in their more usual, everyday lives enact the routines of more or less stable institutions. And it is within the master trends of institutional structures that such people, in their collective behavior, may place their imprint upon an epoch of history.

CHAPTER
XVI

Master Trends

IN reflecting upon the basic transformations of twentieth-century societies, we may first examine those institutional orders in which the distribution of power is most visible. We do not intend by this approach to imply that "power" is the highest value, for men in general or for us; it is simply expedient to approach modern social structures from this point of view, for it is from this vantage point that we may best hope to understand the ground swell of our age. The "revolution of our time," as it is called in contemporary tracts, is certainly most readily discernible in the military, political, and economic orders. Moreover, from the point of view of "social control," "staff controlled" sanctions offer the easiest way to an understanding of the master problems of a society as a whole.

The development of technologies of production and of destruction—from the stone ax to the atom bomb—has now reached a new threshold of efficiency in both the economic and the military orders of the great powers. With these developments, the institutional units which incorporate these technological developments are enormously expanded. In the United States, for example, a handful of corporations centralize decisions and responsibilities that are relevant for military and political as well as economic developments of global significance. For nowadays the military and the political cannot be separated from economic considerations of power. We now live not in an economic order and in a political order, but in a political economy and moreover a political economy that is closely linked with military institutions and decisions. This is obvious in the repeated "oil crises" of the Middle East, or in the relevance of Southeast Asia and African resources for the Western powers. Thus, an American state governor, upon his return from the Far East in 1951, spoke casually of "our tin" and "our rubber" when speaking of French Indo-China, British Malaya, and the Indonesian Republic. In the perspective of the naval powers, the Mediterranean, as well as the North and the Baltic Seas, are but extensions of the Atlantic Ocean. A network of looser or firmer treaties now extends throughout the "Western world," from the eastern Mediterranean to the borderlands of Asia on the Pacific coast.

1. The Co-ordination of Political, Economic and Military Orders

Various tensions and bargains now implement a world drift whose direction in the postwar era has been unmistakably towards an increasing integration of economic, military, and political structures, on both sides of the dividing lines running through Central Europe and Korea. At the same time, ideological and diplomatic, and economic and military conflict has been increasing. This is what is meant by the cold war that is characteristic of a world of nations increasingly polarized between the United States and the Soviet Union.

The enormous range and the destructive capacities of modern weapons has by itself made for a great increase in the power wielded by central decision-making units. This process was already forcefully under way during the depression of the thirties, for at that time the various efforts of central governments to plan rather than drift were inaugurated on some scale. This enhancement of central executive power has occurred, as it were, blindly, and it has been actively implemented by the deliberate centralization policies of public authorities. The result is an ever-increasing bureaucratization.

In each of the two major crises of modern capitalist societies— in world depression and in world war—central planning and regulation and the enforcement of big decisions lead men of power to an increasing awareness of the interdependence, and accordingly of the need for co-ordination, of all major institutional orders. In order to control the ramifications of key decisions in one field— for instance, the universal peacetime draft for an army—the authorities have promptly to consider the cumulative effects in the educational sphere: the decreasing enrollments of institutions of higher learning, the threats of bankruptcy for small colleges, the long-run scarcities of trained professional personnel in strategic

skill-groups, and so on. Or, the ramifications into the economic order: How do the armies' demands for equipment affect industry?
the state's demands for "big hardware" and the public's demands
for consumer goods? How will the draft affect the labor force, in
agriculture, in industry? How about the equality of men and
women—shall both be drafted? If so, in what ratio? at what age?
for how long? What of allies? What is their economic and military
potential? What about their internal cohesion and political reliability?

The tensions of policy alternatives reverberate throughout the
value structure of modern societies. Religious institutions are also
affected, as clergymen enter the discussion with teachers and other
professionals concerned with marriage and population policies.
"Moral problems" thus come to the fore, and decision-making
groups realize that their decisions touch directly or indirectly
upon all institutional orders of society. Accordingly their decisions
must, it seems, be "total."

Under laissez-faire conditions of the nineteenth century the various institutional orders were, so to speak, left alone, and it was
taken for granted that harmony would win out in a process of
dynamic oscillations, of minor frictions and adjustments, that
would end up in a new "equilibrium." Today such a spontaneous
balancing can no longer be assumed, nor can harmony be left to
chance. Hence, the top decisions tend increasingly to be "co-
ordinated" decisions and to ramify throughout institutional orders;
so decision-makers, when speaking of "calculated risks," anticipate
long-range consequences. The decision to "go all out" in an armament race, for example, goes together with purchasing programs
for stockpiling strategically significant raw materials in the hegemony area, and the U.S. demand, as the universal protector of the
Western orbit, to blockade the Soviet orbit. These decisions, in
turn, affect the weaker economies of other nations:

Raw material countries may raise their price levels. Weak im-
porting industrial countries may feel their export opportunities
threatened under conditions of rising costs of production. Debtor
nations may see their relation to creditors badly affected, as well
as fear for their economic, political, and psychological stability,
should mass unemployment emerge. These national fears are due
to cumulative international processes often beyond the control of
the nations involved.

It is because of such specific consequences as these that decisions tend to become total, and the political decisions of parties
and cabinets to become key decisions. Certain goals stand out in
relatively clear focus, as military and economic targets, and the
time required for their realization can be predicted within relatively narrow limits. Up to a point, moreover, their ramifications
into various institutional orders can be assessed. But beyond a
given point, chances have to be taken. It is then that trained and
imaginative judgment seems scarce, is highly premiumed, and leads
to plaintive feelings among executives in political, military, and
business life about the shortage of qualified successors. This feeling, in turn, leads to an increasing concern with the training of
successors who could take over as older men of power retire.

The repeated experience of "boomerangs"—the unintended and
unstated consequences of key decisions—leads to mass disillusionment and to the apathetic withdrawal of groups whose willing
support, or at least readiness "to go along," is indispensible for
implementing expected changes. In postwar Germany, Hitler's
phrase, "The Thousand Year Reich" has become a stock phrase for
deriding his twelve-year rule. The disillusionment of the American
public with Wilsonian idealism shortly after World War I, and with
the starry objectives of the Atlantic Charter, even during the course
of as well as after World War II, also comes to mind. In fact,
one must realize that the mass acceptance of false or insufficient
definitions of reality—and subsequent disappointment—is now a
recurrent feature of the opinion processes and symbol spheres of
the great powers.

Continent-wide publics lack the flexibility of mind which characterizes the ruling few; besides, these masses are expected to have
"faith" in these changing definitions and frequent revisions of
images of reality. For such publics, the rapid succession thus constitutes a process of profound disillusionment, comparable to
changes of creeds in other times. And since, nowadays, these
changes occur within the living experience of a single generation,
the demand for forgetfulness and for learning new definitions of
reality make many men lose the capacity wholeheartedly to accept
publicly sponsored or official definitions of their situation. At the
same time, "the will to believe" may increase, as the successful
mass propagation of demonologies and world conspiracy myths
seems to indicate. Thus, propaganda neurosis on the one hand,

and fanatical superstition on the other, tend to be widely diffused and always to threaten the "small still voice of reason."

The great increase in the volume of official secrets, or secret diplomacy, of security demands, reduces the amount of relevant information available to the mass public. "News behind the news" becomes a ubiquitous advertising slogan, aimed at the suspicious public; "newsletters" are addressed to small circles of decision makers in business, political, and military affairs. The U.S. mass media, under corporate business control, often fail to "represent" public opinion, as is evidenced by the frequent disparity between the stand taken by "the organs of public opinion" and the electorate during presidential elections since 1936.

Instead of free competition and unco-ordinated "adjustments," there are planned "relay systems" which ramify across entire institutional orders. Hence "co-operation" is at a premium, and moreover, co-operation from a multiplicity of leaders all of whom cannot always be informed of the whys and the wherefores of key decisions. Rivalry makes for secrecy; it is, for example, in the nature of modern warfare to launch formless "surprise attacks" and to exploit old-fashioned diplomatic forms as mere means and shadow boxing. Accordingly, there is much competition for superior morale, a competition open to the eyes of world-wide literate groups and their publics, organized as well as in aggregate condition.

The nature of key, national decisions, in summary, involves long range perspectives and targets, and extended and complex means-ends schemes. These decisions are of global scope and they cross institutional orders into which they ramify and which implement them. There is about such institutional mechanics in our time an unheard of "momentum," and the decisions, accordingly, are weighty and grave, and often frightful. They affect no less than the future of mankind.

2. Psychological Aspects of Bureaucracy

All these bureaucratic developments, so central to modern society, may be accompanied by psychological phenomena, which, in brief, result from increased stresses upon the person and from problems he cannot solve by "individual adjustment."

I. An increasing number of employed persons find themselves in a position which does not give them an opportunity to take stock of their whole situation. Their working environment is a mere fragment of a hierarchal structure, on whose total proper functioning they are dependent, even though the total structure and its movements are not intellectually accessible to them. Modern employees—the worker, the salesmen, the clerk—know that they are dependent on the decisions of others, and that few persons have opportunities to attain the key positions from which day-to-day decisions are made. Moreover, the specialized knowledge necessary for decisions makes the ordinary individual's intelligence just as fragmentary as is his environment. He does not choose the ends, for they are set for him; his rational knowledge is of a predetermined character and has to do with means. The traditionalist peasant, in contrast, understands "his business," knows many of the factors which affect him, and the rest he leaves to God or to other supernatural forces.

II. At the same time, the bureaucratic organizations tend to become more and more interdependent, partly because the political community cannot allow for the breakdown of large-scale institutions under private management and motives—such as the profit considerations of the strongest competitor. In an expanding economy of relatively small enterprises, the free market did not lead to such cumulative repercussions in the entire social structure. But in our time breakdowns of industrial corporations or big banks and markets have enormous consequences for all members of society. The government is therefore increasingly obliged to intervene and to support by special political measures whole industries and sectors of social life. This interventionism, in turn, tends further to centralize controls and to increase the interdependence of the large structures.

III. Should crises disrupt the social process, as in the world crisis of the thirties, mass unemployment and world-wide insecurity are among the consequences. Even a "recession" of the American economy causes anxiety in Western Europe. Given the instability and difficulties of the debtor countries, the psychological and political consequences of a major crisis would be unpredictable, but in any event disastrous for democratic regimes based on uneasy coalitions of weak, middle parties. As long as unemployment or bankruptcy was experienced as a selective process eliminating the inefficient and strengthening the efficient, the adversities of crises were ascribed to personal shortcomings. The underprivileged person might seek to extricate himself, and by and large each strove as best he could to find his way out of the strain and duress.

But when in such crises the breakdown is of the scope of the last world slump, individual avenues of escape are insignificant, and the anxieties of underprivileged persons become the basis for collective readjustment. In due course, the unemployed person may give up the hope of finding any job, his former aspirations break down, and with them, the hopes and policies of the family of the breadwinner. In modern society insecurity tends to be experienced not as a personal mishap or misfortune, nor as an irrevocable fate due to supernatural forces nor even to natural forces. And men, full of the tension of insecure positions correctly blame social factors for personal defeat.

IV. It is under such conditions that beliefs in traditional social and political values may be shattered. "Freedom," for example, may be derided as "freedom to starve," and unless democratic leadership succeeds in reconstructing the social order, or in providing substitutes for former institutions, general despair, skepticism, and a debunking type of agitation are likely to spread. This was, for example, the course German society took during the economic crisis of the early thirties.

V. If militantly organized political parties succeed in attracting general attention, if they play successfully on the frustrations of socially descending and disappointed masses, if at the same time they promise "miracles" and "salvation," then fascist-type movements find their opportunity, especially if they couple revolutionary tactics with nationalist propaganda—if they succeed in using frustrations and anger in such a way that scapegoats can be offered. The scapegoat provides for tension release, makes for strong group loyalties, and heightens the belief in the "reality" of the propagandist symbols. It thus makes action, such as terrorist attacks against Jews and working-class organizations, psychologically possible and politically effective.

VI. Such revolutionary or pseudo-revolutionary activities give the fighting individual new aspirations and new self-esteem, now built around his identification with the new organization and its "leader." As the individual breaks away from all formerly held values, cuts off many former social obligations, he feels "free" although, in fact, he is enthusiastically subjecting himself to a rigidly disciplined organization, a political demonology, and a sanctioned image of reality. However, by virtue of the undemocratic character of its organizational pattern, this kind of movement gives the individual feelings of security. He need neither make decisions nor think for himself. He has merely to have faith and carry out the plans and commands of the party. These plans and commands, embodied in "the party line" as defined from on high, often zig and zag in incredible patterns. For Communists all over the world, for example, the last war was an "imperialist war"—during the Stalin-Hitler alliance of 1939 to 1941. Then Hitler was no aggressor and the military offensive presented not "aggression," but merely "the best defense," as though it were a mere tactical question. But with Hitler's attack upon the Soviet Union, the previously "imperialist war" was quickly transformed into a "people's war," and despite the Russian annexation of half of Poland, Romania, Bessarabia and what was formerly Czechoslovak Carpatho-Ukraine, the Baltic states, Königsberg, Finnish Karelia—the Soviet Union by Communist definition never practiced but only fought imperialism. Since the war, the retrospective definition of "all peace-loving nations" (never including neutral countries such as Switzerland, Ireland, and Sweden) excludes the naval democracies of the West and includes all former allies of Hitler once they are inside the Soviet orbit and so reorganized into "People's Democracies." Such are the changing images of reality, defined from on high and officially sanctioned. Deviations from them are conventionally and administratively punished as indicating disloyalty, submission to petty bourgeois or to ultra-rightist or ultra-leftist thoughtways.

The totalitarian party state is not oriented to the pursuit of personal happiness; it demands "sacrifice." Life is serious; "encirclement" is the claustrophobic theme. The Fascist party is concerned with the attainment of political power, with the distribution of spoils, and the reorganization of society for military conquest. With the attainment of political power and the organization of social life in a totalitarian manner, the problems it poses become international. For as long as the party member feels that there is any power which might possibly check his, he remains an aggressive person with the one objective of power.

The frustrated party spreads its psychology of anxiety and its compensatory craving for power. There is a characteristic emotional cycle observable. During the phase of preparatory surprise coups —Hitler, for example, timed them on week ends—the hate campaigns are built to a mounting crescendo. At the same time, intense secrecy places all official personnel and the party machine on guard. The irritability and nervousness of men of responsibility increases. The metropolitan men-in-the-street sense an ominous atmosphere of mounting danger, without being able to discern its source. This sense of ominousness heightens mass anxieties inside and outside the party. Then suddenly, once the coup has been successfully completed, diffuse awareness is replaced by maximum publicity and information; the leader triumphantly proclaims his deed, and the anxieties give way to a public orgy of boisterous *heils,* jubilation, and frenzy. It is then that "internal enemies" are hunted down, rounded up, and thrown into concentration camps.

3. *The Decline of Liberalism*

It is in this world context of total integrations and bureaucratization that we must understand the decline of liberalism as a style of thinking and the rise and spread of totalitarian slogan manipulation and opinion management. For the problems of mass insecurity and of anxiety levels, of mental imbalances and unclear definitions of unstructured situations now form the sociological context of political and economic psychology.

As one of the great thought systems of the Western world, liberalism is rooted in the "enlightenment movement" of the Occidental middle classes and their intellectual vanguards; it incorporates the legacy of Greece and of Rome—a legacy which has been reassimilated by various renaissances since the waning of the Middle Ages.[1]

Liberalism has made its greatest and least questioned headway in the United States. In Europe it has met with older and more entrenched patterns having elaborate defensives of their own. Among these have been Catholic and Protestant orthodoxies, often linked with modern conservative thinking, and anticapitalist intellectuals and parties. From the "right" and from the "left" anticapitalist thinking has emerged: European liberalism has been identified with "the middle." But no such position and no such iden-

[1] See L. T. Hobhouse, *Liberalism* (New York: Holt, 1911); and G. De-Ruggiero, *The History of European Liberalism* (Collingwood Tr., London, 1927).

tification occurred in the United States, where liberalism has become, at least as rhetoric, a common denominator.

This difference between liberalism in Europe and America is due to many factors, but the most important of them is the fact that in Europe capitalist societies developed from older feudal structures, which were never entirely displaced but which, in a number of ways, were transformed and adapted to new societies. The nobility moved from the military camp to the court, becoming an "office nobility"; and to this day nobles play a significant part in the high ranks of ecclesiastic dignitaries in the Roman Catholic Church, of royalty in Lutheran Scandinavian countries, and in the established church of England. Landlordism in Italy and Spain, in France, Great Britain, and Germany, although affected by the complex history of capitalism, has allowed strong feudal elements to adapt themselves and so survive in complicated forms.

The rise of capitalist society in Central Europe and in large areas of Eastern Europe did not involve the transfer of political and military power to the economically most powerful group—the urban capitalist middle class. Because of the failure of the 1848 revolutions, and the complexities of national formations in Italy, Germany, and Japan during the second half of the nineteenth century, princely power, although reduced in prerogative, maintained itself in the status structure and retained its prestigeful influence among intellectuals. The cultural patronage of petty courts and nobles continues to exist in some European societies right into the present.

To all this the United States is the great exception, for here there was no feudal age, and from their beginnings the middle classes combined economic ascendancy and expansion over a continent-wide territory with unhampered dominance of economic wealth and monopoly of status structures. Their monopoly of status was facilitated by their financing of numerous prestigeful institutions: art collections and museums bound intellectual and cultural elites to the "donors" and "philanthropists." Educational institutions, libraries, colleges, universities, and research institutions were impressively endowed, sponsored, and controlled by wealthy "private" citizens, and the dependent personnel became indebted to them; if they were not sycophantic, they were at least grateful.

Wealth in the United States also asserted itself through politics as the ascending middle class became the upper class without having to compromise with ecclesiastic or monarchal elements or with wealthy elites of older standing. Nor did they need to compromise in military, diplomatic, and cultural areas with the standards or traditions of feudal or semifeudal groups clustering around the courts of landed princes and nobles or state university chairs. One has of course to make allowance for the "slavocracy" of the southern plantation society as quasi-feudal, but the Civil War and the reconstruction period eliminated it as a setup not having clear-cut capitalist aspect.

Political and economic power, religious and educational institutions, military and judicial elements as well as status dominance—all these could be vested in the hands of a ruling class of bourgeois extraction and composition. Accordingly, the United States became the great scene for an unadulterated capitalist society and a business civilization built in its image.

The unique situation of a geographical area which allowed continental expansion until the turn of the twentieth century, and the growth of a nation of 5 million into one of 150 million in the short span of 150 years—this made liberalism uniquely fit the reality of American society. For liberalism is "generous": it requires and assumes a friendly universe of equal and open opportunities, and it assumes that men are born "free and equal." Here, the coming of the immigrant coincided with "unlimited opportunities" and a "consciousness of abundance." Liberalism thus found its affirmation in the daily experience of millions of people living in an expanding society.

Instrumental and efficiency values could be and were readily seen as one with moral values. Characteristically, the obvious problem of the double-edged nature of technology—capable of working for good or for evil—was profoundly and insistently impressed upon the American public mind only after the dropping of the atom bomb.

In America the marriage of science and technology, and the joyful reliance upon the values of efficiency, did not entail the destruction or the displacement of cultural legacies, which in Europe aroused the esthetic and nostalgic reactions of men in "romantic agony." Here there was no sense of tragic loss, for on virgin territory such romantic sentiments could at best be attached to the lure of distant horizons and the image of the "noble savage," who, at any rate, upon closer view seemed more savage than noble. The superiority of the white man's advancing efficiency over the primitive ways of the Indian never led to doubts about God-willed steward-ship. Besides, "these illiterate savages" could neither work steadily in the fields nor read the Bible or the catechism; hence all the easier the slogan, "the only good Indian is a dead Indian." Their displacement led to no more travail than that of other preliterate societies on the widening colonial frontiers of the "expansion of Europe."

The widening of economic opportunities and the extension of the territorial setting of United States society went hand in hand and reinforced each other, as did technical progress and the rising levels of skill and education. Entrepreneurial, propertied groups, in urban as well as rural sectors of the society, pulled in the same direction: both have been money-minded groups which took the competitive market for granted.

In this setting, the social costs and liabilities of capitalism could be overlooked, in fact, many of them could be socially defined as ethnic peculiarities of immigrant minorities, and hence not truly American. The anticapitalist sentiments of protesting intellectuals such as John Ruskin or Thomas Carlyle could not perturb the onrushing multitude in its "pursuit of happiness."

The dominance of Puritanism, with its conception of property as "stewardship," cast a religious halo about the successful, and the secularization of Puritanism could easily make for the self-righteous identification of "success" in this world with the complacent sense of being "blessed by God." This was all the more possible as prop-erty was for a long time work-property, and the linkage between such personal virtues as diligence and initiative, persistence and hard work, with property was highly and widely visible. Mass literature, from juveniles to human interest stories and novels, suc-ceeded in publicizing the lore of success and the romance of those who had made it: the titans, the tycoons, the robber barons, the founding fathers, the pioneers, the technological heroes. Such men, standing at the center of popular attention, have provided popu-lar models of aspiration. In American society nothing has been able to rival such affirmations of the efficient, successful heroes of liberalism.

In other countries, Germany for example,[2] the middle-class in-

[2] See Paul Kosok, *Modern Germany* (Chicago: Univ. of Chicago Press, 1933); Max Weber, *From Max Weber . . . , op. cit.*, pp. 363-85.

dustrialists who had economic power did not thereby have status and power in political, educational, or religious orders. For princely power continued, entrenched in Bismarck's constitution of 1870-1918, that underpinned the position of nobles in diplomatic and officer corps, in Protestant church, and student association. Access to such positions was denied the bourgeoisie, which accordingly was forced to adapt feudal and bureaucratic prestige models, to seek intermarriage with nobles, to purchase titles: in short, to renounce liberalism.

The course of Japan is comparable, except in its case, the lower nobility absorbed capitalist business and, in the absence of a productive middle class in the Western style, assimilated the corporate phase of capitalism to the feudal ways of noble and military clan.[3]

In Britain,[4] repeated compromises between landed gentry and court society, on the one hand, and the political and economic ascendancy of the new entrepreneurial class on the other, led to an integrative process in which *rentier* strata of feudal aristocrats and urban patricians could fuse in exclusive clubs and hold their own in navy and army, in "society" and diplomacy. In this they were aided by the "public school" pattern and a widespread system of scholarships which implemented educational opportunities and made for the staying power of feudal elements as well as for the ascending bourgeois elements. The liberal heritage was thus assimilated to the reconstructed conservative thinking of Edmund Burke and his successors.

In Russia, capitalism was tied in with foreign (largely French) political and strategic loans.[5] In the short period from the emancipation of the serfs in 1861 to the revolution of 1917, this capitalism did not allow an economically independent and politically self-reliant middle class to emerge. Moreover, the agrarian problems of Tsarist Russia coincided with the oppressive social evils of early industrialization. The peculiarities of the Russian agrarian commune, and the quasi-religious fervor of the intelligentsia provided

[3] See the excellent monograph, E. Herbert Norman, *Japan's Emergence as a Modern State* (New York: Institute of Pacific Relations, 1946).

[4] See Wilhelm Dibelius, *England: Its Character and Genius*, M. A. Hamilton, tr. (New York: Harper, 1930).

[5] See Leon Trotsky, *The History of the Russian Revolution*, Max Eastman, tr. (New York: Simon & Schuster, 1936).

a barren soil for the ideas of Western liberalism. In addition to the illiterate peasant masses, there was the Eastern Orthodox Church, and the oppressive weight of the Tsarist office and court nobility. There was the anti-Western turn of writers such as Tolstoi and Dostoevski, of the Slavophiles and populists, whether repentant noblemen, or proletarian writers such as Maxim Gorki; and there was the anticapitalist turn of the nihilist, anarchist, and socialist intellectuals, acting as the conscience of their time and people. Accordingly, liberalism as a temper of mind or as a political system had little ground in which to take root.

Since World War I, the international scene, as it bears on the fate of liberalism, has been greatly changed: Nationalist restrictionism and economic protectionism has led to increasing stress and strain.[6] The United States, as well as the dominions and colonies of the British Empire, closed their doors to immigration, and so the great nineteenth-century mobility of populations ceased. Currency policies and protective tariffs fenced off economic areas against unwanted competitors and deadlocked the market system. The rise of large corporations and monopolistic practices made for a new scene, which no longer lent itself to liberal models of social reflection. There was a "scarcity consciousness" in regard to educational and to job opportunities, in regard to migratory opportunities, and even the marriage opportunities for women in the war-decimated nations after the two world wars. "Free and open competition," instead of rationing and planful administration of market processes, now becomes—as in postwar Germany—a mechanism for distributing what is to be had, in which the physically weak, the morally scrupulous, the politically unorganized are pushed to the side. Those who in the eastern areas of Europe have lost everything they once had—their farms, houses, businesses, and skilled jobs—were the last to find jobs for themselves and opportunities for their children in the west. As "new citizens" they are unwanted competitors, walled out by the competitive endeavor of the older residents to build fences wherever possible around preferred opportunities.

Liberalism under such conditions means free competition for all vested groups—from trade unions to businessmen's associations,

[6] See E. H. Carr, *The Twenty Years' Crisis* (London, 1949) and *The New Society* (London: Macmillan, 1951).

from villages to metropolitan communities and new states—to build fences. The highminded endeavors of welfare bureaucracies might soften and mitigate and channel the pressures, but they have not prevented the emergence of irate, embittered mass movements among the "disinherited." Mass unemployment and impoverishment remains a lasting threat, despite the phoenixlike upswing of the Western German economy with American aid.

Such facts can no longer be viewed as temporary or exceptional; in present-day contexts the incongruity of liberal ideologies with modern social facts are glaringly evident. The sense of an open horizon of unlimited opportunities is gone; competition as a fair and equitable way for mating merit and compensation is no longer believed in. The competitive group pressures of society appear to many as "rackets," and freedom takes on the attributes not of rational and moral self-determination among neighbors but of a Hobbesian jungle where the "elastic man," the man without conscience, fends for himself with tooth and claw, a lone wolf in an unfriendly universe.

Such sentiments and feelings of bitter frustration are greatest where "competition among unequals" prevails—in the commodity market, where little and big units, with quite different capital assets and capacities for risk, meet in "free and open competition"; where the little man risks his all and the big corporation risks practically nothing; where economic heavyweights are free to knock out flyweight competitors.

In international relations, the economically strong country transfers the burden of unemployment to weaker countries by maintaining an active balance of trade in its favor, and by attracting whatever capital takes to "flight" from the pressured nation. Thus, in the "family of nations" economic nationalism disintegrates. International trade dwindles, a common currency standard does not exist, weaker nations are indebted to strong creditors, who refuse to accept imports which alone can serve as payment. Hence debtor countries mortgage or sell their land and other capital assets to creditor nations, and are virtually reduced to colonial status.

As in trade, so in war and diplomacy: a weak state may be peacefully carved up—as was Czechoslovakia at Munich by Hitler and Mussolini with the assistance of Chamberlain and Daladier. Strong powers do not deem it honorable to live up to treaty commitments unless it is expedient to do so. In 1914 the Kaiser's chancellor still expressed guilt feelings about the invasion of Belgium and the breaking of neutrality treaties, but great powers now project alleged acts of "aggression" upon the prospective victim, however helpless and weak, of their attack. In the world of nations today might makes right and all is fair in war. And when the shooting pauses, not moral and legal norms but the *de facto* principles of action and power in a world at war is the order of the age.

Industrialized peoples adjust to these changes by building up huge "pressure groups" which emerge out of the upward and downward shifts in economic opportunities for the aggregates of people in common class situations. These pressure groups seek, on various levels, to translate their organized power into policy decisions. The price of bread thus becomes as much a political price as are the rents of tenement houses. "Bloc competition" and "bloc bargaining" replace the competitive scatter of small units; strivings for security replace the sense of joyful individual initiative; feelings of solidarity become more important than self-reliance. Self-help becomes a joke, and "breaking out of line," that is, lack of loyalty to one's organized comrades or colleagues or the "business community" becomes just short of a crime. The term "self-made man" becomes slightly embarrassing; inherited wealth is believed a prerequisite for high status; and the glamour of "the heiress" becomes equivalent if not superior to the majesty of an old-world princess.

In the face of all these changes, Liberalism as an ideology becomes "formalized"; it becomes a political rhetoric which is increasingly meaningless and banal to large masses. The prerequisites for the classic "freedoms" espoused in its name are often simply not available, and hence its classic tenets are easily perverted.[7]

Social and psychological changes of a wide and deep sort thus undermine the moorings of liberalism. In the face of such changes, cynical upper classes may be ready to discard the democratic legacy and allow or support policies that end in a totalitarian society of Fascist or Nazi type. In industrial societies, such move-

---

[7] See John Hallowell, *The Decline of Liberalism as an Ideology* (Berkeley and Los Angeles: Univ. of California Press, 1943). For countertendencies, however, see Morton G. White, "The Revolt against Formalism in American Social Thought of the Twentieth Century," *Journal of the History of Ideas*, Vol. VIII, No. 2, April 1947, pp. 131-52.

ments have arisen at times when the power of labor was declining, as in Italy after the revolutionary upsurge of the post-World War I, and in Germany, as labor's strength was enervated by depression, and unemployment led to mass agony. On both occasions, terrorist organizations were subsidized and turned loose on labor, and the labor press suppressed, as chauvinist frenzy replaced rational public debate. Hero worship drowned the competition in rational ideas and arguments in public. The policy of the street, the assassination of leaders, the orgiastic howling and pogroms against scapegoated minority groups implemented the transitions. A political landslide occurred among the masses, and after some bargaining and compromising, the old elites fused with the ascending political movement, which established its own brand of dictatorship. Society was put on a war footing.

Totalitarianism is an imperialist response to the impasse of corporate capitalism. It is a twentieth-century response, occurring in a time when scarcity consciousness prevails and when to many liberal ideologies seem hollow. Despite its destruction in Central Europe by the last war, neo-Fascist and neo-Nazi tendencies have appeared in Western Germany and Italy. Nobody could call Peron's or Tito's or De Gaulle's program liberal democracy; and nobody can call Franco Spain anything but a fascist dictatorship. In France and Italy close to one-third of the electorate demonstratively and persistently votes Communist. Only the complacent and the uninformed can feel assured of liberal and democratic developments in the world today.

4. Character Structure in a Polarized World

On the one hand, there is the U.S.S.R., the world's greatest land power, extending its sway across the Eurasian land mass, from the Thuringian mountains to the Pacific coast and including in its orbit the vast areas of China. On the other hand, there is the U.S.A., the world's greatest industrial and naval power, including in its continental reach the greatest agricultural production basin on the globe, and rallying the somewhat unstable British Commonwealth of Nations, France and her shaky empire, Western Germany, Italy, and other Mediterranean countries. By their existence and policies, such hegemony powers as the U.S. and the U.S.S.R. define new "in-group" and "out-group" situations within and between nations.

There are, to be sure, anxious endeavors to "build bridges," to find "common ground," to prevent conflict from spreading, to win peace. The British have been eager—and successful in spite of the United States' misgivings—to maintain trade relationships with the Soviet Union and with Communist China. Yet "the war of words," the voting patterns of governmental representatives in the United Nations meetings and other diplomatic conferences, have made the unavailability of "harmonious co-existence" obvious. The big powers have shown a competitive eagerness to integrate their respective alignments. The minor powers, in their fear, have sought protection under the air umbrellas of the leading powers, and such "protection" is of course secured only by the "obedience" of the weak.

All countries are now interdependent, but all countries are also now directly or indirectly dependent upon the dollar or the ruble standard, upon what the United States or the Soviet Union does or fails to do. Each can rely on a "voting discipline" among its minor partners, debtor states, satellites, and protégés. The "United Nations" are disunited and engaged in "cold war." The Eastern bloc uses the legal veto and the Western bloc the *de facto* veto by majority vote; and some powers, great and small, remain outside the "United Nations." There is no undivided court of "world opinion," and in our time, long before a shooting war begins, the propaganda and prestige battles are underway to put the potential enemy in the wrong, to win the sympathy of potential allies, to secure at least benevolent neutrality from the rest. Since industrial nations have become literate, and ever larger masses of people have come into the political order—regardless of constitution—an increasing array of values and institutions has been used for political purposes.

World War II revealed war leaders who would state neither their war aims nor their peace aims, beyond "victory" or "unconditional surrender," which meant the same thing. In fact, since World War I, statesmen, for the benefit of mass sentiments, have vilified one another as war criminals and threatened to hang one another. Since World War II they *have* hanged one another. To be sure, the victors give the vanquished a fair trial before they hang them, but then, soon after the trial, the judges, falling into disagreement, may accuse one another of being "war criminals," and retroactively revise their wartime roles.[8]

Let us consider this polarized world in its military and in its industrial aspects and as we do so, let us keep in mind that these are not far-flung structures alien to the human beings of the twentieth century, but that they are in fact crucial parts of the conditions that make and are made by men and women.

Since the Louisiana purchase and the definition of its north and south borders, the United States has been practically free of military neighbors. Its growth into the mightiest sea power was more or less certain. World War I ended with naval parity between Great Britain and the United States; World War II led to U.S. industrial and naval dominance. Today global strategy for the West is worked out in Washington; Great Britain has become an indebted junior partner.

"The West" represents naval and air power opposed to "the East's" land power. The East cannot hope to conquer the West without sea power; the West cannot hope to conquer the East without land power.

The industrialization of Europe, its urbanization and population growth despite emigration losses during the nineteenth century, made Europe less and less autarchic, more and more dependent upon raw material areas overseas. Hitler shouted, "Germany must export or die," and in fact, this holds for all the industrial countries of Europe. They have to import food and raw materials from outside Europe.

It is this fact that accounts for the efficiency of naval wars of attrition against the central powers during World War I, and against the "Axis" during World War II. Germany's conquest of the larger part of European Russia, of Northern and Eastern Europe, could not compensate for the blockade. Naval blockade, combined with war purchases of what was to be had in neutral countries, proved unbeatably effective weapons of attrition in the

[8] Thus, a Congressional committee of the United States hears testimony of a hooded Polish immigrant, of a Polish officer, of a German general, against Russia to prove Russian war crimes in the forests of Katyn. The Russians resume their early war-time theme of "imperialist powers" being guilty of aggression all along—the military offensive being but a technical question. See the New York *Times,* April 20 and 21, 1952, and Milton R. Konvitz, "Will Nuremberg Serve Justice?," *Commentary,* Vol. I, No. 3, January 1946, pp. 9-15.

hand of the West. The military *coup de grace* could be administered through the invasion of Europe when a weakened military structure was crumbling in the East, and disintegration was aided by a saturation bombing of cities that greatly softened the resources, disrupted railroad communication and the industrial foundations of military strength.

But: this constellation of sea power versus land power, which was elaborated theoretically by Mahan and demonstrated practically to pre-industrial Europe during the Napoleonic age, differs from the present confrontation of American sea power and Russian land power.

The Soviet orbit is not necessarily economically dependent upon outside resources. It contains all the vital raw materials—food, fiber, metal, and oil. And it can—as the history of Russia's industrial development has shown—develop its own resources. To be sure, skill levels are comparatively low, but so are the costs of labor and the levels of mass consumption. There has been and will be "compulsory savings" for the formation of capital, forced upon agrarian masses by bureaucratically planned decisions.

Military power depends upon industrial power, and so the two power blocs of the world are now engaged in an armament race and in an industrial race. The West realizes that the nonindustrialized areas—long exploited as raw-material areas—are socially unstable, economically deteriorating, politically shaky, and ideologically open to Soviet influence. They can be "Western" in orientation only at the cost of industrialization under Western aegis. Africa, India, and the Middle East are crucial, and development projects in Africa such as the Point Four Program—and schemes to develop skills in the Far East—indicate the drift.

Regardless of the enormity of institutional diversity and psychological types, the trend with the widest scope and the most far-reaching ramifications is the industrialization of the world. The key importance, in fact, of the rise of the Soviet Union to great international stature lies in this simple fact: for the first time in the intricate history of the industrial revolution men can now see that this industrialization does not require capitalism as an institutional framework, that it can be accomplished without depending upon private initiative, and that when it is carried out by state bureaucrats, industrialization can even be a more rapid and orderly process than when carried out by private capitalists running private firms for private profits.

Russia has reversed America's industrial sequence: Whereas unplanned industrialization under free, private initiative has proceeded from "light" consumer goods industries to heavy industries, Soviet planning has assigned priority to electric power, metallurgy, and other war-important industries. In Russia, modern industrial civilization did not emerge autonomously as a slow-motion process from medieval guilds and burghers, with the rise of a middle class. Industrialization, in its late nineteenth- and twentieth-century phase of corporate or monopoly capitalism, entered the "backward" agrarian society of Tsarist Russia in the usual forms of political capitalism, governmentally promoted and subsidized.

Under Stalin's leadership, industrialization has been imposed in the great pushes of the "Five-Year plans." Soviet men and women have been rallied behind the party and its plans by propaganda campaigns and excessive orders. An agrarian revolution from above, at the price of a famine costing two and a half million lives, has accompanied this industrialization. But the industrialization has been accomplished, not in any cumulative, competitive, and adaptive way, but in the form of centrally enacted and imposed changes under the leadership of a totalitarian one-party state, engaged in successive campaigns to transform traditionalist agrarian societies, primordial tribes, and congeries of nations in varied stages of cultural development. The last war allowed the Soviet Union to emerge as the world's greatest land power, and this power is now reinforced by Bolshevized Eastern European countries and revolutionized China. For we must remember that Russia lost a war with Japan in 1904-05, and again, with Germany, in 1914-17. The triumphant advance of the Soviet Union and her "indefinite occupation" of Central Europe with a boundary line only eighty-five miles from France has made her victory over Nazi Germany a victory over old Europe. The Nazi drive to the East has resulted in the Soviet drive to the West.

The United States, on the other hand, consummated its industrialization and nation-building in the span of one and a half centuries under conditions that were ideal for the rise of the entrepreneurial middle class under laissez-faire conditions sanctioned by liberalism.[9]

[9] Cf. above, p. 355 ff.

Technologically, the United States may be the fulfillment of the Soviet dream, but this does not mean that the United States is therefore an ideal image and model for the Soviet world. In fact, the Soviet Union has many assets of its own as an industrial leader of borderland areas.

Stalinist communism, in the phrase of G. F. Achminow,[10] is "substitute capitalism." For many peoples of the world the master problem of our time is simply how to overcome "backwardness," which means, how to industrialize and make their populations literate. This world problem of rapid industrialization becomes acute when there is war, or when there is the loss of a war, or when war threatens, or when dependency upon more advanced states becomes for any reason unbearable.

The success of communism, in those areas where it has been successful, may be due to the simple fact that capitalism—seated primarily in Northwestern Europe in the nineteenth century, and in the United States, Europe, and Japan in the twentieth—has not been able to put through this rapid industrialization. It has not been able to industrialize such areas, because it has not put through the "primary accumulation" necessary for building up a productive apparatus among nations composed of the preindustrial masses of the world. But communism—as the shadow of a capitalism that has defaulted—is able to do so by virtue of its public management of investment policies. The communists thus flourish on the failure of capitalists to solve this world historical task.

Everywhere that communists have come to power we find a condition in which, contrary to nineteenth-century expectations, there is no politically effective and economically strong bourgeoisie. In Russia such a bourgeoisie as existed was dependent upon the political commissions of a despotic state and on foreign loans. Wherever capitalism has passed beyond such weakling beginnings and become of sizable stature and deep political entrenchment— as in Britain, the United States, and Germany—communism has not, even during severe depressions, become strong.

The success of communism has not been due to the senescence of mature capitalism; it has been due to its insufficient development.

[10] *Die Macht im Hintergrund: Totengräber des Kommunismus* (Spatenverlag Greunchen, Ulm: 1950). In the following pages, we have drawn upon this interesting although contradictory book by a postwar Russian refugee.

After a hundred years of railroad building in China, the Western nations had not built much more mileage than exists in tiny Belgium. India, enjoying British rule and guidance for over 150 years, has built few cities of more than 100,000 population. Since profits were taken out of these countries, there was no investment capital of sufficient size for the task, and there were not sufficient political guarantees nor will to attract private investment in suitable amounts.

But the Communist Mao Tse-tung may well accomplish "primary accumulations" by transforming his army into a labor force, under military discipline, to do all that is required for the industrialization of China. Mao Tse-tung takes up where the old Confucian emperors left off: his tax policy in labor contributions, however, does not result in the building of big stone walls or imperial tombs, but in the industrialization of China. If his policy is brutal—and it is—one must bear in mind Colbert's use of the French army and the other methods used by European civilizations in their time of primary accumulation.

There are apparent exceptions to the idea of communism as substitute capitalism. There is the voting strength of communism in pre-Hitler Germany, in postwar France, Czechoslovakia, and Italy. France, however, was liberated, after defeat in a six weeks' war, only by her allies, who made her a victor—and the French know it. Italy, especially southern Italy, is still semifeudal in its agrarianism, it lacks raw materials, and it has had to pay dearly for Mussolini's dream of a "Third Rome." Communism failed repeatedly and disastrously in Germany. Only when the Red army stood in the country or close by, as in Czechoslovakia, has communism come to power in a country with a developed capitalist economy.

When it has taken over, communism has co-ordinated all efforts by dictatorial imposition; it has destroyed pluralist and open-ended economic and political endeavors. Fascism gathered the old rulers together, even if they did not like it, and supplemented them by newer, gangster types; communism has replaced the old ruling groups by new ones from below.

In Achminow's view, three conditions are necessary and sufficient for the rise to power of communism within a society:

(1) The society must be on a level of development in which the most urgent national task is the overcoming of the backward-

ness of rural society sweating under the burden of feudal rulers, usurious capitalists, and a national debt. Russia of 1917, and China of between the last two wars certainly fulfill this condition. (2) The existing ruling stratum must be incapable of solving this task. Either the old ruling elements misread the signs of the times and offer desperate resistance to change, or they become cynically corrupt and so incapable of any consistent policy that might solve the tasks they confront. (3) There must be people who are able to take over the management of the state, but who under pre-communist conditions have had no chance to do so. This means a closure policy on the part of the old rulers, or simply the absence of a qualified counterelite.

Whenever these three conditions are met, there is a chance for communist upheaval; the absence of any one of them precludes the victory of communism, although for strategic reasons, of course, the armed force of the Soviet Union could, and might, try to impose it from without.

In the conflict of East and West—of the United States and the Soviet Union—Europe occupies an especially important position, if only because of its cultural, religious, and historical ties with the white populations of the Western Hemisphere. It is also important because of the 250 million population that are settled on this peninsula of Eurasia, which is militarily weak in the neighborhood of a great land power controlling the Baltic Sea and producing atomic bombs. Europe is a major "prize" of the contest of the two great powers. Were Europe to drift or to be shoved into the Russian orbit, Great Britain would be open to atomic attacks at close range, and the addition of skilled populations and of the Ruhr industries to the East might possibly be sizable enough to make the decisive difference. Inside Europe, rival nations and states—which have been variously realigning themselves for centuries and which have known climactic heights of prestige and power—must now redefine their respective positions as well as their hopes and expectations for the world's future.

In almost all orders and spheres, leading policy-makers are having to learn to share European problems and to educate Europeans to the appreciation of American decision-making contexts. Accordingly, we may say that a great process of social and cultural fusion is underway, a fusion comparable only to the spread of Hellenism after Alexander in the Eastern Mediterranean, or to the blending, in the leading urban strata of late antiquity, of the legacy of Athens and Rome under the Caesars. Militarily, economically, and politically, there is going on a struggle for the world, of which there is a portentous psychological meaning: We witness and participate in an historic contest which will decide what types of men and women will flourish on the earth.

Man is a unique animal species in that he is also an historical development. It is in terms of this development that he must be defined, and in terms of it no single formula will fit him. Neither his anatomy nor his psyche fix his destiny. He creates his own destiny as he responds to his experienced situation, and both his situation and his experiences of it are the complicated products of the historical epoch which he enacts. That is why he does not create his destiny as an individual but as a member of a society. Only within the limits of his place in an historical epoch can man as an individual shape himself, but we do not yet know, we can never know, the limits to which men collectively might remake themselves.

Bibliographical Note

In this brief bibliography we list only books in English which we have found profitable and enjoyable in the production of the present volume. Although we do not wish to impose this list on others, we cannot help but feel that as a selection it does suggest the major legacy available to the student of man and society.

We should note that we are constant perusers of *The Encyclopaedia of the Social Sciences* and of the eleventh edition of *The Encyclopaedia Britannica*. Students who wish detail on any of the factual or historical topics we have discussed should first consult these wonderful volumes. Those who wish further listings of books by historical topic or event may consult the Library of Congress file catalogue, to be found in most university libraries. In the following, we cite the latest, or the most convenient, editions available to us.

Albright, William F., *From the Stone Age to Christianity* (2nd ed.; Baltimore: Johns Hopkins Press, 1946).

Bagehot, Walter, *Physics and Politics* (New York: D. Appleton, 1912).

Beard, Charles, *An Economic Interpretation of the Constitution of the U.S.* (New York: Macmillan, 1935).

——, *Economic Origins of Jeffersonian Democracy* (New York: Macmillan, 1915).

Berle, A. A., Jr., and Means, Gardiner C., *The Modern Corporation and Private Property* (New York: Macmillan, 1933).

Borkenau, Franz, *World Communism* (New York: Norton, 1939).

Bovet, Pierre, *The Fighting Instinct*, J. Y. T. Greig, tr. (New York: Dodd, Mead, 1923).

Bryce, James, *The American Commonwealth*, 2 vols. (New York: Macmillan, 1895).

Bücher, Karl, *Industrial Evolution* (New York: Holt, 1901).

Burckhardt, Jacob, *The Civilization of the Renaissance in Italy*, S. G. C. Middlemore, tr. (New York: Oxford Univ. Press, 1945).

Calhoun, Arthur W., *A Social History of the American Family*, 3 vols. (New York: A. H. Clark, 1917-19).

Carr, E. H., *The Twenty Years Crisis, 1919-1939* (New York: Macmillan, 1940).

Cash, W. J., *The Mind of the South* (New York: Knopf, 1941).

Commons, John R., *Legal Foundations of Capitalism* (New York: Macmillan, 1924).

Cooley, C. H., *Social Organization* (New York: Scribner's, 1909).

———, *Human Nature and the Social Order* (rev. ed.; New York: Scribner's, 1922).

Dewey, John, *Human Nature and Conduct* (New York: Holt, 1922).

Dibelius, Wilhelm, *England*, Mary A. Hamilton, tr. (New York: Harper, 1930).

Dorfmann, Joseph, *Thorstein Veblen and His America* (New York: Viking, 1934).

Durkheim, Émile, *The Division of Labor in Society*, George Simpson, tr. (Glencoe, Ill.: Free Press, 1947).

———, *Suicide*, John A. Spaulding and George Simpson, trs. (Glencoe, Ill.: Free Press, 1951).

Earle, E. M., and others, eds., *Makers of Modern Strategy* (Princeton: Princeton Univ. Press, 1943).

Fenichel, Otto, *The Psychoanalytic Theory of Neurosis* (New York: Norton, 1945).

Freud, Sigmund, *The Basic Writings of Sigmund Freud*, A. A. Brill, tr. (New York: Modern Library, 1938).

———, *Civilization and Its Discontents*, Joan Riviere, tr. (London: Anglobooks, 1952).

———, *Collected Papers*, vols. i-iv (London: Hogarth Press, 1946).

———, *General Introduction to Psychoanalysis*, Joan Riviere, tr. (rev. ed.; Garden City, N. Y.: Garden City Publishing Co., 1943).

———, *Group Psychology and the Analysis of the Ego*, James Strachey, tr. (London: Hogarth Press, 1948).

Fromm, Erich, *Escape from Freedom* (New York: Farrar & Rinehart, 1941).

Hauser, Arnold, *The Social History of Art*, 2 vols. (New York: Knopf, 1951).

Hegel, G. W. F., *The Philosophy of History* (New York: Wiley, 1944).

Hendrick, Ives, *Facts and Theories of Psychoanalysis* (2nd ed., rev. and enl.; New York: Knopf, 1939).

Hobson, John A., *The Evolution of Modern Capitalism* (new and rev. ed.; New York: Scribner's, 1926).

Horney, Karen, *The Neurotic Personality of Our Time* (New York: Norton, 1937).

Huizinga, J., *The Waning of the Middle Ages* (New York: Longmans, 1949).

Isaacs, Harold, *The Tragedy of the Chinese Revolution* (London: Secher & Warburg, 1938).

James, William, *Psychology: Briefer Course* (New York: Holt, 1923).

Kardiner, A., *The Individual and His Society* (New York: Columbia Univ. Press, 1939).

Kohn, Hans, *The Idea of Nationalism* (New York: Macmillan, 1944).

Korsch, Karl, *Karl Marx* (New York: Wiley, 1939).

Kosok, Paul, *Modern Germany* (Chicago: Univ. of Chicago Press, 1933).

Kroeber, A. L., *Anthropology* (new rev. ed.; New York: Harcourt, Brace, 1948).

———, *Configurations of Cultural Growth* (Berkeley: Univ. of California Press, 1944).

Lasswell, H. D., *World Politics and Personal Insecurity* (New York: Whittlesey, 1936).

———, *The Analysis of Political Behaviour* (New York: Oxford Univ. Press, 1948).

———, and Kaplan, A., *Power and Society* (New Haven: Yale Univ. Press, 1950).

LeBon, G., *The Crowd* (new ed.; New York: Macmillan, 1925).

Lenin, V. I., *State and Revolution* (New York: International Pubs., 1932).

———, *Two Tactics* (New York: International Pubs., 1935).

———, *What Is to Be Done?* (New York: International Pubs., 1929).

Lippmann, Walter, *Public Opinion* (New York: Macmillan, 1927).

Lukács, George, *Studies in European Realism,* Edith Bone, tr. (London: Hillway, 1950).

Luxemburg, Rosa, *The Accumulation of Capital,* Agnes Schwarzschild, tr. (New Haven: Yale Univ. Press, 1951).

Lynd, Robert S. and Helen M., *Middletown* (New York: Harcourt, Brace, 1929).

———, *Middletown in Transition* (New York: Harcourt, Brace, 1937).

Mannheim, Karl, *Ideology and Utopia,* Louis Wirth and Edward Shils, trs. (New York: Harcourt, Brace, 1936).

———, *Man and Society in an Age of Reconstruction*, Edward Shils, tr. (New York: Harcourt, Brace, 1940).

Marcuse, Herbert, *Reason and Revolution* (New York: Oxford Univ. Press, 1941).

Marx, Karl, *Capital,* 3 vols. E. Untermann, tr. (Chicago: Kerr, 1906-09).

———, *Selected Works in 2 Volumes* (New York: International Publishers, 1933).

———, and Engels, Friedrich, *The German Ideology* (New York: International Publishers, 1939).

Mead, George H., *Mind, Self and Society* (Chicago: Univ. of Chicago Press, 1934).

Mead, Margaret, *Sex and Temperament in Three Primitive Societies* (New York: Morrow, 1935).

Mencken, H. L., *The American Language* (4th ed., rev. and enl.; New York: Knopf, 1936).

Michels, Robert, *Political Parties*, Eden and Cedar Paul, trs. (Glencoe, Ill.: Free Press, 1949).

Mills, C. Wright, *White Collar: The American Middle Class* (New York: Oxford Univ. Press, 1951).

Mosca, Gaetano, *The Ruling Class*, H. D. Kahn, tr. (New York: McGraw-Hill, 1939).

Mumford, Lewis, *Technics and Civilization* (New York: Harcourt, Brace, 1934).

Myrdal, Gunnar, *The American Dilemma* (9th ed.; New York: Harper, 1944).

Neumann, Franz, *Behemoth: The Structure and Practice of National Socialism* (New York: Oxford Univ. Press, 1942).

Nietzsche, Friedrich, *The Complete Works* (Levy ed.; New York: Macmillan, 1896-1930).

Norman, E. Herbert, *Japan's Emergence as a Modern State* (New York: Inst. of Pacific Relations, 1946).

Oppenheimer, Franz, *The State,* John M. Gitterman, tr. (rev. ed.; New York: Viking, 1926).

Ostrogorskii, M., *Democracy and the Organization of Political Parties,* Frederick Clarke, tr., 2 vols. (New York: Macmillan, 1908).

Piaget, Jean, *The Moral Judgment of the Child* (New York: Harcourt, Brace, 1932).

——, *The Language and Thought of the Child* (New York: Harcourt, Brace, 1926).

Powdermaker, Hortense, *After Freedom* (New York: Viking, 1937).

Power, Eileen, *Medieval People* (Boston: Houghton Mifflin, 1924).

Rosenberg, Arthur, *Democracy and Socialism* (New York: Knopf, 1939).

Ross, E. A., *Social Control* (New York: Macmillan, 1904).

Sabine, George, *A History of Political Theory* (New York: Holt, 1937).

Sapir, Edward, *Language* (New York: Harcourt, Brace, 1921).

Schumpeter, J. A., *Capitalism, Socialism, and Democracy* (3rd ed.; New York: Harper, 1950).

Simmel, Georg, *The Sociology of Georg Simmel*, Kurt Wolff, ed. and tr. (Glencoe, Ill.: Free Press, 1950).

Sombart, Werner, *The Quintessence of Capitalism*, M. Epstein, tr. (London, 1915).

Sorokin, Pitirim, *Social Mobility* (New York: Harper, 1927).

———, *Social and Cultural Dynamics*, 4 vols. (New York: American Books, 1937-41).

Speier, Hans, *Social Order and the Risks of War* (New York: Stewart, 1952).

Spencer, Herbert, *Principles of Sociology*, 2 vols. (New York: D. Appleton, 1896).

Sullivan, Harry Stack, *Conceptions of Modern Psychiatry* (Washington: W. A. White Psychiatric Foundation, 1947).

Tawney, R. H., *Religion and the Rise of Capitalism* (new ed.; New York: Harcourt, Brace, 1947).

———, *Equality* (4th ed. rev.; New York: Macmillan, 1952).

Thomas, W. I., and Znaniecki, F., *The Polish Peasant in Europe and America* (New York: Knopf, 1927).

de Tocqueville, Alexis, *Democracy in America*, 2 vols. (New York: Knopf, 1945).

Toynbee, Arnold, *A Study of History*, 6 vols. (New York: Oxford Univ. Press, 1951).

Troeltsch, E., *The Social Teachings of the Christian Churches*, 2 vols. (New York: Macmillan, 1949).

Trotsky, Leon, *The History of the Russian Revolution*, Max Eastman, tr. (New York: Simon and Schuster, 1936).

Vagts, Alfred, *A History of Militarism* (New York: Norton, 1937).

Veblen, Thorstein, *Absentee Ownership* (New York: Viking, 1923).

———, *The Place of Science in Modern Civilization* (New York: Viking, 1919).

Wallas, Graham, *The Great Society* (New York: Macmillan, 1914).

———, *Human Nature in Politics* (3rd ed.; New York: Knopf, 1921).

Weber, Max, *From Max Weber: Essays in Sociology*, H. H. Gerth and C. Wright Mills, trs. (New York: Oxford Univ. Press, 1946).

———, *General Economic History*, Frank H. Knight, tr. (Glencoe, Ill.: Free Press, 1950).

———, *The Protestant Ethic and the Spirit of Capitalism*, Talcott Parsons, tr. (New York: Scribner's, 1930).

———, *The Theory of Social and Economic Organization*, Talcott Parsons and A. M. Henderson, trs. (New York: Oxford Univ. Press, 1947).

———, *The Religion of China*, H. H. Gerth, tr. (Glencoe, Ill.: Free Press, 1951).

———, *Ancient Judaism*, H. H. Gerth and D. Martindale, trs. (Glencoe, Ill.: Free Press, 1952).

Wellek, René, and Warren, Austin, *Theory of Literature* (New York: Harcourt, Brace, 1949).

Index